The Complete MRCGP Study Guide

FOURTH EDITION

SARAH GEAR
General Practitioner
Cheshire

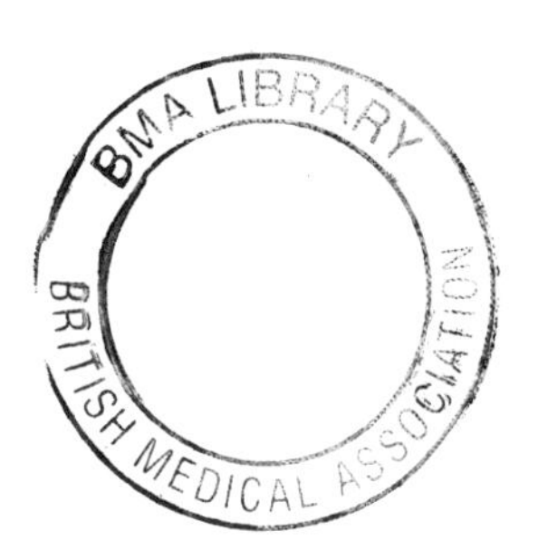

Radcliffe Publishing
London • New York

Radcliffe Publishing Ltd
33–41 Dallington Street
London
EC1V 0BB
United Kingdom

www.radcliffepublishing.com

First Edition 2004
Second Edition 2006
Third Edition 2008

Every effort has been made to ensure that the information in this book is accurate. This does not diminish the requirement to exercise clinical judgement, and neither the publisher nor the author can accept any responsibility for its use in practice.

New research and clinical experience can result in changes in treatment and drug therapy. Users of the information in this book should therefore check the most recent product information on any drug they may prescribe to ensure they are complying with the manufacturer's recommendations concerning dosage, the method and duration of administration and contraindications.

British Library Cataloguing in Publication Data

A catalogue record for this book is available from the British Library.

ISBN-13: 978 184619 563 1

The paper used for the text pages of this book is FSC® certified. FSC (The Forest Stewardship Council®) is an international network to promote responsible management of the world's forests.

Typeset by Darkriver Design, Auckland, New Zealand
Printed and bound by TJ International Ltd, Padstow, Cornwall, UK

Contents

About the author

Dr Sarah Gear graduated in 1995 from Manchester Medical School. She undertook SHO posts followed by the GP vocational training scheme at the North Staffordshire Royal Infirmary in Stoke-on-Trent, qualifying as a GP in August 2001 and successfully gaining the MRCGP the same year.

In April 2002, she became a principal at her former training practice in Madeley, near Crewe.

Acknowledgements

As with the previous editions, the fourth edition of *The Complete MRCGP Study Guide* has taken a lot of work to ensure it is as up to date as it can be before being published. This new edition would not have been possible without the help of family, friends and colleagues. The medical educational courses that are run both locally and nationally are of huge importance to our continuing professional development, as are the online facilities that we are fortunate enough to be able to access.

Special thanks to Gillian Nineham for her initial belief in the project and to the whole team at Radcliffe for the advice and polite suggestions on how to improve my grammar (which has sometimes left me smiling for days!). Without such dedication I would still be printing off individual workbooks for circulation. Thank you.

Introduction

The MRCGP is upon you. How long have you got?

To be a competent GP you need to be well read (a true generalist) and have an open, sensible approach to acquiring knowledge that will fill in any gaps. This book is geared to take you through the Royal College of General Practitioners curriculum statements and give you a comprehensive overview, to help you with your revision for this vocational exam and then test you with an Applied Knowledge Test- and Clinical Skills Assessment-style examination.

This is not meant to be a walk through aetiology, pathophysiology, investigations and treatments – quite the opposite. Its purpose is to save you the colossal amount of time you would otherwise require to cover the same ground, by supplying a large amount of information and then testing your understanding with exam-style questions, all in one place.

The college website (www.rcgp.org.uk) must be consulted. Even if you have sat the exam before, you must read the rules again – they can change, so don't be caught out.

Part of the groundwork at an early stage is to speak to as many people as possible about their learning techniques and approach for the MRCGP. You will find that in most cases people will identify a topic ('learning need'), read around it and then apply that knowledge in their working clinical context. Then they might do a MEDLINE search for current review articles or look in *Clinical Evidence* to ensure there has not been some new, revolutionary information presented that may change the way they would tackle the given subject (i.e. the way they practise).

More enlightened doctors manage to keep up to date with the journals and comics, do their own video analysis and even have a mentor. Thinking about what you want to achieve in general practice from early on in your career will mean you can maximise what you get out of your hospital jobs and training post and how best to work towards passing the MRCGP examination.

Finally, it is important to remember the following points.

- You don't need to know everything (you cannot possibly).
- Learning is easier if what you are learning is topical/relevant.
- It is not how much you know but how you apply that knowledge that matters.

Sarah Gear
January 2012
gear@doctors.org.uk

How to use this book

Probably the worst thing you could do is to try to plough through this book from beginning to end – you would never make it, and even if you did, you would be unlikely to remember much of it.

Use this book, alongside the curriculum guide (www.rcgp-curriculum.org.uk), as a starting point, a guide or for summing up to ensure that you are as well read as you think you are. Flick through and get a handle on the layout and what is included. No doubt there will be parts you know inside out – so don't be tempted to spend too much time on these sections: move on.

Consider the online facilities that you can access free of charge, such as BMJ Learning (http://learning.bmj.com) and Doctors.net.uk modules (www.doctors.net.uk). You can also subscribe to *InnovAiT* (www.oxforde-learning.com/innovait) for examples and practise questions. Such facilities can make the difference between thinking you know something that you have skim-read and really knowing the answers. Information from these sources is well written and peer reviewed before being published.

Set yourself a revision timetable that takes into account this is no longer medical school and you are working for this exam on top of doing your job. Give yourself short, regular breaks throughout each revision session – you will take more in this way.

The curriculum statements allow you to break things down into manageable sections. Each statement should be used together with its supporting questions, as there are points covered in the questions that are not covered in the text – a subliminal message about time management and unnecessary duplication! How much time you have left for revision will depend on the time you allow yourself for each statement (ideally there should be time for more than one statement a night).

Following the curriculum statements is an exam section with practise Applied Knowledge Text questions and Clinical Skills Assessment cases to work through. Some candidates choose to go through this at the beginning and then again at the end of their revision, so they can test their improvement. It really doesn't matter, just get started. Scribble comments and questions on the pages, highlight text, use Post-it notes or completely deface the text. Do whatever you like, but make sure it works for you.

All answers are comprehensive but not exhaustive. If you have left yourself plenty of revision time, take the opportunity to look through the references for sources to consolidate what you have learned.

No book will ever cover everything you need to know, but this one encompasses a huge amount. I hope you find it an indispensable guide to both your GP registrar year and the MRCGP.

General practice is a fantastic career and the MRCGP has always been a worthwhile exam to work for. You will gain an incredible amount from it if you are willing to put in the time and effort.

Enjoy and good luck!

The MRCGP exam

The MRCGP exam involves three areas: the Applied Knowledge Test, the Clinical Skills Assessment and the Workplace-Based Assessment.

Applied Knowledge Test

This is a 3-hour summative assessment of knowledge involving a 200-question paper in a multiple-choice style. You need to apply to the Royal College of General Practitioners in plenty of time and pay the correct fee to be able to sit this. Once the application is accepted you will need to phone the centre of your choice to book in to sit the test. It is computer-based and marked. Approximately 80% of the exam will be on clinical medicine, 10% on critical appraisal and evidence-based medicine, and 10% on health informatics and administrative issues. You would not usually sit this until you are in a level 2 specialty training post.

Clinical Skills Assessment

This is a series of 13 consultations, each being 10 minutes long. These are marked on your data gathering, clinical management and interpersonal skills. You are given a brief summary of a patient and stationed in a single room with the examiner; the patient comes to you.

Workplace-Based Assessment

This utilises a number of different evidence-gathering tools for marking professional competence. These are:

- case-based discussion
- consultation observation tool, COT (in primary care only)
- multi-source feedback, MSF
- patient satisfaction questionnaire (in primary care only)
- direct observation of procedural skills, DOPs
- clinical evaluation exercise (mini-CEX tool) (in hospital posts)
- clinical supervisors' report (in hospital posts).

Don't forget your e-portfolio entries. If you get into the habit of logging things in once a week you won't fall behind; the last thing you need is a panel review by forgetting to get enough evidence on the e-portfolio.

> **Remember, it is important to read the college website and exam instructions about documents that will be needed for identification and other issues. Things often change and you do not want to get caught out.**

The six core competencies

The six competencies outlined as part of the Royal College of General Practitioners curriculum are separate to the Essential Knowledge Statements.

Specific to the GP-consultation:

1 primary care management
2 person-centred care
3 specific problem-solving skills.

The wider perspective:

4 a comprehensive approach
5 community orientation
6 a holistic approach.

These are attitudinal in many ways, but there is also a contextual and a scientific application; your trainer will focus on these in various ways (the knowledge, skill and attitude aspects).

The curriculum is comprehensive and although many issues cross-reference with the Essential Knowledge Statements, where this hasn't been appropriate, I have included any issues that may be of additional help in this section.

General practitioner's workload

The Royal College of General Practitioners printed their updated information sheet on GP workload in 2004. Its findings are briefly summarised as follows.

- There has been an increase in the number of part-time contracts in general practice from 5.4% in 1990 to 22.3% in 2003.
- The average duration of a consultation had increased from 9.36 minutes in 1997 to 13.3 minutes in 2004 (data from the Audit Commission).
- Ninety-seven per cent of patients were able to see a GP within two working days.
- Ninety-eight per cent of patients were able to see a healthcare professional within one working day.

These statistics, and variations of them, are updated periodically by many different surveys.

How should hamsters run? Some observations about sufficient patient time in primary care

BMJ 2001; 323(7307): 266–8

This article summarises the finding that GPs in both the United Kingdom (UK) and the United States (US) believe they have less time for each patient, although statistically this is not the case. Doctors feel stressed because there is now more that can be done within a consultation and for a particular problem, patient's expectations are higher, and there are more external forces impinging on their practice.

There is little evidence to support that doctors are 'running faster' in terms of both patient management and administration, despite the fact that doctors complain more. Reasons why areas of workload have increased are as follows.

- The population has increased by 3%, now 58.4 million (the birth rate is less, so a large proportion is through immigration).
- Life expectancy has doubled over the last 150 years:
  - there has been a 9% increase in the geriatric population in the last decade
  - there has been a 13% increase in the over-75 population in the last decade.
- Infant deaths have decreased.
- Divorce affects one in two marriages (associated social morbidity).
- Families are more spread out (so there is a decreased support network).
- The number of single-parent families has increased.
- Preventive healthcare has added around 23% to the workload.
- Mental health is now more acceptable for patients to present with.
- Most consultations are minor; 15% are life threatening and need to be identified.
- Overall knowledge has increased (the *Oxford Textbook of Medicine* now runs to three volumes).
- There is increased accessibility (telephone and email) to healthcare and surgeries.
- GPs are accountable for practice nurse roles and so forth.
- Advances in information technology.
- There are more part-time GPs.

Derek Wanless (a former NatWest bank chief executive) has published his final report, *Securing our Future Health: taking a long-term view* (the Wanless report). The main points are briefly summarised as follows:

- The current method of funding healthcare, through general taxation, is fair and efficient, so it should not be tampered with.
- Around 70% of the work currently done by doctors could be done by nurses and other healthcare professionals.

The Wanless review

***BMJ* 2007; 335(7620): 572–3**

This is an editorial that summarised NHS performance since 2002. On the positive side there are more staff, less waiting and improved provision in high-priority areas (such as cardiology and cancer). On the negative side, there hasn't been an improvement in productivity (in real terms) and new contracts have come at a high cost. The editorial focuses purely on a before-and-after review, without detailed insight into the collated information, and recognises that more funding is necessary to deliver further improvement.

The new General Medical Services contract (2004) was partly sold as a way GPs could control their workload. However, there are significant penalties for doctors choosing to limit certain services. There are many initiatives to try to improve workload, such as electronic prescribing, nurse practitioners and prescribers, and nursing management for chronic disease reviews. Similarly, there are many issues that are to demand an increase in GP workload in the future, such as Choose and Book, practice-based commissioning and keeping ourselves up to date. An individual's personal work ethic and their time management skills are both factors of workload management that are always important.

Stress and burnout

There are four levels of human functioning: emotional, mental, behavioural and psychological. Burnout is the end-stage response to excessive stress and dissatisfaction. No one is immune to stress; you don't have to be overworked to struggle with it and we need to find a pressure level at which to work that is constructive, not destructive. To do this you need to be self-aware and recognise how it affects you. How you manage it then depends upon whether you think the level of stress is a good or a bad thing. It should be actively managed with your own personal survival plan to prevent burnout in the long run.

Stress is also a physiological response to an inappropriate level of pressure. Noradrenalin increases, which, via the medulla, increases adrenaline production. This in turn increases adrenocorticotropic hormone levels and hence steroid production, which we all know improves your immunity and your ability to deal with stress. When you stop working (e.g. go on holiday), all this falls down and you develop a cold!

People heading towards burnout go through four stages: overwork, frustration, resentment and finally depression (with burnout). It has always been acceptable to complain about stress but it has not been acceptable to have symptoms, as these are interpreted as a sign of weakness. As GPs we need to be aware of the well-being of both our employees and ourselves.

Causes of stress include:

- escalating workload
- frequently imposed change
- patients' expectations
- fear of litigation
- conflict (e.g. between career and family life)
- lack of career structure, and so forth.

Predisposing features of stress in the doctor include:

- type A personality, obsessive personality
- conscientiousness, high personal standards
- reluctance to decline work
- reluctance to delegate
- competitive nature
- fear of failure to match colleagues' achievements.

In the practice they include:

- single handed or dysfunctional partnerships

- professional isolation
- repeated interruptions
- unpredictable work
- long hours, out-of-hours cover
- lack of variety, no challenge
- lack of peer recognition.

In society, predisposing features include:
- increased patient expectation
- shift of work from secondary care
- increasing litigation and complaints
- imposed change and political agendas.

Signs of stress and burnout to look for include:
- poor time keeping and decision-making
- sick leave
- increasing frequency of mistakes
- strained relationships.

What can we do for our employees?

- Understand inappropriate pressures lead to stress; differentiate between pressure and stress.
- Conduct staff appraisals/personal development plans to identify problems.
- Hold practice development sessions:
    - review attitudes to stress
    - audit – establish a baseline, make the issue less confrontational, measure effectiveness of any strategy
    - develop skills at dealing with pressure – assertiveness (not aggressive), increase resilience by creating a balance and developing your own strategy for dealing with pressure, time management
    - look at neurolinguitsic programming – this technique helps understand the structure of how you think and behave, and it uses specific techniques to make your thinking and behaviour more resourceful.
- Be vigilant, observe individuals.
- Develop your own helping skills.

Useful online resources are:
- Mind Tools (www.mindtools.com)
- *Work-Life Balance* (www.nhsemployers.org/Aboutus/Publications/Documents/Work-life%20balance.pdf).

Avoiding burnout in general practice

Br J Gen Pract 1993; 43(376): 442–3

Although published some time ago, this article remains relevant and recommends the following points to keep in mind:

- Trainees should be given realistic expectations of general practice.
- Chose the right job.
- Develop practice support systems as well as personal ones (e.g. groups outside work).
- Be assertive.
- Develop time management skills.
- Be aware of your own response to stress.

Other considerations

Delegate, prioritise, keep up to date, audit, develop practice policies, balance your life (maintain outside interests) and make sure you have a plan for dealing with stress.

Organise your workload with realistic targets. Make sure you take time out to exercise and that you set aside time for your hobbies (i.e. strike a balance between your professional and personal life). Make time to exercise and make time for sleep. And beware caffeine!

Speaking to your trainer and other colleagues often helps get things in perspective and it may provide you with solutions that you may not have considered. Primary care trusts usually have dedicated counsellors for staff use in situations such as this.

How you manage pressure, stress or burnout is up to you, but make sure you do manage it, otherwise someone will take it to task and you will be 'managed' as someone else deems appropriate – not a comfortable situation.

Essential Knowledge Statements

This section looks at the different statements relating to core knowledge in the curriculum. I have resisted the temptation to regurgitate the curriculum skills, outcomes and objectives for you, as these can easily be found on the Royal College of General Practitioners website (www.rcgp-curriculum.org.uk/rcgp_-_gp_curriculum_documents/gp_curriculum_statements.aspx) or, alternatively, in the Condensed Curriculum Guide.

With each statement I have reviewed certain issues you should probably be familiar with because they are either topical or ingrained in what we do. The statements are not meant to be exhaustive, and where National Institute for Health and Clinical Excellence or other guidance is used, I have selected some areas rather than summarised the whole document. I have included the references for you to look at as part of your extended reading.

There is a significant amount of overlap between sections, and some areas are related more to your future job rather than to your current practice. Don't worry about this, as proportionally it will account for a relatively small part of the exam, and the exam will be a fair representation of what the job entails. The final statement, 15.11, should be the one to make you smile; this statement looks at everything not covered in the statements that have gone before and the Royal College's own personal safety net. It is the epitome of what general practice is: anything and everything in medicine, social care and life.

The questions at the end of each statement will either test your interpretation of the information in the text or explore other issues. Each section is ideal for an evening's revision after work, as they are relatively contained areas of work.

Statement 1

Being a general practitioner

The Royal College of General Practitioners curriculum has six domains of competency:

1 primary care management
2 person-centred care
3 specific problem-solving skills
4 a comprehensive approach
5 community orientation
6 a holistic approach.

The three essential applications are:

1 Contextual – the context of the person, family, community and their culture.
2 Attitudinal – actions based on the doctor's professional capabilities, values and ethics.
3 Scientific – a critical research-based approach, maintained through continued learning and quality improvement.

General Medical Council good medical practice: duties of a doctor (2006)

www.gmc-uk.org

This guidance is slightly more modern than the Geneva Convention and was developed because in the job that we as doctors undertake, patients must be able to trust us with their health and their life.

- Make the care of your patient your first concern.
- Protect and promote the health of patients and the public.
- Provide a good standard of practice and care:
  - keep your professional knowledge and skills up to date
  - recognise and work within the limits of your competence
  - work with colleagues in ways that best serve patients' interests.
- Treat patients as individuals and respect their dignity:
  - treat patients politely and considerately
  - respect patients' right to confidentiality.
- Work in partnership with patients:
  - listen to patients and respond to their concerns and preferences
  - give patients the information they want or need in a way they can understand
  - respect their right to reach decisions with you about their treatment and care
  - support patients in caring for themselves to improve and maintain health.
- Be honest and open and act with integrity:

- act without delay if you have good reason to believe that you or a colleague may be putting patients at risk
- never discriminate unfairly against patients or colleagues
- never abuse your patients' trust in you or the public's trust in the profession.

You are personally accountable for your professional practice and must always be prepared to justify your decisions and actions.

World Organization of Family Doctors European definition of general practice

The World Organization of Family Doctors published a new definition of family practice in 2002. An overview of this was published in the *New Generalist* (spring 2003):

The discipline of general practice:

- is normally the first point of medical contact in the healthcare system
- makes efficient use of resources through coordination
- develops a person-centred approach
- has a unique consultation process that establishes a relationship over time
- has a decision-making process based on prevalence and incidence of illness
- manages acute and chronic problems
- promotes health and well-being
- deals with health problems in their physical, psychological, social, cultural and existential dimensions.

The specialty of general practice was summarised as follows.

- GPs are specialist physicians trained in the principles of discipline. They are primarily responsible for provision of comprehensive and continuing care.
- They care for individuals in the context of their family, community and culture. They recognise they have a professional responsibility to their community.
- They exercise their professional role by promoting health, preventing disease and providing cure or palliation.
- They must take responsibility for maintaining their skills, personal balance and values.

The future of general practice

Parliament is responsible for the entire NHS, and Gordon Brown's first major speech regarding the NHS emphasised the role in not only disease management but also prevention and health promotion. General practice is here to provide a primary care service to the whole population, and everyone in the United Kingdom has a right of access to a GP (i.e. the first point of contact with the NHS together with A&E, family planning, NHS Direct, genitourinary clinics and other primary care services).

The role of GPs is demand-led and covers preventive healthcare, acute and chronic diseases, business and personnel management, research, audit, training and teaching, as well as coordination between services for patients and their families.

Over the past years there have been several major changes:

1 2000: NHS Plan.
2 2004: The new GMS Contract.
3 2005: Practice-based commissioning.
4 2007: The Future Direction of General Practice.

The future direction of general practice: a road map

www.rcgp.org.uk/PDF/Roadmap_embargoed%2011am%2013%20Sept.pdf

This is a vision document, mapping the way forward for general practice in a time of rapid change.

The focus is on three main points.

1 Improving quality of the doctor–patient relationship.
2 Developing general practices as learning organisations.
3 Encouraging collaboration between practices.

Interestingly, it cautions against the polyclinics that have received a great deal of media attention recently.

Shaping Tomorrow: issues facing general practice in the new millennium

In 2002, as part of the ongoing development, Chris Mihill of the General Practitioners Committee of the British Medical Association issued this discussion document. It collected views from the profession, from politicians and from patients, addressing topics such as what patients want and what model should replace the 'Dr Finlay, icon of the all-purpose, 24-hour, home-visiting family doctor'. Although there are 12 chapters in the document, I have selected and summarised what I consider to be the most important issues.

My doctor or any doctor?

With regard to access directives, two main patient groups have emerged: the essentially well who value easy access to healthcare with staff able to deal with their problems, and those with chronic diseases who prefer to see their own doctor. In countries where there is little continuity of care (or records) there are higher rates of investigation. Here lies an obvious argument for continuity of both care and records.

Should GPs let go and use the primary healthcare team?

This really focuses on the purpose of the consultation, and although most patients are happy to see a nurse for triage or treatment of a minor illness there is the flip side that no consultation is trivial but, rather, is an opportunity for discovering hidden agendas and health promotion.

Independent contractor status versus salaried service

Independent contractor status is deemed to allow GPs greater control over their working practice, hours and staff, and to act as advocates on behalf of their patients. This is thought to encourage innovation, change and efficiency. However, there is a widely held belief that independence is an illusion. Taking a salaried stance does not mean that you lose your autonomy, or that you can no longer be an advocate for your patient.

A job for life or a portfolio career?

Young doctors want flexible careers, to work part-time, the chance to move between practices or even to mix general practice with other careers.

Gate keeper: is there still a role? Will walk-in centres and NHS Direct change the game?

It is anticipated that in the future this, or another form of triage, will be used in the first instance, with GPs further down the line.

Clinical autonomy, does it have a place any more?

This in a way goes back to the independent contractor status issue in that, whatever your opinion, we live in the world of the National Institute for Health and Clinical Excellence, the National Service Framework, guidelines, protocols, evidence-based medicine and clinical governance.

Primary care groups: working together or professional straightjacket?

Primary care trusts mean increasing accountability and increasing pressure to deliver consistent care in an evidence-based way.

Promoting quality – what makes a good GP? Will revalidation stop bad doctors?

This chapter looks at issues such as quality (which in itself will not mean the same to us all), consistency and increasing the number of GP specialists (i.e. additional GP roles contracted by the primary care trust – patients would then be referred to secondary care from that point).

Future pressures

This looks at what patients want (not what they necessarily need), funding and rationing. Pressure will come from all areas – the elderly, genetics, the Internet, consumerism and patient expectations, all of which will drive standards.

Out-of-hours care/24-hour responsibility

The demand for out-of-hours care by patients has been steadily increasing over the last 40 years. This is reflected by the increase in night visits claimed and the attendance in casualty departments. Deputising services and out-of-hours cooperatives changed the way GPs fulfil their 24-hour responsibility to their patients, and following the new General Medical Services contract, the out of hours cover for our patients is something that we are no longer directly responsible for.

Raising Standards for Patients: new partnerships in out-of-hours care was published in October 2000, followed by the 3-year guidance plan. It made various recommendations including:

- triage through a single call to NHS Direct by 2004 (for all out-of-hours care)

- electronic records that out-of-hours staff can access
- quality assessments of medical staff, organisation and access through clinical governance.

NHS Direct

www.nhsdirect.nhs.uk

NHS Direct is a 24-hour telephone advice line staffed by specially trained nurses and aimed at empowering patients by giving them 'easier and faster information about health, illness and the NHS' (i.e. going some way towards the government's vision of a modernised healthcare system). It now allows single-call access to out-of-hours care (the Exemplar Programme), offering a triage service – and it has been gradually increasing in capacity since 1998. It also has a health website and the facility to ask for information if you are unable to locate it on the site (although it cannot answer specific health queries online), as well as an NHS Direct digital television service.

Positive points included are that it:

- is aimed at reducing NHS workload
- has easy access for patients
- empowers patients
- encourages self-care
- has an accompanying NHS Direct healthcare guide.

Concerns include the following:

- It may fuel workload/demand.
- Issues surrounding continuity of care.
- Missed diagnosis with telephone consultations.
- Will there be adequate integration with out-of-hours cover? If not, this may cause confusion.
- Not equally accessible to all (e.g. deaf, elderly, mentally ill, non-English speaking).

Dr Ian Banks (a GP in Northern Ireland), with the help of an editorial board, wrote the NHS Direct healthcare guide. The literature is designed for use in conjunction with NHS Direct. It gives basic information using narratives and flow charts on health and illness, as well as giving a guide as to when patients should contact NHS Direct for further advice. As well as being a printed booklet, it is available from the NHS Direct website. Again, a large problem is promotion and accessibility to those most in need (e.g. socially deprived or illiterate).

Impact of NHS Direct on general practice consultations during the winter 1999–2000: analysis of routinely collected data

BMJ 2002; 325(7377): 1397–8

The introduction of NHS Direct had no impact on the number of consultations for influenza-like illness and other respiratory infections. NHS Direct was not introduced to increase or decrease the number of consultations but, rather, to make them more appropriate. This was not looked at in the study.

Effect of introduction of integrated out of hours care in England: observational study

BMJ 2005; 331(7508): 81–4

This study was to quantify service integration achieved in the national Exemplar Programme for single-call access to out-of-hours care through NHS Direct and its effect on the wider healthcare system. Outcomes measured were extent of integration; impact on ambulance transport; attendance at A&E, minor injury units and walk-in centres; and emergency admissions to hospitals.

It concluded that most patients made two calls to contact NHS Direct and then had to wait for nurse feedback (29% achieved single-call access). Emergency ambulance transports increased in three of the four exemplars. The overall concern was the lack of capacity within NHS Direct to support the National Implementation Strategy.

Walk-in centres

These have been developed to cover demand and integrate out-of-hours care, to offload some of the burden on A&E departments, to improve access to healthcare professionals and to help reduce GP workload by providing treatment and information for minor conditions.

In the initial period, 40 centres were opened in England. The King's Fund Report released at the end of 2001 called for a halt in the expansion of the pilot programme and for more skills training for nurses. It also suggested improved links with GPs and other healthcare providers.

When trying to determine the efficacy of walk-in centres (and NHS Direct) it is worth bearing in mind that:

- they direct funds from other areas of primary care
- there can be a lack of continuity of care and delay in treatment
- patients are often referred back to their GP
- the service may generate a new demand.

The impact of co-located NHS walk-in centres on emergency departments

Emerg Med J 2007; 24(4): 265–9

This study looked at eight sites with co-located centres and eight controls. As most hospitals had implemented the concept to a very limited extent, there was no evidence of any effect on attendance rates, process, costs or outcome of care.

Impact of NHS walk-in centres on primary care access times: ecological study

BMJ 2007; 334(7598): 838

This study looked at 2059 practices in 56 primary care trusts, over a 21-month study period. It considered the number of people waiting for appointments over 48 hours and the distance from a walk-in centre. The waiting time of less than 48 hours increased from 67% to 87% over the study period and this was not related to proximity of a walk-in centre. The study was re-run to determine whether the improvement was artificial because of the government target to improve access, but results were similar.

Intermediate care

Intermediate care is a new phrase for the old concept of bridging the gap between primary and secondary care. This is not just about providing social care for elderly patients in the effort to free hospital beds; it can encompass various schemes such as mental health, the young chronically ill and so forth. It should not be regarded as a cheap alternative to acute hospital and specialist care.

Intermediate care, by definition, is not part of the current GP contract/General Medical Services. Although much of the medical input is provided by GPs, it does not follow that if no GP cover is available that these patients should be allocated to a GP until they are discharged from their intermediate care bed. It is envisaged that intermediate care beds will primarily be nurse-managed on a day-to-day basis, and GPs would be involved from the diagnostic, management and review aspect. The role of community matrons as part of the intermediate care team is starting to be explored.

For intermediate care/hospital at home to be successful, it is important to set up measurements of success, and to determine the type of patients who are to be cared for and the level of care to be input, as well as determining resource allocation. The paper 'Intermediate care and specialist GPs' calls for the expansion of numbers of GPs and nurses with the necessary educational support to cope with what will become an increased demand.

Nurse practitioners

Nurse practitioners are playing an increasingly large part in the service provision of primary care. Coupled with the ongoing struggle in some areas to fill GP posts, nurse practitioners will continue to expand their role. Their roles are varied, depending upon the skills and experiences of the nurse, but the main areas of input are disease prevention, health promotion, chronic disease management, immunisation (child and travel), smears and family planning. Management of minor illnesses, triage and prescribing are areas of ongoing development but they require specific diagnostic skills training to reduce errors in treatment and advice.

From the GP's perspective, this addition to the team will allow redistribution of workload and will improve access, satisfaction and standards of care. GPs may have more time for more challenging problems and may be able to operate with larger lists.

Possible problems include the following:

- Nurses are not regulated, so who will be accountable? Will it be us as the GP?
- Is a two-tier system being introduced and will GP recruitment suffer further because of this, particularly in inner cities?
- We may lose continuity of care as the GP.
- Nurses may misdiagnose rare but serious conditions, if there is no diagnostic index of suspicion.
- GPs may start to lose their generalist role.
- Protocols and guidelines need to be developed. Who will write these – the GP? Would they then be accountable when the patient dictates a variation from the directive?

- Nurses as a body are already overloaded trying to reach targets with the new General Medical Services contract and National Service Frameworks. Can we really expand their role further, given the current shortfall in numbers?
- Funding and training as well as interest/staffing are areas where needs have to be met.

Safety of telephone triage in general practitioner cooperatives: do triage nurses correctly estimate urgency?

Qual Saf Health Care 2007; 16(3): 181–4

This study used five mystery callers who telephoned four cooperatives to assess whether 118 nurses, using the telephone triage guidelines, assessed the degree of urgency accurately. In 19% of the calls the urgency was underestimated, giving cause for concern regarding safety. It would have been interesting to compare with GPs using the same scenarios!

Impact of nurse practitioners on workload of general practitioners: randomised controlled trial

BMJ 2004; 328(7445): 927

This was a randomised, controlled (before and after) trial of 34 general practices in the Netherlands. Five nurses were randomly allocated to practices to undertake specific duties. Workload was derived from 28-day work diaries and was measured for 6 months before and 18 months after the introduction of a nurse practitioner. They found there was no significant difference in workload for GPs in this short term.

Community matrons

These posts are a logical extension into the community of nurse practitioners aimed at improving health and social care for patients with long-term complex medical problems, the aim being to reduce hospital admissions. As yet there are no data or trials looking at the effectiveness in terms of their brief.

Their role is to include the following:

- Avoid inappropriate hospital admissions.
- Optimise the health and well-being of adults who meet set criteria for being managed within their own home (e.g. falls, non-specific illness, long-term conditions, revolving-door patients).
- They will define the category of patient, develop care plans and evaluate progress.

Nurse prescribing

www.dh.gov.uk

Since the 1990s it has been possible for nurses to prescribe independently from limited formularies. The number of nurse prescribers is slowly increasing and is currently around 8000, reflecting the time needed to complete training.

Prescribing by nurses falls into five different categories:

1 Specific exemptions (e.g. midwives, health visitors and district nurses).
2 Patient specific directives – is a written instruction from a recognised prescriber which is patient specific.

3 Patient group directives – a named drug can be issued for specific clinical situations (all must conform with HSC 2000/026). This is as opposed to a clinical management plan, which is patient specific, not drug specific.
4 Independent nurse prescribers – are deemed competent to assess, diagnose and make treatment decisions and may prescribe from the British National Formulary.
5 Supplementary prescribers – have to be an independent nurse prescriber but have a voluntary prescribing contract working to clinical management plans (patient specific, with no restriction on the condition). Some pharmacists have undertaken this role.

The benefits of nurse-prescribing include the following.

- The prescription can be written by the clinician who sees the patient.
- Nurses can work independently.
- It improves patient safety, the professional seeing the patient is trained to make the decision, and as a doctor signing a script you are not reliant on often inadequate information.
- Safety is helped with use of electronic systems that highlight interactions.
- The full British National Formulary is now available for use within the practitioner's area of competence (since 2006).
- It can free up medical time.

The current drawbacks include:

- A number of GP systems will not accept nursing prescribers and scripts must be a handwritten duplicate.
- There is concern about the safety fears of many prescribers, drug safety and the necessary continuity of patient care.
- Many nurses do not use their skills following the training, lose confidence and so are less likely to initiate scripts.
- The Commission on Human Medicines has expressed concerns over lack of monitoring the initial objective: timely and safe access to medicines.

Pharmacists

The role of the pharmacist in primary care is also increasing. Community pharmacists are an underused resource in the NHS, despite their level of training. The government launched the first wave of its National Medicines Management Programme in October 2001. This project may help the government go some way towards reaching its National Services Framework targets and meeting patient demand; they can also train as supplementary prescribers in the same way as a nurse practitioner.

Following successful pilot studies, and with the new pharmacy contract, repeat prescribing for patients (along with other enhanced services such as warfarin monitoring, services for drug misusers) is to be undertaken by pharmacists and commissioned by primary care. Other areas of pharmacist management that will be considered in the future include lipid management, immunisation, diabetes and weight management.

Repeat prescribing: a role for community pharmacists in controlling and monitoring repeat prescriptions

Br J Gen Pract 2000; 50(453): 271-5

This study looked at conventional repeat prescribing versus pharmacist-managed prescribing. It concluded pharmacist management was feasible. It identifies problems not always seen by GPs (in terms of compliance, adverse drug reactions or interactions) and it could make savings in the drug bill (up to 18%) – that is, it would outweigh the cost of the pharmacist.

Randomised controlled trial of clinical medication review by a pharmacist of elderly patients receiving repeat prescriptions in general practice

BMJ 2001; 323(7325): 1340-3

This trial concluded that a clinical pharmacist can conduct effective consultations with elderly patients in general practice to review their drugs. These reviews resulted in changes in patients' drugs and saved more than the cost of the intervention without affecting the workload of GPs.

The 2001 British Lifestyle Survey (conducted by consumer research firm Mintel) found that the number of people who asked the pharmacist for advice had increased by 25%. Over-the-counter analgesic sales have risen by 41% and sales for remedies for coughs and colds have increased by 10%, all over the last 10 years.

Being a general practitioner: questions

For questions 1–5 answer true or false.

Effective teamwork requires which of the following?

1 Information systems.
2 Professional divisions.
3 A blame culture to get to the bottom of things and understand shortcomings.
4 Goals and objectives.
5 Appropriate leadership.

Being a general practitioner: answers

1 **True** Communication lines are important.
2 **False** Professional divisions usually create obstacles.
3 **False**
4 **True**
5 **True**

Statement 2

The general practice consultation

The consultation. You can't ignore it, it is central to what we do every single day and has always been important. To be an effective doctor, communication skills are of paramount importance, and for these to be evident there has to be an inclination to engage with your patient. Harry Brown described the consultation as a 'complex series of interactions that have to be analysed and assessed quickly'; although we become accustomed to doing this rapidly it is in itself a huge area of risk.

With your trainer you will be doing this indirectly all of the time as part of your video work and consultation observation tools. Once you are familiar with the different models you could use the frameworks to help structure consultations in a positive way, especially if you feel that your usual style isn't working, or when analysing a consultation that has gone wrong.

What I have tried to do for this statement is to give a brief summary of some of the more commonly used models. Of course, this is no substitute for reading the original texts from cover to cover, but this is probably a little easier to digest.

It is worth noting that the formal history-taking part of clinical management, if used prematurely, can stifle the patient's agenda. A patient's initial narrative is an important part of the consultation. It has been proved, contrary to popular belief, the majority of patients will not go on to talk indefinitely, but will usually stop within 1 minute. Allowing patients to get their problem off their chest uninterrupted greatly increases satisfaction on all sides.

General reflections

Getting it right in the consultation: Hippocrates' problem; Aristotle's answer

Dr John Gillie, Occasional Paper 86, Royal College of General Practitioners

This paper considers many thoughts and approaches to medicine, decision-making, ethical values and philosophies that have developed, mainly over the last 50 years, but drawing on work 2000 years old (given the understanding that human nature has changed little over that time).

Among other analyses, Gillie considers Toon's analyses of several models of general practice, and McWhinney's 1996 description of the four main ways general practice differs from other specialties. These can be briefly summarised:

1 It defines itself in terms of relationships, especially the doctor–patient relationship.
2 We tend to think in terms of individuals rather than generalise.
3 We have an organismic approach (i.e. consider the whole) rather than mechanistic (i.e. the part).
4 It is the only major field that transcends the division between mind and body.

This will in no way be a quick read, but it would be worthwhile.

Reflections on the doctor-patient relationship: from evidence and experience

Br J General Pract 2005; 55(519): 793–801

Moira Stewart considers general practice 'whole-person medical practice', with the understanding that doctor–patient relationships evolve over time and with shared experiences (with a common goal of diagnosis and cure).

The six interactive components of the patient-centred methods discussed are summarised:

1. Exploring disease and the patient's illness experience.
2. Understanding the whole person.
3. Finding common ground.
4. Incorporating prevention and health promotion.
5. Enhancing the patient–doctor relationship.
6. Being realistic.

The paper concludes that without general practice there would be more confusion, fear and doubt.

Calgary–Cambridge guide

This 1996 model can be summarised as follows:

1. **Initiating the session:**
   - establishing a rapport
   - identifying reasons for consultation.
2. **Gathering information:**
   - exploration of the problem
   - understanding the patient's perspective
   - providing structure for the consultation.
3. **Building the relationship:**
   - providing the correct amount and type of information
   - aiding accurate recall and understanding
   - achieving a shared understanding
   - shared decision-making
   - negotiating a management plan.
4. **Closing the session:** final summary.
5. **Contracting:** establish a plan or contract with the patient.
6. **Safety netting:** similar to Neighbour's model.
7. **Final check:** before moving on.

Stott and Davis model

Stott and Davis published this four-part model in 1979 that would probably be the way many of us deal with a consultation, certainly on the face of it.

Management of presenting problem	Management of continuing problem
Management of health seeking behaviour	Opportunistic health promotion

Neighbour model

This is a popular five-point check model from 1987. It consists of the following steps:

1. **Connecting** – establishing a relationship; this needs rapport-building skills.
2. **Summarising** – 'What I am hearing is …'; this needs the ability to listen and skills to facilitate effective assessment.
3. **Hand over** – responsibility is given to the patient; this needs good communication skills to hand over the responsibility for management as it involves negotiating and influencing (to a certain extent).
4. **Safety netting** – 'Have I missed anything?' and instructions for follow up if . . .; this needs predictive skills to suggest contingency plans for the worst-case scenario. Ability to mentally file one consultation so there is no effect on the next patient's consultation.

Pendleton model

This is otherwise known as the 'social skills model'. It has seven tasks.

1. To define the reason for the patient's attendance including the following:
   - the nature and history of the problems
   - their aetiology
   - the patient's ideas, concerns and expectations
   - the effects of the problem.
2. To consider other problems:
   - continuing other problems
   - at-risk factors.
3. To choose with the patient an appropriate action for each problem.
4. To achieve a shared understanding of the problems with the patient.
5. To involve the patient in the management of their case and to involve them in acceptance of appropriate responsibility for it.
6. To use time and resources appropriately.
7. To establish or maintain a relationship with the patient which helps in the achievement of other tasks.

Balint model

This is a psychological model of the doctor–patient relationship, formed in part by the understanding that doctors have feelings and that these have a function within the consultation.

Balint explains that a patient's problem will have psychological and physical components and that these will be interlinked. Indeed, psychological problems may manifest themselves clinically. Individual doctors vary in their awareness of these points, but they can be trained to be more sensitive and aware.

Important features of Balint's model include the following:

- The doctor as a drug.
- The child of a patient may be brought in with a trivial problem for the patient to make contact (i.e. the child as the presenting complaint).
- Elimination by appropriate examination.

- Collusion of anonymity.
- 'The Flash'.

Berne's transactional analysis

Berne, *The Games People Play*, London: Penguin Books; 1968

This model looks at the roles that patients and doctors take within the consultation, and it identifies three ego states.

1. Parent: critical or caring.
2. Adult: logical.
3. Child: dependent.

This is a useful model for analysing why consultations go wrong. Often a doctor will flit between the adult and parent states, and the patient will flit between the adult and child states (and the parent state, to a lesser degree). Imagine a consultation in which both the doctor and the patient assumed the role of 'child'. I'm sure you would agree it is likely to be dysfunctional.

There are many variations on Berne's ego states. Peter Tate considered how people perceive themselves with a health belief model and identified three types of patients: (1) the internal controller (a person in charge of their own health); (2) the external controller (they do not believe they are in control); and (3) the powerful other (they do not believe they are in control but they are not fatalists either).

Middleton agenda model

This is a four-point dynamic model where the patient's agenda is paramount. It is not task-oriented.

1. **Patient's agenda**: this includes the ideas and reasoning that underlie the problems presented.
2. **Doctor's agenda**: this includes risk factors, continuing problems, public health agenda, partnerships and personal agendas.
3. **Communication skills**: these can be chosen to reconcile the agendas (e.g. facilitation and negotiation).
4. **Negotiated plan**: this includes management of problems and health promotion.

Patients' perceptions of GP non-verbal communication: a qualitative study

Br J Gen Pract 2010; 60(571): 83–7

We sometimes forget that patients are very astute and will often come back reflecting how you looked or how things went based on the non-verbal aspects of the consultation (and usually indicative of the type of day where there are more patients than there is time). This qualitative study looked at 24/36 patients who reported a total of 48 non-verbal clues: tone of voice, eye contact and facial expression. Keep things like this in mind when you look at your watch for the date!

Confidentiality

The success of the doctor–patient relationship is dependent on a number of factors. Confidentiality ('secrecy and discretion') has a therapeutically significant role, and has been fundamental to our code of practice since before the Hippocratic oath. Without its assurance patients may be reluctant to give doctors the information they need in order to provide good care. Information learned about a patient belongs to that patient (even after death) and they have the right to determine who has access to it.

Confidentiality: NHS Code of Practice

www.dh.gov.uk

This document is for people working in the NHS and it:

- introduces the concept of confidentiality
- describes what a confidential service should look like
- describes the main legal requirements
- support tools for sharing/disclosing information
- lists examples of disclosure scenarios.

Disclosure to a third party, the Data Protection Act

A doctor's legal obligation of confidentiality is best seen as a public not a private interest (i.e. the obligation is not absolute and in some situations the law allows or even obliges doctors to breech confidentiality). You are advised to discuss issues with your Defence Union if there is any ambiguity surrounding the need to disclose the information being requested.

Examples where a doctor must breech confidentiality include termination of pregnancy (Abortion Act 1967), notifiable diseases (Public Health Act 1984), births and deaths (Births and Deaths Registration Act 1953) and forms for Incapacity Benefit. The police can request names and addresses (but not clinical details) of persons alleged to be guilty under the Road Traffic Act 1988.

Examples of circumstances where doctors have discretion to breech confidentiality include imparting information to other members of the healthcare team, a patient driving who is not fit to drive (the General Medical Council advises informing the Driver and Vehicle Licensing Agency), and where a third party is at significant risk (e.g. the partner of an HIV-positive patient who is unaware of the diagnosis and risk).

Consent and confidentiality go hand in hand and it is good practice to seek the patient's consent to disclosure of any information wherever possible, whether or not you judge that a patient can be identified from the disclosure.

The Human Rights Act 1998, the Data Protection Act 1998, the Crime and Disorder Act 1998 and the Common Law Duty of Confidentiality all enable agencies to share information without consent with regard to children at risk of harm. Any person arguing that their medical information has been unlawfully disclosed is likely to argue the right to a private life under Article 8(1) of the Human Rights Act.

Access to Health Records Act 1990

A patient has the right to see his or her medical records, obtain copies of these records and have records explained.

Limitations to this right include the following:

- This act only applies to records after 1 November 1991. Records before this date are included if they are needed to understand later notes.
- A doctor can deny access to a patient's medical records if it is believed serious harm to the patient's physical or mental health will result from seeing records.
- A doctor should ensure that confidentiality of other people is maintained.

The doctor's duties in accessing health records

- The doctor should enable the patient to see the records (or copies) within 21 days, or 40 days for records that are more than 40 days old.
- The doctor may charge a reasonable fee for copying records and time spent explaining records.
- The doctor should make corrections if the original data is incorrect.

Confidentiality and the Caldicott report

Following the review by the Caldicott committee of patient-identifiable information (December 1997), the Caldicott report was issued. The report was commissioned in light of publication of *The Protection and use of Patient Information* in 1996, because of concerns about the way patient information is used in the NHS and the need to ensure confidentiality is not undermined.

The report has 16 recommendations:

1. Every dataflow, current or proposed, should be tested against basic principles of good practice. Continuing flows should be re-tested regularly.
2. A programme of work should be established to reinforce awareness of confidentiality and information security requirements amongst all staff within the NHS.
3. A senior person, preferably a health professional, should be nominated in each health organisation to act as a guardian who is responsible for safeguarding the confidentiality of patient information.
4. Clear guidance should be provided for those individuals/bodies responsible for approving uses of patient identifiable information.
5. Protocols should be developed to protect the exchange of patient identifiable information between NHS and non-NHS bodies.
6. The identity of those responsible for monitoring the sharing and transfer of information within agreed local protocols should be clearly communicated.
7. An accreditation system that recognises those organisations following good practice with respect to confidentiality should be considered.
8. The NHS number should replace all other identifiers wherever practicable, taking account of the consequences of errors and particular requirements for other specific identifiers.
9. Strict protocols should define who is authorised to gain access to patient identity where the NHS number or other coded identifier is used.
10. Where particularly sensitive information is transferred, privacy enhanced technologies (e.g. encrypting identifiers or 'patient identifying information') must be explored.

11 Those involved in developing health information systems should ensure that best practice principles are incorporated during the design stage.
12 Where practicable, the internal structure and administration of databases holding patient identifiable information should reflect the principles developed in this report.
13 NHS number should replace the patient's name on Items of Service Claims made by GPs as soon as is practically possible.
14 The design of new systems for transfer of prescription data should incorporate the principles developed in the Caldicott report.
15 Future negotiations on pay and conditions for GPs should, where possible, avoid systems of payment that require patient-identifying details to be transmitted.
16 Consideration should be given to procedures for GP claims and payments which do not require patient identifying information to be transferred, which can then be piloted.

If you only remember five points from the Caldicott guidelines, remember that information should be treated as follows:
1 held securely and confidentially
2 obtained fairly and efficiently
3 recorded accurately and reliably
4 used effectively and efficiently
5 shared appropriately and lawfully.

Assuring the confidentiality of shared electronic health records

***BMJ* 2007; 335(7632): 1223–4**

This editorial was written following the recent loss of patient information (of 25 million people) and looks at the security issues that arise with our increasing move to centralise huge amounts of data from multiple sources. Although centralisation is thought to be advantageous from a patient safety point of view and for overall general security when protecting the data, there is still a great degree of concern over the NHS Care Record Service.

The difficult patient

This is an inevitable problem for us all and happens for different reasons (doctor, patient and/or external factors). 'Heartsink' patients form a different group of people to frequent attenders, they have been defined (by Groves, 1978) as patients who most physicians would dread having to treat as they engender negative feelings.

As early as 1951, Groves defined four types of difficult patient:
1 **Dependent clinger**: grateful but seeking reassurance for minor ailments.
2 **Entitled demander**: complaining about imagined shortcomings in service provided.
3 **Manipulative health rejecter**: has symptoms the doctor cannot improve.
4 **Self-destructive deniers**: refuses to accept their behaviour affects their disease and will not modify habits.

Heartsink patients are often over-investigated or referred unnecessarily, particularly if they are seeing several GPs and no one doctor takes responsibility for that patient. It is important, for your own sanity (as well as it being in the patient's best interest), to develop coping strategies and a sensible, thorough approach to heartsink patients.

Coping strategies

- Recognising your own feelings.
- Accept that heartsinks will occur.
- Review patient's notes.
- Set goal limits for the patient.
- Assume ownership of a problem and review regularly.
- Set limits for the patient (e.g. when you expect to see them again).
- Challenge inappropriate demands.
- Peer group meetings/Balint groups with other doctors.
- Consider alternative sources of therapy (for your patient).

Heartsink patients: a study of their general practitioners

Br J Gen Pract 1995; 45(395): 293–6

Mathers looked at the heartsink patients' GPs and found that GPs who had a low job satisfaction and no post-graduate qualifications reported more heartsink patients. It is important to recognise this association for our own self-preservation. If we are stressed we start to lose our coping mechanisms and start heading towards burnout.

Angry patients

We come across this in many ways for many reasons: a patient that has had difficulty getting an appointment, feels someone has been rude to them or that there has been a mistake or shortfall in the service provided. It may come in the form of a letter, in a consultation or across the reception desk. It may be anticipated but it may be totally unexpected and although it would be mainly verbal outbursts, sometimes there may be physical elements.

With the current MRCGP exam, the most likely way you will have to deal with this will be in the Clinical Skills Assessment. Practise it in your training practice and consider the following thoughts below to try and diffuse the situation. Remember patients get angry for lots of reasons and respond differently to techniques to try calm things down; feel your way gently and acknowledge the effect it has on your own levels of adrenaline.

Handling aggressive patients

BMJ Careers 12 August 2006

This article by Anita Houghton looks at non-violent communication to deal with anger and considers three main rules.

1. Resist your instinctive responses (the fight-or-flight mechanism) – try not to be defensive or confrontational.
2. Remain calm; manage your own mental and emotional state.
3. Be curious about their feelings and needs.

In your own surgery a number of these cases will be expected before they happen and your team will have ways of checking that all is well, such as a well-timed phone call or interruption, and there are always the alarm bells if you find yourself in a dangerously aggressive situation.

Continuity of care

Access and continuity have both long been identified as being important factors, the problem being that the more swift the access the less likely the ability to maintain continuity.

Continuity of care in GP surgeries: valued by many but hard to deliver

New Generalist 2007; 5(3): 53–5

George Freeman explains a programme he has been working on to determine what patient's priorities are. There is some criticism of Darzi's plans for polyclinics and lack of foresight as to the importance and preference of continuity. Continuity can be segmented into: information, management and relationship. The article is thoughtful and gives a robust overview of current thinking, definitely worth reading.

The work is based on a qualitative paper (*Br J Gen Pract* 2006; 56(531): 749–55) interviewing 31 patients to look at service use.

The general practice consultation: questions

1 Which of the following is correct regarding the folk model of illness (1981)?
   a. It was written by the medical anthropologist Helman Folk as part of his PhD thesis.
   b. It is not a sapiential piece of work.
   c. It suggests that when a patient comes to see a doctor they are seeking the answer to six questions.
   d. The Stott and Davis model is a more up-to-date model applicable to today's method of consultation.
   e. Is a model that deals with the role of doctor and patient in the parent, adult and child context.
2 Which of the following would be a good summary of the triaxial model?
   a. The roles of parent, adult and child personas.
   b. Physical, psychological and social terms of a patient's problem.
   c. A sapiential, moral and charismatic anthropological approach.
   d. A sociological approach to history, diagnosis and management of the issues.
   e. An informative, catalytic and supportive approach to the patient's problem.
3 The health belief model is which of the following?
   a. A three-point model.
   b. A four-point model.
   c. A five-point model.
   d. A six-point model.
   e. A 12-point model.
4 Which of the following is not a reason to breach confidentiality?
   a. A patient who is driving 2 months after having an unexplained daytime fit.

b. In the case of a termination of pregnancy.
c. When completing an Incapacity/Disability Benefit form.
d. When requested by the police to provide details on a patient arrested for death by dangerous driving who is blaming his medication.
e. A patient with human immunodeficiency virus.

5 The Expert Patients Programme is about which of the following?
a. Allowing patients to self-medicate for their condition with confidence.
b. Is the individual support for patients provided by healthcare workers?
c. Group education for patients to help them self-manage and understand their condition.
d. Groups of patients coming together to form action groups and to develop pathways that are patient-oriented.
e. Groups organised to enable patient to fully understand their legal rights within the NHS today.

The general practice consultation: answers

1 c The folk model of illness was written by the medical anthropologist Cecil Helman in 1981 (after Stott and Davis) and is not related to Bern's transactional analysis that focuses on the parent/adult/child roles in a consultation. Helman believes that patients want six questions answered when they attend:

- What has happened?
- Why has it happened?
- Why has it happened to them?
- Why has it happened now?
- What would happen if nothing were done about it?
- What can/should be done about it?

2 b The triaxial model was written in 1972 and encouraged doctors to think of the patient as a whole: emotional, family, social and environmental effects. It specifically refers to physical, psychological and social terms.

3 b The health belief model is a four-point model around the decision of a patient to consult:

- The individual's general interest in health matters, which may correlate with personality, social class or ethnic group.
- How vulnerable or threatened a patient feels to be towards a particular disease.
- The individual's estimation of beliefs of treatment weighed against cost, risk and inconvenience.
- Trigger factors, such as alarming features, advice from family or friends, messages through the media, disruption of work or play.

4 d These are very general comments. The Driver and Vehicle Licensing Agency should be informed (i.e. confidentiality breeched) in the scenario with a fit. Notifiable diseases (Public Health Act 1984) and termination of pregnancy (Abortion Act 1967) both need to be declared through the proper channels (i.e. breech of confidentiality). The police can request name and address details of patients but they cannot request clinical details without patient consent and usually legal representation.

5 c Expert Patients Programme (www.expertpatients.co.uk/course-participants/self-management-life).

Statement 3.1

Clinical governance

Highlighted to the public in a Labour government White Paper was the point that the NHS will not tolerate anything less than the best. This was and is to be achieved in a no-blame, questioning, learning culture.

Where revalidation is a professional-based measure to ensure high standards of care, clinical governance has more of a management and quality base, being accountable to the government through the primary care trusts. It is aimed at improving the quality of services offered in the NHS and safeguarding high standards, as well as creating an environment in which clinical excellence will flourish.

There are many facets to governance but our working knowledge is on a day-to-day basis with National Institute for Health and Clinical Excellence guidance use, audit, medicine management teams and local quality initiatives with associated monitoring and feedback.

The government has done for medicine as it did for teaching and created beacon practice status for those 'most worthy'. These practices demonstrate high standards in access, patient care, health improvement and so forth. They are paid a nominal £4000 a year and in return are expected to promote their way of working, mainly through 12 open days per year at the practice for others to learn by example.

Each GP has a responsibility to provide a high quality of care and to audit this. Patients need to be confident that their doctor is up to date and is offering effective treatment. Clinical governance is an effective tool for monitoring and improving quality of care in general practice.

Making clinical governance work

BMJ 2004; 329(7467): 679–81

This discussion opens with the statement that clinical governance is 'by far the most high-profile vehicle for securing culture change in the new NHS'. The main points made are as follows.

- Clinicians should be at the heart of clinical governance.
- Failing to take account of the scope of the clinicians' work will result in their disengagement of management.
- Integrated care pathways are needed for common conditions.
- Healthcare professionals need support and systematic evaluation of their performance.

Commission for Health Improvement

www.chi.nhs.uk/ratings/

This is a body representing the government; it is made up of GPs, nurses and laypeople, to look at clinical governance at the local level every 4 years. They can report underperformance to the Health Secretary. They will investigate mainly organisational systems.

There are new proposals suggested in the National Health Service Reform and Health Care Professions bill where the Commission for Health Improvement will be able to recommend that the Health Secretary takes special measures against failing GP practices. This bill also created an office within the Commission for Health Improvement to collect and publish statistics on primary care services and give patient groups the right to inspect all GP premises.

Significant event analysis

This process of significant event analysis (SEA) is known by various names including significant event audit, critical event audit or analysis, and significant event review. It can include examples of when things go right as well as wrong. It can be clinical or non-clinical and it can involve anyone in the team, the point being that such events are powerful motivators for change and the questions that may be raised could identify a previously unidentified learning need. SEA should be felt to be a positive experience by all those involved.

How can SEA be organised?

- Decide who is to be involved (e.g. doctors, nurses, receptionists, administration/office staff) for specific SEA.
- How are they to be organised (e.g. regular meetings, triggered by specific cases)?
- The time interval after the event should not be too long, otherwise momentum is lost and details are forgotten; this is especially important if new ideas are to be implemented.
- The meeting should be free of interruptions.
- A suitable environment is needed. Sometimes it is beneficial to be outside the work place.
- Set ground rules (e.g. confidentiality and anonymity).
- Appoint a chairperson and a scribe for appropriate record keeping.
- The agenda may include the following points:
  - Why has the significant event been chosen?
  - What do people want to achieve by analysing it?
  - What are the facts of the case? (These are often circulated before the meeting.)
  - What issues are raised (e.g. care, communication)?
  - What went well?
  - What went badly and how can things be improved? (Shortcomings could be highlighted and things that are amenable to change, rather than personal attacks. Comments should be constructive.)
  - What actions should be taken? (Formulate a plan, prioritise points, decide upon a time scale, consider how success can be determined.)

Medical/clinical audit

Audit definitions have evolved somewhat from Maurin's thoughts in 1976, in terms of it being a general counting exercise, to the modern-day government's definition in *Working for Patients*, which defines audit as 'the systematic critical analysis of the quality of medical care, including procedures used for the diagnosis and treatment, the use of resources and the resulting outcome and quality of life for the patients' (i.e. it is a much more active approach).

Donabedian identified three major categories in 1982:

1 Audit of **structure** – delivery of care (e.g. appointments).
2 Audit of **process** – how patients are treated (e.g. looking at prescriptions).
3 Audit of **outcome** – what ultimately happens (e.g. mortality, morbidity).

In *Duties of a Doctor*, the General Medical Council describes audit as an essential professional responsibility. The Royal College of General Practitioners Information Service (No. 17) published an information leaflet on medical audit in March 2001 (www.rcgp.org.uk).

Audit is a means by which we can look systematically and critically at our work, the final stage of evidence-based medicine. It is not research (research is done to find out what best practice is). Audit is a measure of performance against a predetermined standard. It can highlight problems, encourage change, reduce errors and demonstrate good care. Audit is increasingly part of clinical governance and will become an integral part of revalidation. Help with audits can be found in primary care audit groups and medical audit advisory groups.

The audit cycle:

- Ask the question – the reason for your choice of audit.
- Identify the criteria – evidence based.
- Set the standards – identify the criteria and set the standard to be audited against.
- Prepare and plan the audit.
- Observe practice/collect data.
- Compare with set standards.
- Implement changes.
- Reassess and conclude after a specified time.

The other frequently used approach is a PDSA: Plan, Do, Study, Action.

Complaints

A complaint is an expression of dissatisfaction that requires a response. The number of complaints against GPs has doubled in the last 10 years, and handling of complaints has become part of the new General Medical Services contract. Handling complaints well puts things right for the individual who has received (either real or perceived) a poor service and allows those services to be improved. Resolving issues at an early stage is the ultimate aim. The Medical Defence Union estimates that 90% of complaints are resolved at practice level.

Main complaints encountered in general practice are:

- delay or failure to make a diagnosis, or an incorrect diagnosis
- failure to visit
- surgery appointment times/availability

- staff attitudes/rudeness
- inadequate examination
- refusal to refer.

If an individual wishes to make a complaint this should be done within 6 months of the incident, or within 6 months of finding out that there was something to complain about. The general consensus is that a complaint should be made within 1 year.

The NHS complaints procedure has three stages:

1. Local resolution (with or without an independent lay conciliator liaising between the two parties).
2. A convenor who can request an independent review or refer back for local resolution.
3. The Ombudsman (Health Service Commissioner).

Complaints procedure in primary care

Following the Wilson report in 1994, *Being Heard*, the complaints procedure was revised in 1996 and is now in the process of being updated again. This is happening following a response document, *Reforming the NHS Complaints Procedure: a listening document* (which is available from www.dh.gov.uk), and the General Medical Council have published several booklets that explain the complaints procedure and how to raise concerns.

All practices should have a written and publicised complaints procedure explaining who patients should speak to and what to expect (required as part of our contract).

In the event of a complaint:

1. The nominated person or deputy should interview the complainant and again explain the procedure.
2. Complaints must be acknowledged within 2 working days, or at the time if verbal.
3. The complainant should receive a written response within 10 working days (20 if it is a hospital complaint).

The response should:

- summarise the complaint
- explain the patient's view of the complaint
- apologise, if appropriate
- describe the outcome and steps taken
- explain the next step, how to contact the health authority/primary care trust if the complainant is still unhappy with the outcome.

If someone other than the patient makes the complaint, ensure that consent is obtained from the patient. Be clear and concise and try to avoid medical terminology. If you do have to use technical terms, ensure they are explained clearly.

Practices should:

- keep separate complaints file

- include complaints statistics in the contract report, and for revalidation in the future
- hold practice meetings on complaints and how to manage them.

The NHS complaints procedure is not about tackling disciplinary action, which would need to be investigated by a professional disciplinary body having been referred by the primary care trust to a disciplinary panel. Disciplinary measures can only be taken if a GP has failed to comply with their terms of service. Furthermore, the procedure does not deal with claims for financial compensation, private healthcare treatment or events about which an individual is already taking legal action.

The Independent Complaints Advocacy Service in the NHS body will help patients or families who wish to lodge a complaint against the NHS. The Patient Advice and Liaison Service is there to help patients, arbitrate and assist if they wish to make a complaint.

If all routes have been exhausted and the patient still does not have the response they were looking for, then the Parliamentary and Health Service Ombudsman would be their next step (www.ombudsman.org.uk).

Revalidation: professional self-regulation and recertification

www.gmc-uk.org and www.rcgp.org.uk

Although plans for revalidation have been in progress since 1998, the fifth report of the Shipman Inquiry in 2004 and other recent cases (such as the Bristol case) have meant that the process of ensuring fitness to practice has become much more public. Sir Liam Donaldson published *Good Doctors, Safer Patients*, and a recent White Paper, 'Trust, assurance and safety: the regulation of health professionals in the 21st century' (2007) which re-enforces the government stance on driving revalidation forward.

Revalidation will be an episodic process (probably 5-yearly) to show fitness to practise to the professional regulator (the General Medical Council).

There will be a:

- relicensing process based on generic standards
- recertification process that will apply to specialists or general practitioners to show they meet standards that apply to their specialty
- suspension and retraining process in the event of failure.

The responsibility of basic competence is that of the individual doctor; it always has been and always will be, and there will always be other factors that allow incompetence and poorly performing professionals to be brought to our attention (e.g. prescribing data, complaints, new contract fulfilment, referral types – not specifically quantity but quality and so forth). One of the difficulties highlighted by various editorials is how to make revalidation stimulating and worthwhile for the majority of doctors while also being sensitive enough to pick out those who are performing poorly.

A revalidation party produced *Revalidation for Clinical General Practice* for the Royal College of General Practitioners. It anticipates that revalidation will be related to a number of different systems, e.g. clinical governance, accredited professional development, appraisal, General Medical Council performance procedures and so forth.

The criteria identified for revalidation to work are:

- **It should be understood by the public and be credible.**
- **It should identify unacceptable performance.**
- **It should identify good performance.**
- **The profession should support it and it should support the profession.**
- **It should be practical and feasible.**
- **It should not put any GPs or practices at an advantage or disadvantage.**

Revalidation should be a continuous summative process with an episode submission and assessment of fitness to practise, having been through an annual appraisal process. Evidence should be drawn from the doctor's day-to-day practice.

Where are we with revalidation/recertification?

In Autumn 2007 Mayur Lakhani published an article in the *New Generalist* about the framework of recertification. He outlines four pillars:

1 Essential general practice.
2 Managing continuing professional development.
3 Modern professional practice in the specialism (performance).
4 Professional standing relicensure (standards).

There are several reasons why revalidation has been postponed. The Chief Medical Officer is conducting an enquiry into the General Medical Council's role, following concerns raised by the fifth Shipman report. It is thought that initial changes may have been brought about because of the cost of revalidating 30 000 doctors a year and the duplication of current systems with little evidence that it would stop another Shipman.

A way forward

BMJ 2005; 330(7503): 1326–8

This article, written by Lakhani, outlines ten guiding principles for revalidation. It includes the recognition that revalidation is summative, needs clear criteria, needs lay involvement, must be in addition to appraisal and clinical governance and should include local certification. It also advocates that reliability of information should be ensured, there should be alternative routes for revalidation, a tighter definition of a managed clinical environment and that the standards should be consistent across the whole medical profession (where possible).

Clinical governance: questions

1 Which of the following options best describes the assessment of structure, process and outcome?
   a. SEA.
   b. Significant review analysis.
   c. Audit.

d. Revalidation.
e. Research.

2 In an NHS complaint to the Health Service Ombudsman about an alleged missed diagnosis, which of the following would you expect him to advise?
a. A referral to a solicitor for independent advice.
b. A request for primary care trust involvement for arbitration.
c. A referral back to the practice for local resolution where possible.
d. A hearing with their representative to assess the facts of the case.
e. A referral to a convenor who can request an independent review and refer back for local resolution.

Clinical governance: answers

1 c This is the process described by Donabedian.

2 c Local resolution is the first step; although a convenor can be involved, that wouldn't normally happen at this stage.

Statement 3.2

Patient safety

Medical error

To err is human. It is also the title of a report published in the United States several years ago that put patient safety on the international agenda. Individual mistakes are inevitable whether or not humans are involved, and they are usually caused by alignment of different factors. Complacency will always be unacceptable.

Reducing medical mishaps is fundamental in improving quality. 'First do no harm' is part of the Hippocratic oath, but harm is done every day, and it needs skill to translate these negative events into useful information. For this to happen there needs to be some sort of reporting to enable system changes that will improve patient safety; for this to be successful it is recognised that there needs to be a no-blame culture. Liam Donaldson wrote that when something goes wrong people want to know who knew what, when did they know and what did they do about it. Averting your gaze or opting for a quiet life is not the correct thing to do, and it gradually loses the respect of your peers. It is important to remain non-judgemental while making preliminary investigations, as things may not be what they seem.

Doctors tend to overestimate their ability to function flawlessly under adverse conditions such as fatigue, time pressure and high anxiety. Aviation and other non-medical, hands-on industries have developed incident reporting where the focus is on near misses. There are incentives for voluntary reporting, confidentiality is ensured and the emphasis is on data collection, analysis and improvement rather than a punitive approach.

Gaps in continuity of care that lead to near misses or harm can be described at three levels:

1. individual people
2. stages
3. processes.

Understanding and reinforcing our ability to bridge these gaps can achieve increasing safety. Despite all the defences, barriers and safeguards that are inbuilt, mistakes will continue to happen, so the aim should be on minimising the risks at each stage.

For example, system changes to improve patient safety would include:

- reducing complexity and having a systematic approach
- optimising information processing with awareness of workload
- automating wisely (i.e. use IT to support human operation rather than because it is available)
- using constraints to restrict certain actions and double-check critical processes

- mitigating the unwanted side effects of change (e.g. test on a small scale to try to predict problems that may occur by monitoring outcome)
- training in safety issues for all staff
- regular audit.

Examples where this approach has been successful are seen in the pharmaceutical industry with drugs and anaesthetic attachments.

The 'error-prevention movement' has accelerated and major changes are occurring in the way that we think about and carry out our daily work. There is an undercurrent of more slowly evolving cultural change in our learning, responsibilities and ability to admit fallibility.

For risk assessment (i.e. near-miss reporting) to be successful, incidents need to be: analysed in an organisational way, rather than on a personal basis, creating a culture that is open and fair; formal protocols need to be developed to ensure systematic, comprehensive and efficient investigations; training needs to be part of the developing programme for it to be a standardised and effective tool, and there needs to be support for patients, family and staff.

Should systems reporting be voluntary?

An example of voluntary reporting is the Safe Medical Devices Act 1990. Reporting is fundamental in the broad goal of error reduction. Non-punitive, confidential, voluntary reporting programmes provide more useful information about errors and their causes compared with mandatory reporting:

- There is no fear of retribution.
- The depth of information is the key to understanding the problem. If reporting is forced then the primary motivation is self-protection and adherence to requirement, not to help others avoid making the same mistake.

As things change in the future, in the name of continuous quality improvement, it must be remembered that the person who makes the mistake needs help too, a point that is all too easy to forget and is often overlooked.

Patient safety: safer by design

***BMJ* 2008; 336(7637): 186–8**

Tonks walks us through the reasons why thousands of patients are harmed. She quotes from a Department of Health report that the NHS is 'complex, chaotic and clueless about design ... the consequence being a significant incidence of avoidable risk and error'. There is an idea that we break rules to make patient's lives easier: a 'conspiracy of benevolence'. Although design skills will help reduce error, it should be used with open-mindedness.

Although this chapter is based on clinical issues, it is important not to overlook that as a GP partner you have a legal responsibility to your staff and their working environment, from working at high levels and risk avoidance to the provision of appropriate ambient temperatures in the work place. The government Health and Safety Executive (www.hse.gov.uk/) and the Advisory, Conciliation and Arbitration

Service (www.acas.gov.uk) are both helpful sites, although probably beyond the scope of what you will need for the MRCGP.

National Patient Safety Agency

www.npsa.nhs.uk

The role of the National Patient Safety Agency (NPSA) is to promote an open and fair reporting culture, collecting, collating, categorising and coding adverse incidents. This helps to look for and identify patterns and trends and then to act on identified risks.

The NPSA was established in July 2001 to improve patient safety by running a national reporting system to log adverse clinical events and near misses, so lessons can be shared and learned from in a blame-free way. GPs have to report all incidents where a patient has been, or could have been, seriously harmed. This comes following *A Commitment to Quality: a quest for excellence*, a document published in June 2001.

The NPSA document *Doing Less Harm* applies the reporting rule to all incidents, including anaphylaxis and unexpected death in the surgery (both of which are categorised as red). Other incidents will be categorised as green, yellow and orange, depending upon severity.

In 2005 the NPSA introduced the *Being Open Policy*, a further document encouraging healthcare professionals to be frank about their mistakes. This was introduced to all NHS organisations in June 2006. There are three main issues to this policy:

1. The principle is that when something goes wrong be open, apologise, investigate, learn and provide support.
2. Patient safety investigations are disclosable in a court case, but the benefits of being open could outweigh the costs.
3. There should be exemption from disciplinary action when reporting incidents with a view to improving patient safety.

The World Alliance for Patient Safety

The World Health Organization launched this in Washington, DC, in October 2004, with a number of important actions intended to reduce harm caused to patients. These included the following:

- The global patient safety challenge – focusing on healthcare-associated infection.
- Patients for patient safety – involving patient organisations in Alliance work.
- Taxonomy for patient safety – ensuring consistency of concepts, principles and terminologies.
- Research for patient safety – promoting existing interventions and coordinating international efforts to develop solutions.
- Reporting and learning – generating best practice guidelines for existing and new reporting systems.

The National Reporting and Learning System for adverse events and near misses was launched alongside the report to encourage healthcare professionals to report incidents on a confidential basis.

Medication and safety

Building a safer NHS for patients: improving medication safety was launched in February 2004. It is a paper that looks at causes and frequency of medication errors and sets out a framework for a common quality of care throughout the NHS (taking further steps to achieve the aims of the Chief Medical Officer's report, *An Organisation with a Memory*). It estimates that potentially serious errors occur between 1 in 1000 and 1 in 10 000 times per script, most of which is identified before any harm is done. The report considers medication processes generally, high-risk patient groups, high-risk drugs and organisational changes.

The Commission on Human Medicines replaced the Medicines Commission and the Committee on Safety of Medicines and has the following responsibilities:

- advise ministers on licensing policies
- have overall responsibility for drug safety issues
- advise on appointment of other professional bodies serving the Medicines and Healthcare products Regulatory Agency (MHRA)
- hear initial appeals from drug companies when a licence has been rejected.

The MHRA circulates updates, cascades areas of risk and advertises the yellow card reporting system (www.mhra.gov.uk/Safetyinformation/DrugSafetyUpdate).

Within the British National Formulary (BNF) and online there is a reporting system for all side effects and interactions that may occur, especially with regard to newer (black triangle) drugs on the yellow card (www.yellowcard.mhra.gov.uk), nd public health departments have ongoing vaccination surveillance programmes for all vaccines.

Other safety issues and thoughts

- Update records appropriately (e.g. information regarding drug allergies).
- Prioritise workload to minimise risk for patients.
- Use everyday tools at your disposal to minimise risk: your computer system to flag up drug interactions and coded allergies, General Practice Notebook (www.gpnotebook.co.uk/), Best Practice (http://bestpractice.bmj.com), coffee break with colleagues and so forth.
- Consider significant event analyses inhouse; this is all clinical governance.
- Consider follow-on audit to identify other patients at similar risk.
- Consider involving the extended healthcare team in identification of problems (e.g. your local pharmacist).
- Be aware of your own limitations – PUNs and DENs again (the patient's unmet needs and the doctor's educational needs).
- Keep up to date.
- Make sure you take your holiday and use your study leave!

Patient safety: questions

1 If you see ▼ next to a drug in the BNF, what does it mean?
   a. This is a drug with new features and it is being intensively monitored by the MHRA.

b. This is a new drug to the market and it is contraindicated in pregnancy.
c. This is an immunosuppressant drug with potentially toxic side effects.
d. This symbol is only ever seen next to new drugs to the market and you should report all suspected adverse reactions.
e. This symbol means that the drug has been withdrawn because of concerns over side effects and adverse reactions.

2 Healthcare professionals and coroners are encouraged to report suspected adverse drug reactions to which of the following groups?
a. The Health Secretary.
b. The local Medicines Management Team.
c. The BNF.
d. The Drug Safety Research Unit.
e. The MHRA.

For questions 3 and 4, see the BNF recommendations for rifampicin prophylaxis.

Rifampicin 600 mg every 12 hours for 2 days; child 10 mg/kg (under 1 year, 5 mg/kg) every 12 hours for 2 days

Rifadin®(Aventis Pharma) PoM

Capsules, **rifampicin** 150 mg (blue/red), net price 20 = £3.81; 300 mg (red), 20 = £7.62. Label: 8, 14, 22, counselling, see lenses above

Syrup, red, **rifampicin** 100 mg/5 mL (raspberry-flavoured). Net price 120 mL = £3.70. Label: 8, 14, 22, counselling, see lenses above

3 The correct dose and total number of tablets required for a 37-year-old woman for prophylactic treatment is:
a. 600 mg daily, 8 × 300 mg capsules.
b. 600 mg daily, 16 × 150 mg capsules.
c. 1200 mg daily, 8 × 300 mg capsules.
d. 1200 mg twice daily, 16 × 300 mg capsules.
e. 1800 mg daily, 24 × 300 mg capsules.

4 The correct dose for a 2-year-old child weighing 15 kg is:
a. 25 mg twice daily for 2 days.
b. 75 mg twice daily for 2 days.
c. 75 mg daily for 2 days.
d. 150 mg daily for 2 days.
e. 150 mg twice daily for 2 days.

5 One of your staff complains that the air conditioning is too cold and that it is causing neck stiffness. What is your responsibility as an employer?
a. Perform a risk assessment measuring the temperature, as it should not fall below 16°C.
b. Perform a risk assessment measuring the temperature, as it should not fall below 11°C.
c. Provide hot drink facilities.

d. Provide appropriate clothing to enable staff to keep warm, so all staff will be happy.
e. Stop the use of the air conditioner until staff can agree on use.

Patient safety: answers

1 a This can apply to any drug; it could be new, have had a change in licence, there may be a new delivery system or it may have a new combination of active substances. You should report (or the patient can) all suspected adverse reactions, even if it is not clear that the medication has caused the problem, on the yellow card system. The MHRA will review all the data, often within 2 years, although there is no set time period.

2 e Through the yellow card system. The Drug Safety Research Unit collects information in a different way, provided voluntarily by GPs when they send through a green form. The patient's details are gained through the prescription pricing authority (where scripts go after being dispensed).

3 c The correct dose and total number of tablets for a 37-year-old woman: 2 × 300 mg bd for 2 days = total of 8 × 300 mg capsules.

4 d Work out the correct dose and amount of syrup needed for a 2-year-old child weighing 15 kg: 10 mg/kg × 15 = 150 mg bd for 2 days; 150 mg = 7.5 mL bd for 2 days = total of 30 mL. What does PoM mean? Prescription-only medication.

5 a This question is included to reflect the importance of employee rights and work place health and safety, as well as patient safety. The Health and Safety Executive site discusses some of the issues around thermal comfort, as it can be a passionate topic among employees (www.hse.gov.uk/contact/faqs/temperature.htm). The general consensus is that temperature should not usually fall below 16°C (13°C degrees if physical work is expected). You could also look at seating position, reason for the air conditioning being used (check the heating isn't on at the same time!) and flexibility in uniforms to enable staff to dress according to temperature.

Statement 3.3

Clinical ethics and values-based practice

Understanding the law helps us deal with disputes, a proper understanding of medical ethics will help us work in true partnership with our patients.

Dr Cox, 8 November 2001

Medical ethics

Medical ethics is a source of anxiety for many, especially when approaching exams like the MRCGP. The Hippocratic oath first outlined an ethical approach to medicine, and the General Medical Council requires that medical ethics be a core subject in the medical curriculum. Try not to be daunted by the subject; most of what you need you already know, but it is now a case of formulating a way of thinking and talking about ethical principles, using an ethical model that you can apply to a given situation.

Medical ethics applies to all areas in medicine, including end-of-life decisions, medical error, priority setting, biotechnology, education, consent and confidentiality.

MEDICINE October 2000 Vol. 28, 'Ethics and Communication Skills'

This provides an excellent narrative, not only on ethics but also on communication skills. I have summarised some of the points regarding ethics.

Simply applying an algorithm cannot solve questions on ethical values. If we are to practise medicine in a way we think is right, we must:

- clarify what value judgements are relevant in a specific clinical situation
- be aware of the relevant issues
- subject our views to critical analysis to ensure they are logical and consistent
- adapt or change our views in the light of such analysis.

In addition we must practise medicine in a legal framework.

The four principles approach

1. Respect for **autonomy** (self-rule): help patients to make their own decisions, and respect that decision even when you do not agree.
2. **Beneficence** (do good): this entails doing what is best for the patient, but who is the judge of what is best? This may conflict with autonomy.
3. **Non-maleficence** (avoiding harm): in most cases this does not add anything to the principle of beneficence.

4 **Justice**: this incorporates time and resources, truth and fairness in a legal context.

Refining and implementing the Tavistock principles for everybody in healthcare

BMJ 2001 323(7313): 616–20

The Tavistock group published their original five principles in 1999, having been brought together by the *BMJ*. The principles are not evidence based but are meant to serve as an ethical framework for those working to improve medical error, and they give doctors another way of considering the ethical basis of decisions we have to help patients make.

The ethical concepts of the Tavistock group can be summarised as follows:

- **Rights** – people have a right to health and healthcare.
- **Balance** – care of individual patients is central, but the health of the population is also our concern.
- **Comprehensiveness** – in addition to treating illness, we have an obligation to ease suffering, minimise disability, prevent disease and promote health.
- **Cooperation** – healthcare succeeds only if we cooperate with those we serve, one another and those in other sectors.
- **Improvement** – improving healthcare is a serious and continuing responsibility.
- **Safety** – do no harm.
- **Openness** – being open, honest and trustworthy is vital in healthcare.

The Declaration of Helsinki (revised for the fifth time by the World Medical Association) was adopted in 1964 and gives widely accepted ethical principles for medical research involving human subjects. It is not clear whether this declaration has any real legal standing, or whether it is just to serve as a guide. The UK Clinical Ethics Network is there to offer educational and practical support for clinical ethics groups.

Consent

The ***Good Practice in Consent Implementation Guide: consent to examination or treatment*** is a 50-page document produced by the Department of Health's Good Practice in Consent Advisory Group. The guide summarises legal requirements and good practice requirements regarding consent. Consent is a process – as you take your patients through initial examination, investigation and treatments – not a one-off event.

The *12 Key Points on Consent: the law in England*, a useful resource, is available online (www.dh.gov.uk/en/Publicationsandstatistics/Publications/PublicationsPolicyAndGuidance/DH_4006131). The document is relevant to all healthcare professionals, including students. It briefly touches on consent issues for the use of organs or tissues after death although this is being reviewed. It is worth noting that law changes depending upon different test cases brought and that the European Human Rights Act will have some effect on English law.

The British Medical Association ethics department published the *Consent Tool Kit* (the fifth edition is available online: www.bma.org.uk/images/

consenttoolkitdec2009_tcm41-193139.pdf), aimed at improving the understanding and the practice of obtaining valid consent by providing doctors with answers to some questions that may arise when seeking consent.

Similarly the General Medical Council have *Seeking Patient's Consent: the ethical considerations*, and *0–18: guidance for all doctors* (for children). Consent under the Mental Capacity Act is discussed in Statement 13.

The approach taken to consent is fundamental to the doctor–patient relationship and highlights an individual's ethical viewpoint to a patient's autonomy. Tony Hope wrote a good ethics-based piece on consent in *Medicine* (October 2000). He points out a useful, quick three-point check on legal validity:

- Is the patient properly informed?
- Is the patient competent to give consent?
- Did the patient give consent voluntarily (without coercion)?

From a legal point of view, consent provides patients with a power of veto. Without consent a patient could successfully sue a doctor for battery. Technically, touching another person without consent constitutes battery (i.e. the patient does not need to have suffered harm). Similarly a doctor could be found negligent if they have not given the patient certain relevant information to allow the patient to give informed consent.

The fact that a person comes to see a doctor or is admitted to hospital does not imply consent to any examination, investigation or treatment. In giving or refusing consent it is important that the patient understands the reasons behind treatment, the associated risks and benefits and the consequences if they refuse treatment (even the issuing of a prescription requires consent). It does not matter how the patient gives consent. It can be written, verbal or non-verbal, and a signature does not prove consent is valid. Documentation of information given and consent received is important.

In UK law, the term 'informed consent' does not exist: explicit consent is required. Legal duties are defined by statute (e.g. the Children Act 1989 and the Human Rights Act 1998) and by common law (which is general principles from specific cases). There is also guidance on the use of chaperones, which should be offered when any intimate (breast, genital or rectal) examination or procedure is to be carried out. Practices are advised to have a chaperone policy in place. This is following the Ayling report (2004) by the Department of Health.

Fraser guidelines

Confidentiality is important in all patients, but young patients often think that their parents can access their records and that they have to be over 16 to see a health professional and receive treatment without their parents. This is not the case.

A young person can consent to treatment if:

- the young person understands the doctor's advice
- the doctor cannot persuade the young person to inform his or her parents, or allow the doctor to inform parents that he or she is seeking contraceptive advice

- the young person is very likely to begin, or continue having, intercourse with or without contraceptive treatment
- unless he or she receives contraceptive treatment, the young person's physical or mental health (or both) are likely to suffer.

The Bolam principle

The Bolam principle is central to understanding our duty of care as applied to consent issues (and negligence). Bolam was a patient who received electroconvulsive therapy that resulted in a fractured jaw. Bolam sued (in 1957) and the outcome was such that 'a doctor is not guilty of negligence if he has acted in accordance with the practice accepted as proper by a responsible body skilled in that particular art'.

Mental Capacity Act 2005

www.legislation.gov.uk/ukpga/2005/9/contents

The Mental Capacity Act 2005 is covered in Statement 13.

Clinical ethics and values-based practice: questions

1 What would be the appropriate course of action in a 15-year-old girl requesting contraception?
   a. Contact her parents to confirm they are agreeable.
   b. Encourage her to talk to her parents, or a responsible relative, and do not prescribe the pill until she has managed to do this.
   c. Encourage her to talk to her parents, or a responsible relative, and only issue condoms for use until she has been able to do this.
   d. Encourage her to talk to her parents, or a responsible adult, and involve social services if she is not able to do this.
   e. Encourage her to talk to her parents, or a responsible adult, providing her with contraceptive cover in the meantime.

Testamentary capacity is dependent on a number of factors that in our role as general practitioners we are often called upon to confirm, given that an increasing number of wills are contested after a testator's death. For questions 2–6, indicate whether each statement is either true or false.

2 If a person is suffering from delusions they are automatically considered as being incapable of testamentary capacity.
3 A testator must be able to understand both the effect of making a will and the extent of their estate.
4 The 'golden rule' should always be observed, no matter how straightforward matters may appear.
5 It is important for a medical practitioner to review all wills where a person has made serial wills over the last years of their life.
6 Answers should be recorded verbatim in the medical records when assessing testamentary capacity.

Clinical ethics and values-based practice: answers

1 **e** This is a Fraser competency question – a relatively straightforward one.

2 **False** Only if the delusion influences the testator in making a particular decision.

3 **True**

4 **True** This is where a medical practitioner witnesses a will, having satisfied himself of the capacity and understanding of the testator.

5 **True** Time-consuming though this may be, it may reveal impairment of memory, judgement and even delusions.

6 **True**

Statement 3.4

Promoting equality and valuing diversity

Equality and diversity training is something that, as well as being available through the NHS, is underpinned by all of our training. From a management perspective it can mean taking an active role in helping people understand how their behaviour affects others. It is important to recognise all of the options we have available for communication with patients, from translators (www.languageline.co.uk) to specialist nurses (using communication aids such as dolls and pictures) and hearing loops for the hard of hearing.

This chapter has the scope to cover the Human Rights Act 1998, the Sex Discrimination Act 1986, the Employment Rights Act 1996, the Maternity and Parental Leave, etc. Regulations 1999, the Sex Discrimination (Gender Reassignment) Regulations 1999 and racial equality issues (visit www.equalityhumanrights.com for more information). Although a comprehensive understanding of all of these acts and caveats is not a realistic expectation, there will be certain issues that crop up that you can use to highlight the gaps in your knowledge and discuss with your practice manager or colleagues.

Equality Act 2010

www.homeoffice.gov.uk/equalities/

This Act bans unfair treatment and allows more equal opportunities of all in the work place.

Disability Discrimination Act 1995

www.legislation.gov.uk/ukpga/1995/50/contents

Divided into eight parts, parts II (Employment) and III (Discrimination in other areas) are the main sections affecting general practice. Part II looks at everything from the job application (you can no longer specify age, although age is still implied when certain qualifications are needed for a specific post) to the help and assistance that would be needed for a person to be able to fulfil a role. Part III is related to your premises, access to buildings, width of doors, automatic doors and positioning of consultation rooms and facilities.

Medicine and the Internet

With specific reference to equality and diversity, you must remember that not everyone has access to the Internet or a computer – sometimes this is too easy to forget.

It is accepted that the Internet can improve communication and access, both among professionals and between professionals and patients. One of the biggest problems with information on the Internet is that there is no quality control/regulation – that is, there is no guarantee the information is reliable – which means that we as GPs may need to guide our patients. The Health On the Net Foundation (HON, www.hon.ch/) is an international non-governmental organisation that provides a database of evaluated health material; you can search for information through this site. Any website health information that displays the HON logo means that the site has been developed in accordance with the foundation's guidelines. Worldwide online Reliable Advice to Patients and Individuals, a project led by HON, has been developed to enable comparison of health/medical documents in any format with this interconnected knowledge base – another step towards the certification of quality online information.

NHSnet

As part of a government directive, all GP practices should be connected to NHSnet, a private wide area network service used by the NHS. There are plans for health records to be networked, allowing doctors 24-hour access. This inevitably raises data protection issues, as addressed in the Caldicott report commissioned in 1997. Appointments (the ability to choose and book), X-ray and pathology requests are online, and pharmacists will be able to accept prescriptions electronically.

Only its users limit the potential applications of NHSnet. At whatever speed things are implemented, the systems used need to have been thought through in terms of confidentiality (patient and doctor), data protection and litigation issues. They also need to be quick, user-friendly and accurate.

Promoting equality and valuing diversity: questions

> **SALARIED GENERAL PRACTICE POST**
>
> Come and join our forward-thinking practice.
>
> - EMIS system and 10 200 patients
> - Maximum Quality and Outcomes Framework points achieved
> - Eight clinical sessions, one admin and one personal development
>
> We are looking for a motivated, experienced salaried GP aged 32–37 years, with a view to partnership.
>
> Call our practice manager on 0845 642345.

1 Consider this job advertisement. Is it legal?
   a. Yes
   b. No
   c. Almost
2 In an older practice with consulting rooms on lower and upper levels, which of the following is a statutory requirement with regard to access?
   a. A lift (or chairlift) should be installed for patients who are unable to use the stairs.

b. The doors to the building should be automatic.
c. All branches of a surgery should have disabled access to the main building.
d. Upstairs consulting rooms should be decommissioned because of disability discrimination.
e. A lift (or chairlift) should be installed if you have a member of staff who is unable to reach the upstairs rooms because of the nature of their disability.

3 When consulting with a person who is hard of hearing, which of the following is readily available?
a. An NHS signer.
b. An NHS lip-reader.
c. An acoustic horn.
d. A loop system.
e. A megaphone.

Promoting equality and valuing diversity: answers

1 b In an advert like this you can almost get away with using experience as a prerequisite, but you cannot specify age (or gender). However, the hours are legal, unfortunately!

2 c Lifts are ideal; chairlifts are probably more of a hazard. There is no great problem as long as there is access and as long as there are downstairs consulting rooms to use. Because of new building laws, if a new build was commissioned then a lift would need to be included. The access to surgeries can be a simple removable ramp; however, as surgeries go through their usual renovation processes many alter their permanent access to become user-friendly for everyone.

3 d Practically we probably all talk louder, jot things down and make sure we are facing our patients so they can lip-read. If using a loop, make sure the hearing aid is on the correct setting.

Statement 3.5

Evidence-based practice

Introduction

Evidence-based medicine was coined as a buzz phrase in the early 1990s. It has increased our awareness of research studies and improved our knowledge base within the profession as a whole. This can give our patients the confidence that we are up to date and that we are giving them appropriate advice.

Research findings (the evidence) are almost never black and white, and often they only look at a specific point at the expense of other issues (e.g. resources) in a specific clinical environment. This leaves us as the clinicians (who are not the best at interpreting studies) with the dilemma of how, or indeed if, we should use certain findings.

Sources of evidence are diverse, but the gold standard is held as a meta-analysis of randomised controlled trials. The Cochrane reviews are one point at which to access such information; however, even their validity has been questioned and The Cochrane Collaboration took steps to improve the quality of its reviews following a paper in 2001 that highlighted some minor problems.

There are many good websites for evidence-based medicine, including:

- National Institute for Health and Clinical Excellence (NICE) (www.nice.org.uk).
- Best Practice (www.bestpractice.bmj.com).
- Evidence in Health and Social Care (www.evidence.nhs.uk).

To be able to ascertain that guidance is reputable, the NHS evidence issues a Kitemark that highlights the most trustworthy. NICE has gained this accreditation.

Bridging the gaps in evidence based diagnosis

BMJ 2006; 333(7565): 405–6

This is an interesting article about making a diagnosis and reliance on valid evidence for tests that help us reach decisions that are based on many factors. It discussed the '4S' test of accuracy described by Haynes that looks at levels of organisation of evidence from research (*see* illustration on next page).

Obviously all this takes a huge amount of time and what we need practically to be able to implement work is concise and easily available information.

Parachute approach to evidence based medicine

BMJ 2006; 333(7570): 701–3

The parachute adage (i.e. you don't need a randomised controlled trial to tell you that testing parachutes is necessary to prevent death) is expanded on in this US article. The concern is that, because of the length of time it takes to get statistically

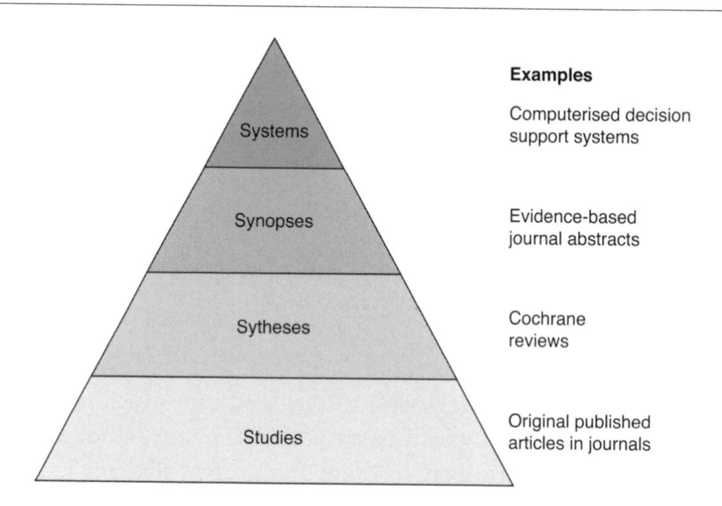

significant numbers, waiting for publication of randomised controlled trials before implementing new interventions can actually cost lives. The authors of this article advocate taking research to the problem and write that in making decisions, risk, benefit and local conditions should be taken into account, not just ideals.

Validation of the Fresno test of competence in evidence based medicine

BMJ 2003; 236(7384): 319–21

The Fresno Medical Education Programme in California has developed this test. It is a tool for assessing knowledge and skill (ability) in teaching evidence-based medicine and it can identify the strengths and weaknesses of curricula and individuals. It has a standardised grading system and it seems to be valid, although the authors point out that familiarity may have led to unrealistic scoring.

Guidelines

Guidelines are defined as systematically developed statements to assist practitioner and patient in making decisions about appropriate healthcare for specific clinical circumstances (Field and Lohr).

The aims of producing guidelines usually include the following:

- to assist decision-making
- to improve quality of care, effectiveness and outcome
- to standardise medical practice.

Guidelines need to be produced in an evidence-based way that acknowledges limitations such as resources, staffing and the local population for whom the guidelines are intended. They are thought of as a simple way to get evidence out into practice, improving quality of care in an equitable way. Despite this there are so many guidelines changing so frequently that even when looking at NICE guidance in isolation a *BMJ* article found that one in six trusts were not adhering to them.

Guidelines in practice, considering their role

Are they useful?

- Are they relevant in a clinical context?
- Are they user-friendly?
- Are they evidence based?

Appraisal of guidelines takes place through the NHS Appraisal Centre for Clinical Guidelines prior to national implementation.

Implementation

- The people who will be using the guidelines should have a sense of ownership, and should preferably be involved in the development (if not, then they should be involved in auditing and making amendments at a later stage).
- Local facilitators should help with the process of implementation.

Legal implications

- Guidelines can be used in court by an expert witness (not in place of) to demonstrate standards of care.
- Non-compliance to clinical guidelines does not mean that care is substandard.

Compliance

It can be difficult to comply with guidelines as they are not written for individual patients, but rather they reflect a consensus opinion based on the current evidence without making it apparent that they take into account uncertainties, or ethical or cultural issues which may arise in clinical management.

Potential benefits of guidelines

Potential benefits for the patients include:

- improved consistency of care
- empowerment to make informed choices.

Potential benefits for healthcare professionals include:

- improved quality of clinical decisions (although to a variable degree)
- as they are evidence based, they improve knowledge, highlight gaps and through audit improve quality of care.

Potential benefits for healthcare systems include:

- efficient use of resources
- distributive justice (i.e. ethical issues relating to rationing)
- improved public perception of equality.

Potential problems and drawbacks of guidelines

- They may be incorrect/flawed/biased or they may conflict with other professional groups.
- They can be time-consuming to implement and use.

- They are written for populations, not individuals.
- They will increase the overall resources needed (e.g. statins in cardiovascular disease).
- They need regular review to keep them up to date and usable.
- They do not address the complexity and uncertainties of medical practice.
- There are a vast number in use that we must be familiar with.

Clinical practice guidelines and quality of care for older patients with multiple comorbid diseases: implications for pay for performance

JAMA 2005; 294(6): 716–24

This is a paper that looked at following guidelines for major conditions (hypertension, ischaemic heart disease, diabetes, chronic obstructive pulmonary disease and osteoarthritis) in a hypothetical case and found that although the hypothetical patient would be eligible for 12 medications, none of the guidelines modified their directives or discussed issues relating to co-morbidity.

Thou shalt versus thou shalt not: a meta-synthesis of GPs' attitudes to clinical practice guidelines

Br J Gen Pract 2007; 57(545): 971–8

Adherence to guidelines is variable. This meta-analysis looked at 17 qualitative papers and it found that guidance was followed to differing degrees depending upon whether it was prescriptive (encouraging a certain type of behaviour and innovation) or proscriptive (discouraged certain treatments or behaviours, which in rationing may affect the relationship with our patients). Another reason identified was differing patient needs (see the paper discussed above and lack of consideration noted for co-morbidities in most guidelines).

National Institute for Health and Clinical Excellence

www.nice.org.uk

NICE was launched in England and Wales in 1999 and aims to produce guidance in three areas of health in order to get the most from the resources available:

1 Health technologies, both new and existing, including drugs, treatments and procedures.
2 Clinical practice – appropriate treatment and care of people with specific diseases and conditions.
3 Public health – promotion of good health and prevention of ill health.

It was created to produce guidelines for health professionals and must ensure its advice is based on rigorous analysis of all the available evidence, both clinical and economic. The group also seeks advice on social, ethical and moral questions from the citizens' council, a team of individuals, representative of the population of England and Wales. Their decisions are advisory, not mandatory, but local health organisations are obliged to review their management against guidelines as they are published. There is a requirement to provide funding within three months for medicines and technologies recommended by NICE.

As part of NICE there is a Referral Practice Project Steering Group, which is responsible for the recently published guidelines.

Following the controversial reversal of its decision on zanamivir, since April 2001 all evidence has to be open. However, there is still a concern that NICE may be influenced by industry or patient organisations.

Resource allocation NICE work

BMJ 2006; 332(7552): 1266–8

This discussion paper looks at where NICE is at currently, how decisions are made, and examines some of the influences it is under. At the time of writing there were 86 guidances and there had been 25 appeals (meaning that some subjects have been appraised several times. At the current rate there are around 20 appraisals a year, so logistically only a minority of new treatments are covered.

The House of Commons Health Committee conducted an enquiry into NICE (January 2002). This considered to what extent the institute has provided independent, clear and credible guidance and also whether it had enabled patients to have faster access to drugs known to be effective, and whether guidance is accepted locally and acted upon. The Health Select Committee and the Consumer's Association have criticised the work of NICE as flaws have been found in guidance issued.

Many independent authors consider that it is a matter of time before NICE guidance becomes mandatory and they continue to discuss the serious concerns as to how statistical tools are decided upon and the ultimate conclusions reached.

One of the most significant human rights issues is that NICE have released a statement that in the future they recommend against treating patients who smoke. Their current thought is that age and lifestyle factors that may have caused disease shouldn't influence guidance on use of interventions unless they are likely to affect the effectiveness of the intervention.

National Service Frameworks

National Service Frameworks (NSFs) were proposed in the 1998 White Paper, 'A First Class Service: quality in the new NHS,' as part of the government's agenda to drive up quality and reduce unacceptable variations in health and social services across the United Kingdom. They have been proposed as accompaniments to NICE and identified as priorities in *Modernising Health and Social Services: national priorities guidance for 1999/2000–2000/01.*

Standards will be set by NICE and NSFs, delivered by clinical governance and underpinned by self-regulation and lifelong learning. The Commission for Health Improvement, the National Performance Assessment Framework and National Survey of Patients will be used to monitor the NSFs. Performance will be assessed through a small number of national milestones and high-level performance indicators.

There will be advances and changes during the implementation of the NSFs. Therefore they will have to evolve if they are to stay relevant and credible in such a changing environment. Similarly, the need for learning and development (organisational, professional and personal) is recognised.

Objectives of NSFs are as follows:

- To address problems that affect quality of NHS care.
- To tackle variations in:
  - agreed standards of care
  - data collection and audit
  - local provision of national services
  - funding and resources
  - involvement with non-NHS agencies.

Critical reading

At the risk of sounding like a secondary school teacher, your ability to assess the quality of the work published will only improve if you practise. If you decide to take the MRCGP, critical appraisal will form part of the applied knowledge test (multiple-choice questions), not to mention your daily job. You may not read whole papers very often but you need to learn the skill to assess whether it is worth taking your time to read papers that may change your practice.

It is well recognised that we are clinicians, not statisticians, and although it is important for day to day work looking at journals to have a simple critical appraisal template that you can apply to articles, it is never usually necessary to appraise articles from scratch. There are some excellent books on appraisal of research – since the written part of the MRCGP is no longer, this has probably less of a specific focus. I have included here some basics (from first principles) on reading a paper and statistics, which you will hopefully find of help. Another good reference is Trisha Greenhalgh's book *How to Read a Paper: the basics of evidence based medicine.*

READER: an acronym to aid critical reading by general practitioners

Br J Gen Pract 1994; 44(379): 83–5

R: Relevance

- to general practice
- to your environment
- general awareness

E: Education

- behaviour modification
- challenges to practices and beliefs

A: Applicability

- own environment
- generalisability

D: Discrimination

- quality of the study
- type of study: descriptive/randomised controlled trial
- sample size
- selection
- controls

- bias
- results
- statistics
- conclusions

E: Evaluation
- reflection

R: Reaction
- implementation

Remember to always try to be positive about a study first.

Template for critical appraisal

1. **Summary**
   - Concise statement of topic and conclusions.
2. **Introduction**
   - Is there a clear outline?
3. **Methods and design**
   - Are the selection and sample size appropriate?
   - Strengths, limitations.
4. **Results**
   - Is presentation clear?
   - Are results both clinically and statistically significant?
5. **Discussion**
   - Are statements true?

Keele University model

This method will help you get the important information from each section (i.e. to summarise the paper).

- **Is it of interest?**
  - Look at the abstract, title, authors and so forth.
- **Motivation, why was it done?**
  - Look at the introduction, is it clear?
  - Who funded the research?
- **Design, how was it done?**
  - Look at the methods: sample, recruitment, numbers, collection of data.
  - Measurements: are they valid/reliable?
  - Analysis: what statistics were used?
  - Any ethical problems or bias?
- **Results, what did it find?**
  - Look the at results: are data described, do the numbers add up and so forth?
  - Was statistical significance assessed?
  - Were all the data used?
- **Conclusions, what are the implications?**
  - Look at the discussion.

- Has anything been overlooked?
- Are the findings relevant?

◆ **Anything else of interest?**

- For example, references.

Appraisal of a paper

1. Is the hypothesis clearly described?
2. Are the outcomes measured clearly described? If these are first mentioned in the results section, then the answer to this is no.
3. Are the characteristics of the group (e.g. inclusion/exclusion criteria) clearly described?
4. Are the interventions clearly described?
5. Are the main findings clearly described?
6. Does the study provide estimates of random variability in the data for the main outcomes?
   - If the data are non-normally distributed, the interquartile range should be quoted.
   - If the data are normally distributed, the standard error of the mean, standard deviation and confidence intervals should be used.
7. Have important adverse events been reported?
8. Have the characteristics of patients lost to follow-up been reported?
9. Have actual probability values been reported (e.g. $p = 0.04$, rather than $p < 0.05$)?

External validity

10. Were the subjects representative of the population?
11. Were the staff and facilities representative of the treatment that the majority of patients would receive?

Internal validity, bias (think selection and information)

12. Was the study blinded?
13. Were the statistical tests used appropriate (e.g. non-parametric tests should be used for data that is not normally distributed)?
14. Was compliance with the intervention reliable?
15. Were the main outcome measurements to be used reliable?

Implications of the study (the final part of appraisal of a paper)

16. What is the general importance in light of other research?
17. Can you extrapolate from the study group to general practice?
18. Is the size of the result observed important? The answer may be no, even if the results are statistically significant.
19. If you conclude that the results are important, what are their implications?
    - for patients
    - for general practice (workload, financially, education, resources, other members of the primary healthcare team)
    - wider issues: ethics, right to choice.

Qualitative research

The approach is similar to quantitative appraisal.

- Focus on methods (e.g. interview techniques and settings) (source of internal bias), as well as the role of the researcher and their qualifications.
- Look at the quality control measures used (e.g. content analysis, grounded theory).
- In qualitative research the conclusions and discussions are not usually separate.

Statistics

This is covered in Statement 3.6.

Communicating risk

This is covered in Statement 5.

Evidence-based practice: questions

Risk of fracture in people aged 70 years and over by levothyroxine use

Levothyroxine use	Cases [n (%)]	Controls [n (%)]	Adjusted odds ratio (95% confidence interval)
Current versus remote use	20 514 (92.3)	96 528 (88.3)	1.88 (1.71–2.05)
Current use			
medium (0.044–0.93 mg/day)	10 907 (53.2)	49 798 (49.5)	2.62 (2.50–2.76)
high (>0.93 mg/day)	6521 (31.8)	23 756 (23.6)	3.45 (3.27–3.65)

1 For the table regarding risk of fracture, which of the answers would best describe the results?
   a. Having been corrected for other risk factors, higher doses of levothyroxine increased fracture risk.
   b. Patients with a lower thyroid-stimulating hormone level had an increased risk of fracture.
   c. Patients receiving a dose of 50 µg/day of levothyroxine were at a higher risk of fracture than those receiving 25 µg/day.
   d. A patient receiving a dose of 75 µg is at a lower risk of fracture than a patient receiving a dose of 100 µg of levothyroxine per day.
   e. A patient aged 50 receiving 150 µg/day of levothyroxine is at greater risk of fracture than a patient receiving 75 µg/day.

Although behavioural therapies are important in smoking cessation, pharmacological therapies are also used as first-line therapies. Consider the statements in questions 2–6 and match them to the correct options listed as follows.

a. Varenicline
b. Nicotine replacement therapy
c. Buprenorphine
d. Nortriptyline

2 This nicotine receptor partial agonist has been developed from a laburnum seed extract.
3 What is known to lower seizure thresholds and should not be prescribed with antidepressants?
4 What may cause hypoglycaemia, so it should be avoided in diabetics?
5 What would be the best choice in pregnant women?
6 Extending the use of what may be effective at preventing relapse?

Evidence-based practice: answers

1 **d** You can't tell from the table what issues have been corrected for, and the data shown are for patients over 70 years. This table is an extract from the article 'Levothyroxine dose and risk of fractures in older adults: nested case-control study' (*BMJ* 2011; 342: d2238). It did not use other risk factors, reason for thyroxine at time of starting (i.e. if following thyroid cancer then the thyroid-stimulating hormone dose would need to be suppressed significantly) or thyroid-stimulating hormone levels. It found that patients aged 70–105 on levothyroxine were up to three times more likely to fracture (by up to three times in higher doses).
2 **a** These questions are adapted from the *BMJ* article Managing Smoking Cessation (*BMJ* 2007; 335: 37).
3 **c**
4 **c**
5 **b** There is a theoretical risk that nicotine may harm the baby. This has not been shown in three meta-analyses.
6 **b** It is too early to know in buprenorphine and varenicline.

Statement 3.6

Research and academic activity

Many practices, especially the teaching practices that many of you will be currently in, will be affiliated with a university and their research department, often contributing to the trials that are taking place by helping with patient selection, development of trial protocols and so forth.

A lot of what is covered in this part of the Royal College of General Practitioners curriculum overlaps with Statement 3.5 (Evidence-based practice) and Statement 3.3 (Clinical ethics and values-based practice) so it is not repeated here. The Data Protection Act 1998 (available along with other useful links at the Information Commissioner's Office, www.ico.gov.uk) and holding of information pertaining to the patient is of paramount importance in research.

Ethics approval

For validity all trials need ethics approval before starting.

The Research Ethics Committee (Centre of Research: Ethical Campaign, www.corec.org.uk/) provides help and advice in the planning stages as well as across the board.

Statistics

Statistics is about gathering, communicating, analysing and interpreting information. In medical statistics we tend to use inferential statistics, in that we draw conclusions from a sample drawn from the population.

You need to have a fundamental understanding of the basics when critiquing papers, embarking on research or auditing yourself. Although this section is rather functional, I will attempt to put the theory in very simple terms and to explain things that may otherwise be somewhat unclear. It is then a matter of actually reading the statistical analyses in papers to gain further understanding and using articles in the *BMJ* and other journals to improve your knowledge. Since first writing this chapter I have discovered Dr Chris Cates's excellent website (www.nntonline.net), which I would recommend. There have also been several articles broken into bite-size chunks and published recently in the press.

There are two distinct types of data:

1 **Qualitative data**: descriptive information.
2 **Quantitative data**: numerical information.

Quantitative data can be either continuous (e.g. 0.1–44 kg, all values within the span are possible), or it can be discrete, usually obtained by counting (e.g. 0, 1, 2, 3, and so on and so forth, such as the number of moles on the skin or shoe size).

Bar chart

A bar chart is a graphical representation of values/numbers.

- The height of the column is proportional to the frequency it represents.
- Each column should have the same width.

Pie chart/pie diagram

This is a circle divided into sectors at angles that are proportional to the frequency of the data they represent.

Measures of location

Mode

This is the most commonly occurring value. It assumes that the modal class is divided into the same ratio.

Time taken to critique a paper (minutes)	People (n)
0–9.9	4
10–19.9	7
20–29.9	9
30–39.9	6
40–49.9	5
50–59.9	3
60–120	9

The mode is time 20–29.9 minutes, *not* 60–120 minutes, as this modal class is longer.

You can have more than one modal class.

Median

This is the middle value of data once it has been placed in numerical order.

e.g. 3 4 5 6 7 **7** 8 8 8 10 15
The 7 in bold is the median.

e.g. 0 1 2 4 5 5 6 7
The median is halfway between 4 and 5, so it is 4.5.

Mean

This generally means the average.

$$\text{mean} = \frac{\text{sum of the values}}{\text{no. of values}}$$

The mean and median are a measure of symmetry or lack of it.

In a normal (Gaussian) distribution the mode, median and mean all have the same value.

Positively skewed

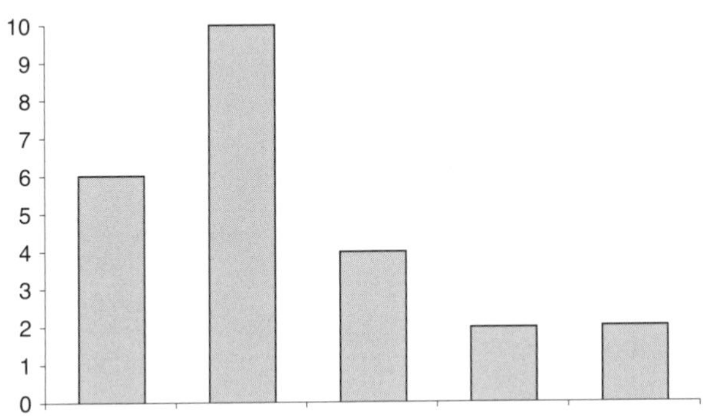

Negatively skewed

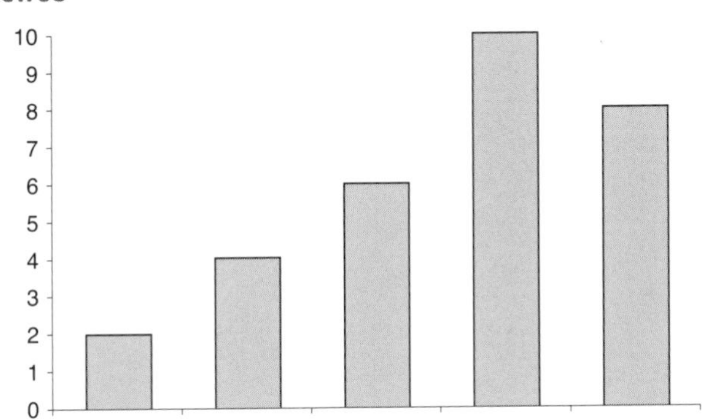

Measures of dispersion

Range

This is the difference between extremes (i.e. the largest and the smallest). It does not take into account anything about the distribution of the data.

Quartile spread

- The median is halfway through the data.
- The point halfway between the lower extreme and the median is the **lower quartile**.
- The point halfway between the median and the upper extreme is the **upper quartile**.
- The difference between the upper and lower quartile is the **interquartile range**.

Standard deviation

- Whereas range and interquartile range relates to the median, standard deviation (SD) relates to the spread about the mean.
- The SD uses all values and is therefore sensitive to outliers (i.e. extreme values).

SD = square root of the variance

$$\text{Variance} = \frac{\text{sum of the square deviations from the mean}}{n}$$

In a normal distribution:
- 65% of values lie within 1 SD.
- 95% of values lie within 2 SDs.
- 99% of values lie within 3 SDs.

Probability
This indicates the degree of likelihood of an event happening, or the uncertainty of an event occurring.

$$\text{Probability of an outcome} = \frac{\text{no. of events in the outcome}}{\text{total no. of possible events}}$$

For example, the probability of rolling a 6 when throwing a dice is 1/6. The probability of throwing a 6 followed by another 6 is:

$$1/6 \times 1/6 = 1/36$$

(i.e. probability of a *and* b, then multiply).

The probability of throwing a 6 or a 4 is:

$$1/6 + 1/6 = 2/6 = 1/3$$

(i.e. probability of a *or* b, then add).

Errors
There are two types of error.
1. **Random error**: the sample mean deviates from the true mean despite the sample being representative.
2. **Systematic error**: the sample is not representative (i.e. there is bias).

Hypothesis test and p-value
This is a test of significance.

The first step is the statement of null hypothesis:

> 'There is no difference between the two groups under study.'

(That is, postulate the hypothesis that the intervention will have no effect.)

The second step is conducting a test of statistical significance based on the null hypothesis:
- Student's t-test
- chi-squared test.

The third step is the production of a p-value from the statistical tests. The p-value is the probability of the result occurring by chance if the null hypothesis were true. If the p-value is small then it is unlikely to have occurred by chance (i.e. it is a significant result). Usually $p < 0.05$ indicates a significant result. If $p < 0.01$ the result is highly significant (i.e. likely to have occurred by chance in <1% of cases).

It is important to appraise a study before taking the p-values as meaningful, as it may be irrelevant in the following cases:

- poor design of trial
- bias
- trial affected by confounding factors.

If there is a small sample size then the statistical analysis may be unable to detect a significant difference when there may be one; this is referred to as the power of the study.

Confidence intervals

Confidence intervals (CIs) are another way of assessing the effects of chance. It is a way of communicating the level of uncertainty, and it can be calculated for various statistical analyses (e.g. odds ratios, relative risks, risk difference, sensitivity, specificity and so forth).

- There is an upper and a lower value and, assuming the study was not biased, the true value can be expected to lie between these two values.
- Most studies use 95% CIs or 95% confidence limits – this is usually 2 SDs either side of the mean.
- The wider the range of the CI, the less certain/significant the results are. The more people there are in the study, the smaller the interval will be.
- If the CI range includes zero the result is not statistically significant.
- If the results are expressed as a ratio then a CI including 1 is not statistically significant.
- The results are visual.

Risk

Measure of risk

New cases = incidence

Existing case = prevalence

$$\text{Incidence} = \frac{\text{new illness episodes}}{[\text{population at risk during a specific period of time}]} \times 10^{a}$$

$$\text{Prevalence} = \frac{\text{no. of individuals with existing disease}}{\text{population size during specific time period}} \times 100\%$$

Measures of association

Risk is calculated by comparing what happens to different groups of people and runs from zero to 1.

Consider populations split into two sub-populations:

population 1 = population exposed to risk factor

population 2 = population not exposed

Both populations have an associated risk of disease.

$$\text{Probability of disease/death} = \text{risk (R)} = \frac{\text{no. with the disease}}{\text{no. at risk of disease}} = \frac{d}{n}$$

$$\text{Risk difference (RD)} = \text{Risk1} - \text{Risk2} = \frac{d1}{n1} - \frac{d2}{n2}$$

$$\text{Relative risk (RR)} = \frac{R1}{R2} = \frac{d1/n1}{d2/n2} = \frac{d1 \times n2}{d2 \times n1}$$

$$\text{Absolute risk (AR)} = \frac{R1 - R2}{R1}$$

AR and RR are figures used to assess the strength of a relationship between a disease and any factor that might affect it. RR is relatively meaningless, AR is more important to understand for us to be able to impart meaningful information to our patients.

$$AR = \frac{[\text{no. of events that occur in the treated and control group}]}{\text{no. of people in that group}}$$

The AR reduction (ARR) is the difference between the control group (ARC) and the treated group (ART).

$$ARR = ARC - ART$$

RR (or the risk ratio) in randomised controlled trials and cohort studies, or relative odds in cohort or case controlled studies, is the ratio of ARs of the disease between the two groups.

RR < 1, then intervention reduces the risk of the outcome being studied.
RR = 1, then the treatment has no effect on the outcome being studied.
RR > 1, then the intervention increases the risk of the outcome being studied.

Odds

Odds are a way of representing probability in a different way to risk. They are defined as the ratio of the probability of an event happening to that of it not happening (i.e. risk) and values run from zero to infinity.

Odds ratio

The odds ratio (OR) is a measure of effectiveness of a treatment, an estimate of relative risk.

$$OR = \frac{\text{odds in the treated group}}{\text{odds in the control group}}$$

OR < 1, effects of the treatment are less than those of the control treatment.

OR = 1, effects of the treatment are no different from the control treatment.
OR > 1, effects of the treatment are greater than the control treatment.

The effects can be good or bad.

Diagnostic testing

	Disease positive	Disease negative	Total
Test negative	a	b	a + b
Test positive	c	d	c + d
Total	a + c	b + d	a + b + c + d

$$\text{Sensitivity} = \frac{\text{no. test positive and disease positive}}{\text{no. disease positive}} = \frac{a}{a + c}$$

$$\text{Specificity} = \frac{\text{no. test negative and disease negative}}{\text{no. disease negative}} = \frac{d}{b + d}$$

Positive predictive value = the probability that an individual diagnosed test positive will be true positive

$$= \frac{a}{a + b}$$

Negative predictive value = probability that an individual diagnosed test negative will be a true negative

$$= \frac{d}{c + d}$$

Number needed to treat

The number needed to treat (NNT) is the number of people you would need to treat with a specific intervention (e.g. aspirin for people having a heart attack) to see one occurrence of a specific outcome (e.g. prevention of death).

$$\text{NNT} = \frac{1}{\text{ARR}}$$

If using a percentage, this value can be multiplied by 100.

So, the smaller the ARR, the higher the NNT.

Cates's website allows you to produce a visual representation of NNT if you have basic statistical information.

This can be applied as NNH – the number needed to harm.

The number needed to screen: an adaptation of the number needed to treat

J Med Screen 2001; 8(3): 114–15

This paper suggests that estimates of NNT should carry a health warning. The concept of preventing one event should be compared with the more likely probability that several people benefit by having an event delayed by a few years. For example, an antihypertensive drug that reduces the incidence of stroke by 30% can be interpreted in two ways: (1) the drug prevented 30% of strokes (with no effect on the other 70%); or (2) all strokes in the treatment group were delayed by 3 years.

Other statistical terms

Bias

This is the deviation of the results from the truth, a one-sided inclination of the mind.

- **Publication bias** is seen where studies with positive results are more likely to be published.
- **Selection bias** is where there are systematic differences between sample and target populations.
- **Information bias** is where there are systematic errors in measurement of outcome or exposure.

Hazard ratio

Is the statistical term used to describe the RR of complication due to treatment based on a comparison of event rates.

Heterogeneity

This term is used when there is no overlap of the trials used in a meta-analysis.

Homogeneity 'similarity'

This term is used to state that all trials on the plot have an overlap of CIs (i.e. in a meta-analysis).

Meta-analysis

This is a paper looking at and summarising a number of original research papers in an attempt to answer a question. The methodology of the search (i.e. not confined to English, using more than one search engine, including unpublished trials) is a good indicator as to the validity of the results.

Validity

This refers to how rigorous a study is.

- **Study validity** is the validity with respect to internal and external bias.
- **Internal validity** is the degree to which conclusions internal to the study are legitimate.
- **External validity** is the degree to which conclusions generated from the sample could be generalised to the target population.

Study designs

Experimental

Randomised controlled trials have a minimum of two groups, to which patient allocation is random; one of the groups is the control (i.e. the non-experimental group).

Observational

Cross-sectional survey

- Sample frame is observed at one particular time.
- Gives prevalence estimates.
- Cause and effect are difficult to establish.

Cohort study

- Longitudinal follow-up of two or more cohorts (groups) with recorded exposure to a risk factor.
- Provides comparative incidence estimates between exposed and non-exposed groups.
- There can be surveillance bias.

Case-controlled study

- Used to compare two groups when prevalence is low.
- ORs are used for analysis.

Forest plot

This is a pictorial representation of odds ratios in the form of horizontal lines. They represent the 95% CI of each trial, with a vertical line representing the point where

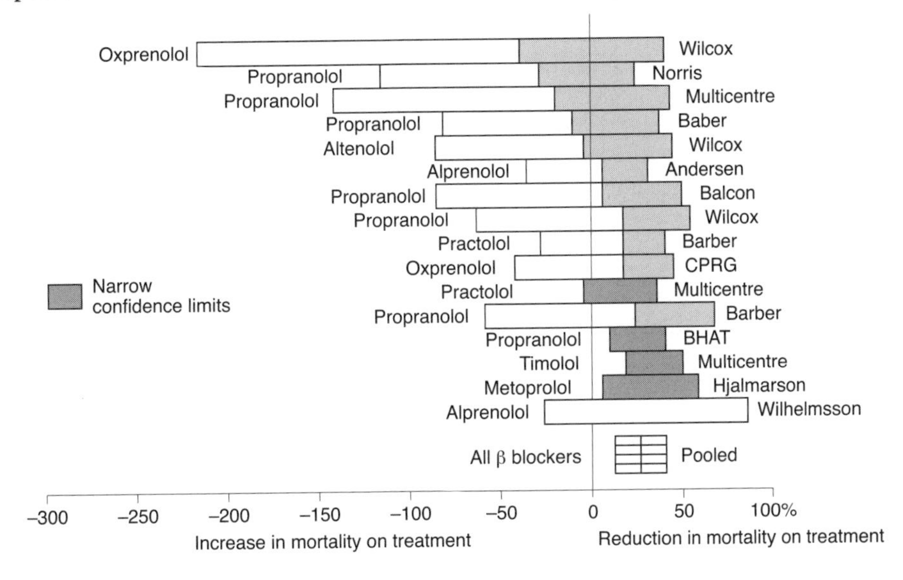

Image from 'Forest plots: trying to see the wood and the trees' (*BMJ* 2001; 322(7300): 1479–80)

the study intervention would have no effect (i.e. if the horizontal line crosses the vertical line then the result is not significant).

Funnel plot

This is a graph/scatter plot where each study is represented by a dot, the position of which depends on the size of the effect of the intervention (on the horizontal axis) and the study size (on the vertical axis). This type of representation is used to examine bias in meta-analyses. For example, there may be an assumption that asymmetry may be due to publication bias (certainly not necessarily the case).

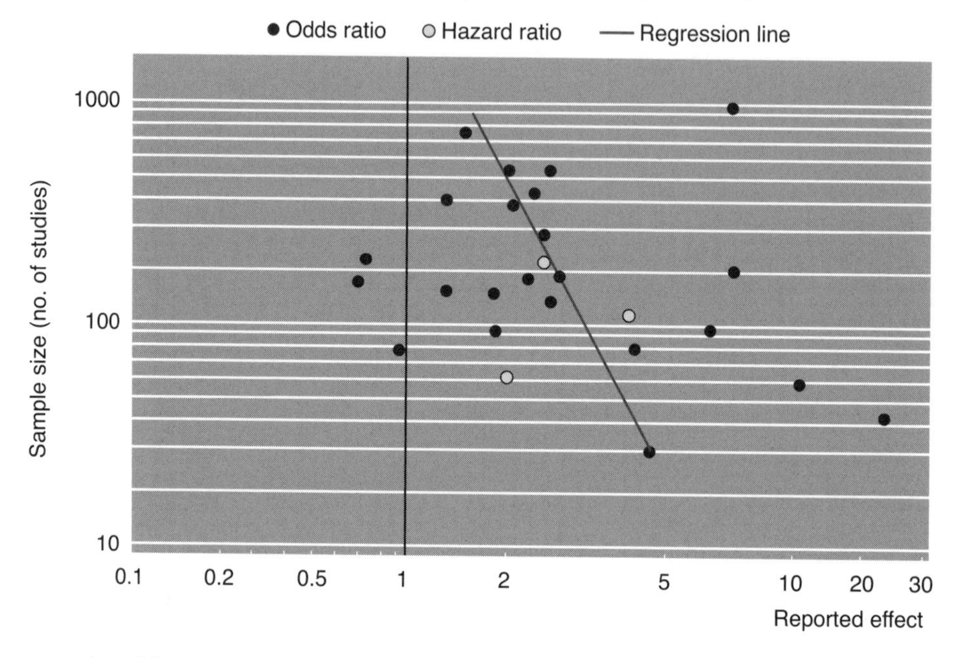

Image from 'The case of the misleading funnel plot' (*BMJ* 2006; 333(7568): 597–600)

Research and academic activity: questions

For questions 1–5 in relation to statistical analyses of significance, answer true or false.

1 The 'null hypothesis' is the test proving there is no difference between two groups.
2 The p-value is a measure of significance generated from tests such as Student's t-test.
3 p-Values are unaffected by trial design.
4 A CI of 97% is based on results that are 2 SDs from the mean.
5 A CI expressed as a ratio that includes zero is statistically significant.

For questions 6–10 choose the most appropriate answer from the following list of options.

	Screening test positive	Screening text negative
Problem present	29	42
Problem absent	64	364

a. 29/93
b. 29/71
c. 42/71
d. 42/408
e. 64/93
f. 64/428
g. 364/406
h. 364/428
i. 29
j. 42
k. 64
l. 364

6 Positive predictive value.
7 Negative predictive value.
8 Specificity.
9 Sensitivity.
10 False negative.

Research and academic activity: answers

Statistics questions come up regularly in *InnovAit*, the *BMJ*, *Pulse*, *GP* and other circulars – practise them!

1 False It is the hypothesis that there is no difference that you then go on to disprove.
2 True A p-value of <0.01 is highly significant.
3 False May be irrelevant, depending on the design (e.g. is a sample size too small?).
4 False This would usually be a 95% CI.
5 False A ratio could not include zero. If the ratio is >1 then the result is not significant.
6 a
7 g
8 h
9 b
10 j

Statement 3.7

Teaching, mentoring and clinical supervision

As part of your e-portfolio you will have come across the area to log your teaching experiences. This can be applied in many ways in practice, such as:

- alongside an audit – with cascade of information 'teaching' to your colleagues
- taking the lead with clinical meetings
- presentation of topics or new guidelines that impact on practice
- involvement with medical student teaching, either sessions or joint surgeries.

It is always important to understand your audience; carry out a needs analysis, both for your own needs and for the needs of those you may be teaching. This can be quite formal, involving a learning styles questionnaire such as the Honey and Mumford options that are available to purchase online (www.peterhoney.com) or more fluidly through your own learning and observation log. It is important to reassess needs regularly and set your course appropriately.

In your own personal assessment you will recognise areas that need development in various ways, such as:

- the curriculum
- PUNs and DENs (patient's unmet needs and doctor's educational needs)
- case-based discussions
- the consultation observation tools applied by your training practice
- letters, referrals, significant events and audits
- articles and circulars
- passing comments made in meetings, by colleagues or patients.

Recognise these and e-portfoliorise them regularly with outcome and completion plans. Don't allow yourself to get behind.

Teaching methods and the role of teachers

Royal College of General Practitioners curriculum

www.rcgp-curriculum.org.uk/PDF/curr_3_7_Teaching_Mentoring_Clinical_Supervision.pdf

Method	Process	Role of teacher	Relevant authors
Didactic	Telling	Passing on knowledge	Many authors
Socratic	Questioning	Facilitation through awareness-raising questions	Neighbour 1992
Heuristic	Encouraging	Promoting learner autonomy and self-directed learning	Kolb 1984 Knowles 1990 Brookfield 1986
Counselling	Exploring	Encouraging self-awareness, discovery and reflective practice through exploring feelings and examining assumptions by using discussion and judicious challenge	Schön 1987 Heron 1990 Bolton 2001

Tips for planning an in-house educational session

Adapted from GP update by Martyn Hewett, February 2009

- Aims – overall of the session.
- Outcomes – be clear about the take-home message, this may need to be adapted as you go through the session.
- Leadership – think about your timings and the direction.
- Methods – PowerPoint, video, cases, small group teaching, snowballing.
- Resources – what equipment you will need.
- Constraints – such as sensitive topics.

Feedback

This is often based on Pendleton's rules, and overall it is about being respectful.

Describing behaviour observed rather than interpretation of that behaviour, and using specific examples for this, is more likely to result in changes for the positive. This is often enough, although in some cases it is important to come straight to the point; for example, if watching a video when a very obvious dysphagia is being described but not heard or acted upon by the consulting doctor, then this needs directly addressing.

Written feedback (e.g. following a tutorial presentation) can be useful if questions are framed in a way that allows you to adapt and develop, also allowing space for comments.

Other resources for learning

The e-Learning for General Practice website (www.e-GP.org.uk), a joint project between the Royal College of General Practitioners and e-Learning for Healthcare, is a useful resource.

Statement 4.1

Management in primary care

The curriculum requires that you are familiar with the following skills:
- appraisal
- delegation – tasks delegated should be SMART (specific, measurable, agreed, realistic and time-bound)
- leadership
- management – such as chairing a meeting, organising projects
- negotiation
- team-work.

It also helps you to be familiar with looking at process of change through SWOT analyses (strengths, weaknesses, opportunities and threats). General advice regarding different approaches to aspects of business can be found on the Businessballs website (www.businessballs.com).

The General Medical Council has published *Management for Doctors* and it also features in *Good Medical Practice.*

The General Medical Services contract

Your contract, your future

www.gpcwm.co.uk/gms2/f_regulations.htm

The contract is between the primary care trust and the practice (i.e. there will be no individual lists) and is for essential and additional services. The contract will safeguard premises, allowing for improvement and development in the interest of quality patient care. The final version was signed up to and launched originally in April 2004.

Investing in general practice: the new General Medical Services contract

The basis of the new General Medical Services (GMS) contract was to:
- provide new mechanisms to allow practices greater flexibility to determine the range of services they wish to provide
- reward practices for delivering clinical and organisational quality and for improving the patient experience
- facilitate the modernisation of practice infrastructure including premises and IT
- provide for unprecedented and guaranteed levels of investment through a gross investment guarantee
- support the delivery of a wider range or higher-quality services and empower patients to make the best use of primary care services
- simplify regulatory regime.

More flexible provision of services

All GMS practices will provide essential services and a range of enhanced services. Practices have the opportunity to increase their income through opting to provide a wider range of enhanced services.

Primary care trusts are responsible for ensuring patient access is not compromised and by 31 December 2004 full responsibility for out of hours (6.30 p.m.–8 a.m. weekdays, all weekends, bank holidays and public holidays) was taken over. This included GP cooperatives, NHS Direct/24, Walk-in centres, paramedics, pharmacists, GP services in A&E, commercial deputising services and social work services.

How does the money flow?

- Protected Global Sum: this will be paid directly to the practice from the primary care trust for essential and additional services, and is based on practice list size.
- Enhanced Services Payments: this money will come from the primary care trusts and includes development money.
- Wisdom and Experience Payments: these are for more senior doctors and will come from the primary care trusts.
- Quality and Outcome Payments covers:
  - infrastructure, e.g. premises, IT, staff
  - chronic disease frameworks and organisational achievements
  - aspiration – declared by the practice at the beginning of the year
  - reward – paid at the end of the year if aspirations are met.

Categorisation of services

Essential services

These are provided by every practice and the patient initiates the service.

This includes:

- management of patients who are ill
  - relevant health promotion
  - appropriate referral
- general management of patients who are terminally ill
- chronic disease management.

Additional services

Most practices would be expected to provide these but could opt out if necessary (e.g. staff shortages):

- cervical screening
- contraceptive services
- vaccinations and immunisations
- child health surveillance
- maternity services (intrapartum care would be an enhanced service)
- minor surgery.

Enhanced services

These are essential or additional services delivered to a higher specific standard, as well as innovative services. These will allow primary care trusts to invest in areas such as routing home visits, patient transport, services for violent patients and so forth.

There will be:

- national direction with specifications and benchmark pricing that all primary care trusts must commission
- national minimum specifications and benchmark pricing, that are not directed
- locally developed services.

Breadth of care will be rewards through holistic care payments.

This categorisation would allow GPs to:

- control their workload
- receive guaranteed resources
- opt out of additional services if they are unable to provide them
- offer innovative services.

New services will only ever be introduced when the necessary additional resources have been provided.

At the beginning of the financial year the practice will receive a proportion of the quality payment for the standard aspired – the aspiration payment (payment per point). Once the standard has been achieved the practice will receive the remainder – the achievement payment.

Exception reporting will be in place to ensure practices don't lose payment as a result of factors outside their control; this will be subject to investigation as part of fraud visits. Similarly, certain categories of patients will be excluded (e.g. those who are terminally ill, those on maximum medication, newly diagnosed patients and so forth).

As part of this original document, global sum payments were to be calculated on the Carr–Hill allocation formula. There were problems with the weighting of this, especially for practices with accurate practice lists. The allocation formula for the global sum was applied to the registered practice population from 1 April 2004. As a result of this, and concerns over income, a minimum practice income guarantee for the first few years was confirmed but has since been adjusted.

Effect of the new contract on GP's working lives and perceptions of quality of care: a longitudinal survey

Br J Gen Pract 2008; 58(546): 8–14

This longitudinal postal questionnaire survey in the United Kingdom was conducted over 19 months and looked at reported job satisfaction (seven-point scale), hours worked, income and impact of the contract. In 2004 there were 2105 doctors who replied; in 2005 there were 1349. Mean overall job satisfaction increased from 4.58 out of 7 in 2004 to 5.17 in 2005. The greatest improvements in satisfaction were with remuneration and hours of work. Mean reported hours worked fell from 44.5

to 40.8. Mean income increased from an estimated £73 400 in 2004 to £92 600 in 2005. Most GPs reported that the new contract had increased their income (88%), but decreased their professional autonomy (71%), and increased their administrative (94%) and clinical (86%) workloads.

Personal Medical Services

Personal Medical Services (PMS) is an alternative to GMS. The NHS Plan expected 30% of GPs to move to PMS by 2002 and all single-handers by 2004. This expectation was to change with the launch of the new GMS contract (nGMS) which was to encompass some aspects of PMS. Recently PMS practices are being offered minimum practice income guarantee to switch to GMS contracts.

The Conservatives introduced PMS in the National Health Service (Primary Care) Act 1997 following the introduction of the initial concept in the 'Choices and opportunities' White Paper. It went live in April 1998 with a core contract doctors had to fulfil. The contract was scrapped in favour of a broad framework with outcomes and targets to be agreed locally.

The intention of PMS was to address local service issues and pilot new ways of delivering and improving services by allowing local flexibility. The emphasis is on local funding for local issues that will hopefully attract GPs into areas with recruitment problems.

PMS contracts have recently been renegotiated. It covers what people would normally expect from GMS but delivery can be different. The focus is on competitive services, achieving targets and a minimum of three audits per year. PMS providers will be accountable for delivery of NSFs and other key national clinical governance requirements (risk management, audits, workforce planning and so forth).

Introduction to Personal Medical Services is a GPC publication that covers the original aims of PMS:

- promoting of persistently high-quality services
- providing opportunities and incentives for primary care professionals to use their skills to the full
- providing more flexible employment opportunities
- addressing recruitment and retention problems
- reducing the bureaucracy involved in the management of primary care provision.

PMS had a variable reception. As happens with all new developments, the initial money available (especially for growth) was quite substantial, but this is no longer the case. Also, interestingly, the PMS core contract for third-wavers is much more directive.

The King's Fund Study, 'Current thoughts on PMS so far', was published in October 2001. It concluded that PMS had so far been disappointing.

'Personal medical services pilots: modernising primary care?' states 'there is little strong or consistent evidence of a 'PMS effect' on quality.

A PMS contract is not enforceable by law but both parties are subject to binding arbitration by the Secretary of State for Health.

Benefits of personalised medical services

- It is locally negotiated so can reflect local circumstances.
- There was less management bureaucracy at the time it was launched.
- It enables flexible employment opportunities, with further opportunities and incentives to develop skills.
- There is improved integration of primary healthcare teams.
- More services available for patients.
- It addresses some recruitment and retention problems in general practice.
- It promotes consistently high-quality services.
- It is practice based, not a contract with an individual doctor (i.e. illness, maternity leave and so forth); much like the new GMS contract.
- PMS practices have the right to alter the quality and outcome frameworks if agreed with the primary care trust.

Drawbacks of personalised medical services

- It is local not national, so is not aligned with national pay reviews.
- There is no agreement on pensions.
- There is annual renegotiation of the contract that is then fixed for a year, which may compromise income.
- The local medical committee statutory levy is not automatically taken.
- Funding for growth reduced with each new wave.
- Discrepancies in earnings (where there is significantly more income than in GMS is being looked into (i.e. to determine if there is provision of a better service for patients).

Alternative Provider Medical Services

Alternative Provider Medical Services contracts allow primary care trusts to amend contract details more swiftly at local level, and terminate more easily. These contracts are usually negotiated every 3 years and can include registered and non-registered patient care. The risk of this type of contract for the provider is often significant as compared to other contracts.

Practice-based commissioning

www.bma.org.uk and www.dh.gov.uk

This is, very simply, how services are commissioned for healthcare. The Public Health Resource Unit (www.phru.nhs.uk) is a site worth dipping into for understanding on this topic.

Implementing the Vision was a report in 2000 by the NHS Alliance that called for multi-level commissioning (the budget having been created following the recognised need in the NHS Plan). In 2002 the Alliance published *Refocusing Commissioning for Primary Care Trusts* and then in 2004 *Practice Led Commissioning: a no nonsense guide*. They have been very keen from the outset to let PBC be seen as distinct from fund-holding by describing it in the following ways:

- It is based on partnerships at many levels so encourages teamwork (there is no personal gain to be made from savings) and re-investment for the good of all.

- The proposal is a clinical vision about what we want to achieve for our patients by improving quality of services.

As the role of planning and provision of health services is developed, practices will be expected to manage the commissioning of services, budgets and an element of risk associated with this (although they would not be held directly responsible for any overspend as budgets are still legally held by the primary care trusts). An Audit Commission report has described the uptake of commissioning as being patchy.

MedEconomics (April 2005) published a special edition on PBC, with a 10-stage approach to PBC (page 30):

1. Find out all you can about it.
2. Discuss it with everybody.
3. Plan what you will commission.
4. Decide which services you will commission jointly.
5. Agree the budget with the primary care trust.
6. Sign on the dotted line.
7. Allow for patient choice.
8. Recoup your initial costs and management expenses.
9. Monitor your budget.
10. Use efficiency gains.

Dr Jenner (in *Doctor*, January 2005) discusses the new guidance and how it has moved from original thoughts in the following areas:

- Inevitability of PBC – there are no targets, but by 2008 all practices ideally should have been involved in PBC.
- Incentives for practices – there will be no cap (previously 50%) on the amount of savings.
- Accountability for practices is to follow national priorities – national and local targets must be delivered (including choose and book, access, waiting list initiatives and so forth).
- Single practice or locality commissioning – the new guidance tips the balance in favour of locality groups (the King's Fund suggests that you need a patient population of 30 000 to manage a total healthcare budget over 3 years).
- Budget setting – these will be set at 2003/4 levels of referral (to avoid the initial increase seen in fund holding where referrals were boosted in the first year to increase budgets) and then move to a shared formula.
- Risk management – practices are not financially responsible for overspends; this lies with the primary care trust, who can intervene if it is thought the commissioning group has overspent.
- Arbitration – the strategic health authority can convene a panel of two GPs, one practice manager and the primary care trust finance director to resolve issues.

Implementing practice based commissioning

BMJ 2007; 335(7631): 1168

This *BMJ* editorial looks at the Audit Commission report from the second year of PBC, given that it is central to the government's reforms. GPs have a better understanding of the financial consequences of their decisions following the involvement and are more engaged in managing use of secondary care (all for a cost of around £98 million so far).

Patient group directives

These are written instructions for the supply and administration of medicines by professionals other than doctors (e.g. pharmacists, nurses, health visitors).

Their development came about following changes to the Medicines Act in 2000, the overall aim being to improve patient care. They are a recognised necessity with the advances in nurse prescribing. The process of drawing up a patient group directive can be time-consuming, needs to be well thought out and involve a multidisciplinary team. For example, pharmacists issuing emergency contraception not only need to be competent in assessing need and explaining related issues but there needs to be a way for effective reimbursement for cost of the drug.

The patient group directive needs to be detailed, and once it is written it must be reviewed by at least one professional advisory group prior to circulation to practices. As with any published document, it should be dated and have a plan for review.

Each directive must include the following:

- the name of the business to which it applies
- the date it comes in to force and is due to expire
- a description of the medicines to which it applies
- the class of health professional who may supply or administer the medicine
- signature of the doctor, dentist or pharmacist and appropriate health organisation
- the clinical condition to which it applies
- patients to be excluded
- when further advice should be sought, and more ...

Appraisal

www.appraisalsupport.nhs.uk/

Appraisal is a formative and developmental process. It is about identifying developmental needs as part of a personal development plan and at the time of writing does not have a performance management role. It is a yearly requirement that was introduced in April 2002. As a GP you will be expected to have an annual appraisal (± revalidation) and may be involved in appraising other doctors or staff.

GP experiences of partner and extended peer appraisal: a qualitative study

Br J General Pract 2005; 55: 539–43

This paper explored different views to approaches that could be adopted for appraisal. Sixty-six GPs took part in the study (46 had a partner appraisal and 20 an external appraiser). This was followed up after 6 months by a questionnaire and 13 GPs were interviewed in depth.

It was felt that clarification in the role of appraisal and revalidation was needed. Given the potentially charged nature of appraisal, there was a risk of collusion between appraiser and appraisee, which may lead to a superficial appraisal.

Personal development plans

The need for personal development plans (PDPs) has been recognised and evolved from the shortcomings of 30 hours of undirected Postgraduate Educational Allowance (PGEA), as well as media attention of recent medical scandals (e.g. Bristol case and Shipman). Revalidation will require us to demonstrate our learning, which we will have to map out according to our own individual needs. These will in turn be determined by priorities that are dictated by the influences around us such as national expectations, primary care groups, practice and personal needs.

Good Medical Practice in General Practice has been published by the Royal College of General Practitioners and states that an excellent GP:

- is up to date and regularly reviews their knowledge
- uses these reviews to develop practice and PDPs
- uses a range of methods to monitor and meet their educational needs.

A First Class Service is a 1998 government publication that states lifelong learning will give NHS staff the knowledge necessary to offer the most effective and high-quality care to patients. Continuous professional development programmes need to meet both the learning need of the individual, to inspire public confidence in their skills and also meet the wider developmental needs of the NHS.

The NHS Plan, published July 2000, is about staff working smarter, not harder. All doctors employed within the NHS have been required to participate in annual appraisals and clinical audit since 2001.

Advantages of PDPs include:

- personal satisfaction
- personally relevant
- more flexible than the PGEA system
- aspirations are achieved
- helps personal reflection
- fulfils contract requirements
- improved patient care
- more cost-effective.

Disadvantages of PDPs include:

- it may lead to isolation
- there may be a loss of objectivity
- it may be overwhelming
- it needs a support network or mentor
- it needs more time investment than PGEA
- for self-motivated learners it can be seen as time wasting and unnecessary
- it may lead to a reinforcement of skills that are already adequate.

Writing a personal/practice development plan

In addition to a PDP, when working in a GP setting/partnership, there will be a requirement for a practice development plan. This is based upon the same principles as a PDP.

Identifying learning needs

These represent the gap between the way things are now and the way they should be or how you want them to be in the future. Learning needs can be identified by keeping lists, reviewing referrals, conducting audits, significant event analysis, asking colleagues, i.e. 360° appraisal (known as the 'Johari window').

Setting learning objectives

Objectives may involve knowledge, skills, attitude and so forth. Success can be looked at by reflection, feedback, audit, reduction in demand and so forth.

Identifying resource implications and time scales

This means that plans should be achievable.

Seeking evidence of achievement

A formal PDP is one stage of a continuous process. The evidence can be used to make a learning portfolio (i.e. a long-term record of past experience and future aspirations) containing workload logs, case descriptions, videos, audits, patient surveys, reflection, significant event analysis and so forth. This is the 'cradle to grave' idea.

Although the plan has now been formalised, conscientious doctors have been doing this for years, as it is the fundamental principle that underpins adult learning, educational theories and learning cycles. We all want to develop and work within an effective team, improve clinical care, plan constructively and provide mechanisms of accountability. PDPs are a starting point for this that will also help us bid for resources in the future.

Freedom of Information Act 2000

This act came into force on 1 January 2005, replacing the Open Government Code of Practice, and it is not just applicable to healthcare. It means that GPs (as well as other public services) are obliged to respond to requests for information that is held (in any format), within 20 days (although this is negotiable at the time of request). A fee would not usually be charged for any work that needed to be carried out to produce the information (there is a limit of £450 per request, where appropriate).

There are 23 exemptions (reasons information would not need to be supplied) that would fulfil either of the following two types of exemption:

1 Absolute exemptions (e.g. court records, legal prohibition, information accessible by the applicant by other means, security issues, personal information and information provided in confidence.
2 Public interest test, e.g. commercial interests (this includes your private income), environmental information, health and safety, audit results, internal relations and information intended for future publication.

Management in primary care: questions

1 Team work: BW Tuckman's theory of team formation encompasses which of the following approaches?
   a. The Team, The Individual and The Task.
   b. Mind Mapping of Elemental Plans and Focus.
   c. Assertiveness as opposed to aggressiveness.
   d. Forming, Storming, Norming and Performing.
   e. Arbitration of organisational disagreements.

2 Assuming that you are in partnership and responsible for team members, what is the most appropriate action when an alleged instance of bullying is reported to you?
   a. Instant verbal warning issued to the person accused of bullying.
   b. Instant written warning issued to the person accused of bullying.
   c. Instant dismissal of the person accused of bullying.
   d. A witnessed meeting of both parties to discuss the issues.
   e. Nothing, it is important not to inflame this type of situation as it will usually settle down.

For each of questions 3–6 regarding team traits, select the single most appropriate answer. Each answer can be used once, more than once or not at all.
   a. The Facilitator.
   b. The Motivator.
   c. The Workhorse.
   d. The Finaliser.
   e. The Researcher.
   f. The Innovator.
   g. The Nurturer.
   h. All of the above.

3 Which of the above best describes the trait needed for a functional team?

4 This person would have the impetus to get the team moving on a problem.

5 This person would be most aware of the interpersonal needs of the team.

6 This person has a good overview of a situation, is able to clarify and guide team members.

7 The ABC model of practice-based commissioning includes which of the following points in its characteristics?
   a. There are penalties for non-compliance and failure to produce the information – the maximum penalty for a lead GP would be 2 years imprisonment. Most practices will have prepared a publication scheme prior to the act coming into force, so that for a number of enquiries could be referred to the website.
   b. We in turn can use the Freedom of Information Act 2000 to benefit our patients. Dr Saul published an article in *Pulse* (September 2007) where he used the act to establish why a patient had been refused bariatric surgery despite meeting all the National Institute for Health and Clinical Excellence criteria, and then challenge that decision appropriately.

c. Is measured by demand.
d. Supports pathway development for commissioned services.
e. Is research based rather than Audit based.
f. Progresses through the ABC part of the model up to M.
g. Is explicit in its roll to privatise the NHS.

Management in primary care: answers

1 d In this theory the Forming stage is working out other team members (new team members at later stages can take the team back to this beginning), followed by Storming and true characteristics. Norming is the establishment of standards of behaviour (if management style is highly directional then you can develop a dependent team). Finally Performing is the final stage that has been added to the theory as it has developed. Team, Individual, Task is based on 'Action Centered Leadership', John Adair, a Sandhurst lecturer. Mind mapping is an approach to learning described by Lorna Israel from the United States.

2 d It is important not to jump to any conclusion as in many cases it is a situation revolving around communication and misunderstanding. It is important to understand the facts, be clear in the issues and arbitrate if there is a disagreement between the two parties.

Ultimately there is a job to do and both parties must be able to work together without it impacting on the rest of the team.

The government site (www.acas.gov.uk) is very useful and there are independent companies that specialise in employment law and offer insurance against a claim for unfair dismissal.

3 h

4 b

5 g

6 a The Workhorse is the person who can be relied upon to get things done, the finaliser does exactly that – finalises in a time scale, the researcher underpins the elements with the necessary knowledge (thank you IT and the Internet, making life so much easier) and the innovator is the person with the new ideas who is often solitary but enthusiastic.

7 b This is adapted from an article on ABC Commissioning in Guidelines in Practice 2011; 14(1): 27–32. The ABC is an outcome-based approach to commissioning that although evidence based is important to audit current services/models as well. It incorporates current National Institute for Health and Clinical Excellence commissioning tools which include the drive towards cost savings and require regular reassessment. There are thoughts that the brief has passed on the unpopular roll of privatisation of the NHS to GP commissioning bodies.

Statement 4.2

Information management and technology

NHS Connecting for Health

www.connectingforhealth.nhs.uk

The National Programme for IT (www.doh.gov.uk) is being implemented across the United Kingdom. The programme's goal is to improve access to information and to develop a more traceable service activity within the NHS.

There are several major changes planned that should improve our ability to deliver for our patients, with the main ones as follows.

- NHS Care Records Service (including Spine): clinical records will be available to out-of-hours doctors and will be jointly used by those professionals caring for patients (this should allow us to make better clinical decisions and reduce risk). This is not yet available and has been put on hold in its current form.
- Electronic prescribing service: pharmacists will manage repeat prescribing rather than repeats being requested through GPs. Again, this should improve satisfaction and safety. It should also reduce the number of fraudulent scripts.
- Health Space: patients will be able to book appointments (GP and hospital) online – this is already available in some practices – and they will be able to view a summary of their personal records. It is anticipated that access to records and email contact with health service provides will be rolled out.
- PACS centralised electronic storage of images such as X-rays and scans will be available and accessible.

There will be several measures to ensure that records remain confidential.

- Smart cards: you will only be able to access the NHS Care Records Service using a smart card.
- Legitimate relationships: only clinicians directly involved in a patient's care will be able to access these records.
- Role-based access: for example, a receptionist would have more restricted access then a GP, who would have full access.
- Sealed envelopes: patients will be able to request that certain information be withheld from the shared record.
- Audit trails and alerts: alerts would trigger irregular access and patients can request to see who has accessed their records. Caldicott guardians would be responsible for monitoring this.

Confidentiality and connecting for health

Br J Gen Pract 2008; 58(547): 75–6

This editorial has been written with the feeling that doctors may come under fire regarding confidentiality because of concerns of centralisation of health data, unlawful access to medical records and lawful access to records (such as police wanting to see a suspect's files). As well as this there is what Ross Anderson calls 'mission creep', where Whitehall plans to make use of the records once they are easily available. The Big Opt Out is a campaign dedicated to these issues (www.thebigoptout.org).

European Computer Driving Licence Programme

www.ecdl.org

This is a scheme to allow all NHS staff to train online and be examined over seven modules of basic skills to European Computer Driving Licence standards. The scheme was developed in Finland in 1988 and is now an international non-profit organisation. Over 200 000 people in the United Kingdom are now registered.

Information management and technology: questions

1 Which of the following best describes the European Computer Driving Licence?
   a. It is composed of three modules: basic introduction, word processing and spreadsheets.
   b. It is a 1-day course on computer familiarisation.
   c. It is a seven-module course.
   d. It is a necessary qualification for work in primary care.
   e. It is mandatory for work in primary care.

Information management and technology: answers

1 **c** The seven modules comprise basic concepts, using the computer and managing files, word processing, spreadsheets, databases, presentations, information and communication. It is not necessary or mandatory, but if people have little computer knowledge it can be very helpful.

Statement 5

Healthy people: promoting health and preventing disease

Health promotion is the process of enabling people to increase control over, and to improve, their health. It moves beyond a focus on individual behaviour towards a wide range of social and environmental interventions.

World Health Organization

This section overlaps with many of the other statements, sometimes in subtle ways, covering many issues. It covers public health, the skill of communicating risk, social and environmental effects, immunisation, screening, smoking and alcohol and drug use.

Screening

Technically screening is a form of secondary prevention, i.e. identifying pre-symptomatic disease before significant damage is done. Examples of primary prevention would include immunisation and water sanitation. Tertiary prevention is about limiting complications (e.g. in diabetic care).

When establishing a screening programme you need to consider the ethics of not just the test but the implications of positive and false positive results. Increasing numbers of studies are looking at the negative effects of screening. For example, a normal cholesterol result may mean that a patient's diet subsequently lapses because they feel justified in indulging more often. Another example would be the psychological implications of being given a positive result in, say, chlamydia through screening that is in fact truly negative.

The UK National Screening Committee is responsible for advising the government on the merits of screening for a particular disease and health problems (www.screening.nhs.uk). As part of their reports they focus on policy, summarise current screening and set out thoughts behind conditions that are not yet screened for and the arguments behind why they do not form part of the national screening programme under the NHS.

The Wilson and Jungner 10 screening criteria

1. Is the disease an important public health problem?
2. Is there an effective treatment for localised disease?
3. Are facilities for further diagnosis and treatment available?
4. Is there a latent or early symptomatic phase of the disease?
5. Is the screening technique effective?

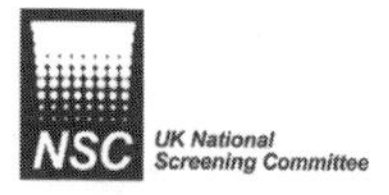

NHS Screening Timeline

NHS Screening Programmes

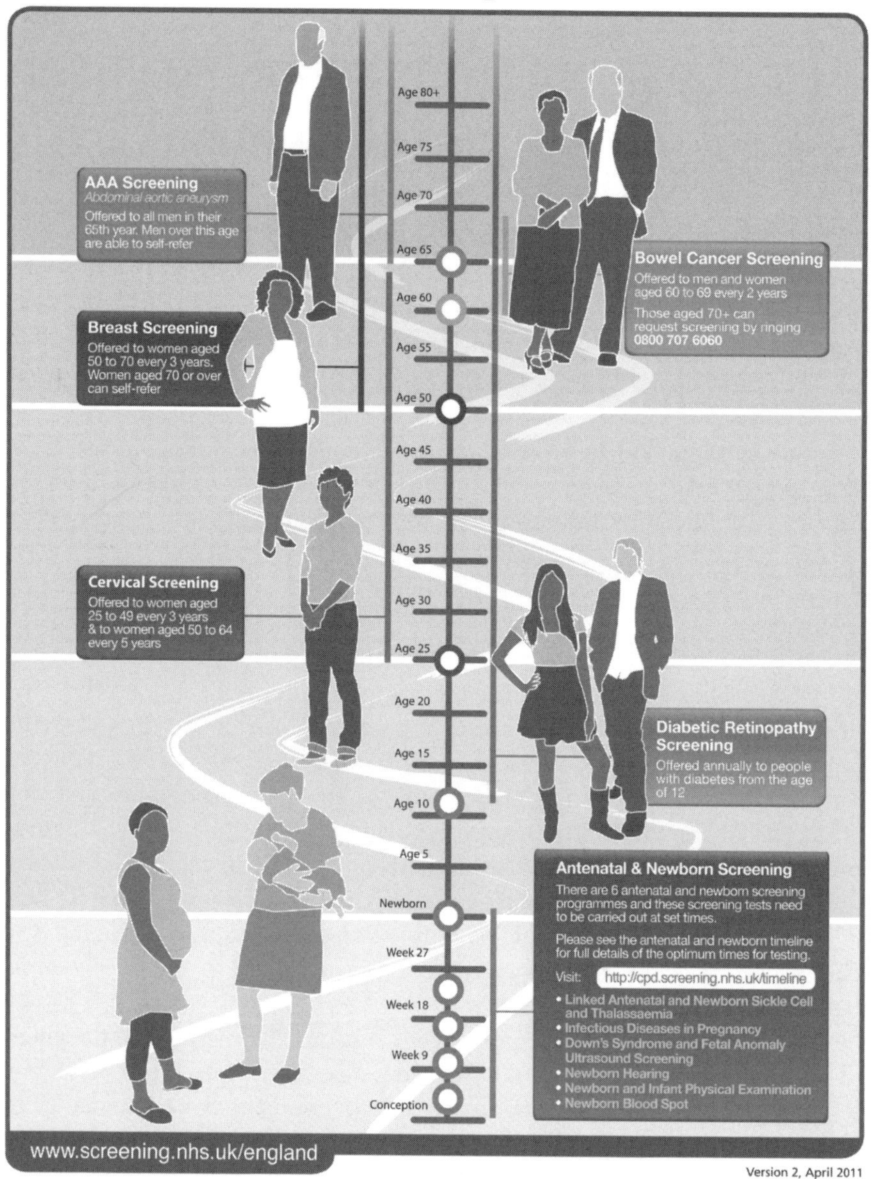

6 Is the screening test acceptable to the patients?
7 Is the natural history of the disease known?
8 Is there a strategy to determine which patients should and should not be treated?
9 Is the cost of screening acceptable?
10 Is effective treatment available and does early treatment give a favourable prognosis?

Gaining informed consent for screening: is difficult; but many misconceptions need to be undone

BMJ 1999; 319(7212): 722–3

In this editorial the author discusses some of the detrimental effects of screening, such as anxiety, false alarms, false reassurance, unnecessary biopsies and associated risk, overdiagnosis and overtreatment. Because of these implications the issues around gaining consent, emphasising the importance of sharing decision-making and a patient's autonomy are all of paramount importance and should be considered.

Communicating risk and evidence to patients

We communicate levels of risk to patients and colleagues throughout most of our working day, for example in prescribing medication, explaining side effects, consenting a patient for a procedure and so forth. The words we use to describe risk affect perception, which in turn may affect compliance with treatment, which in turn may affect success of a treatment and outcome.

Interpretation in words or figures

Verbal	Frequency	Probability
Very common	>10%	>1 in 10
Common	1%–10%	1 in 100 to 1 in 10
Uncommon	0.1%–1%	1 in 1000 to 1 in 100
Rare	0.01%–0.1%	1 in 10 000 to 1 in 1000

A patient's perception of risk is often very different from the health professional explaining that risk. Health professionals who have been trained in using decision aids (e.g. statistical aids such as percentages or probabilities, or visual aids) are able to change the context of their consultation.

Supporting decision-making can involve several stages

Clarify the decision by:

- explaining the problem
- discussing the evidence base
- acknowledging the patient's role in decision-making
- describing benefit and harm (avoid probabilities and try to use absolute, rather than relative, risk).
- understanding the patient's attitudes to the benefits described
- considering how important the treatment is to the patient and how confident they are in making the decision.

When should you involve patients in treatment decisions?

Br J Gen Pract 2007; 57(543): 771–2

This October 2007 edition of the *British Journal of General Practice* included three papers on patient involvement. This editorial reflects on various points. For true shared decisions patients must be given appropriate information about their condition, treatments, outcomes and uncertainties and doctors must be skilled in communicating risk. There are many available tools to help decision-making (the Patient Decision Aids Research Group has a useful site (http://decisionaid.ohri.ca/) where you are able to download material). It concludes by emphasising the 2006 *Good Medical Practice* advice that doctors should listen to their patients and respect their preferences.

Cervical cancer screening

www.cancerresearchuk.org

Cervical cancer screening is offered nationally for all women aged 25–65 years. Women who have never been sexually active or who have never had a male partner do not need screening, although it is still offered.

Since 2003 liquid based cytology has been the test of choice in the UK. It has reduced the need for repeat smears from 9% to 2% since being introduced.

Age in women (years)	Frequency of routine screening
Under 25	No screening
25-49	Every 3 years
50-65	Every 5 years
Over 65	No further screening

The outcome from the results is based on recommendations from the laboratory as shown.

Normal	Recall as per protocol depending on the age
Inadequate smear	Repeat 3 months
Mild dyskaryosis	Repeat 6 months
Moderate dyskaryosis	Colposcopy
Severe dyskaryosis	Urgent colposcopy
Columner atypia	Colposcopy and hysteroscopy

Regarding human papilloma virus testing of women with borderline or low-grade cervical abnormalities in hospital laboratories, if the test is negative the screening will remain at 3 or 5 years depending on age. If it is positive there will be more regular screening (this is currently offered to all women) for borderline abnormalities and colposcopy for low-grade changes.

Ovarian cancer screening

www.nice.org.uk/nicemedia/live/13464/54268/54268.pdf

There is no proven role for screening but methods would include Ca125 and transvaginal ultrasound scanning. In some areas women with one or more first degree relatives with ovarian cancer may be offered a yearly Ca125 and ultrasound scan.

The Medical Research Council launched a 10-year trial (UK Collaborative Trial of Ovarian Cancer Screening) of 200 000 post-menopausal high-risk women looking at transvaginal ultrasound scan versus Ca125 on a yearly basis to try and establish effectiveness of each method in terms of their impact on mortality, morbidity and cost.

Yale University have isolated 35 proteins that are significantly higher in women with ovarian cancer and are currently validating the use of four (leptin, prolactin, osteopontin and insulin-life growth factor 2).

The prostate, lung, colorectal and ovarian trial enrolled 78 216 women aged 55–74 and randomised them to undergo either annual screening (Ca125 for 6 years and transvaginal ultrasound scan for 4 years) or usual care in the United States. They were followed up for 13 years. Ovarian cancer mortality was not reduced (*JAMA* 2011; 305(22): 2295–303).

Breast cancer screening

www.screening.nhs.uk/breastcancer

The NHS breast screening programme was introduced in England and Wales in 1988 on the recommendation of the Forrest Committee. Approximately 19 million women have been screened in the UK and 117 000 cancers have been detected with mammography.

Age women (years)	Routine screening
<50	Not invited
50–70	Every 3 years
>70	Not invited but can opt in

It is estimated that the NHS screening programme saves 1250 lives per year in England (it is worth noting that a 2007 Cochrane review didn't feel there was enough evidence to determine whether screening did more harm than good) and a trial published in the *Journal of Medical Screening* (2010; 17: 25–30) found that for every woman treated for breast cancer unnecessarily, the deaths of two other women from the disease are prevented.

Salivary tests are being developed to measure genetic markers of cancer. Although these will not replace mammography for many years the tests so far predict breast (and oral) cancers with 95% accuracy.

The Leningrad and Shanghai studies are large randomised controlled trials that have both failed to demonstrate a reduction in mortality from breast cancer or increased detection by teaching self-examination.

Mammography has been shown in a Swedish randomised controlled trial to reduce mortality by up to 40%, the benefit being greatest in 50- to 70-year-olds. Compared with symptomatic breast cancers, screen-detected cancers are smaller and are more likely to be non-invasive. If they are invasive they are more likely to be better differentiated and node negative.

It has been calculated that for every 2 million women screened one extra cancer after 10 years may be caused by the radiation delivered to the breast from mammography.

No increase in anxiety has been found in women invited to attend for screening unless there is a need for recall.

Hormone replacement therapy reduces the sensitivity of mammography (from 77% to 65%) and is associated with more false positives.

Maximising benefit and minimising harm of screening

BMJ 2008; 336(7642): 480–3

The opening sentence of this article states: 'All screening programmes do harm; some do good as well, and, of those, some do more harm than good at a reasonable cost.' It summarises the secrets of successful screening as: a total quality approach from the outset; clear objectives and standards; single national protocols to help compare results and identify trends as well as a dataset with well-understood definitions; data must be complete and of good quality; and there should be a clear reference point, such as a randomised controlled trial.

Breast cancer risk assessment tool

This is a tool developed by the National Cancer Institute to calculate 10-year risk of breast cancer, including age, age at first menstruation, age of first live birth, number for first degree relatives with breast cancer, number of previous biopsies (positive or negative) and one biopsy with atypical hyperplasia. There are ongoing studies to look at validity and whether the statistical model can be improved. This can be looked at online (www.cancer.gov/bcrisktool/breast-cancer-risk.aspx). The Gail and Tyrer–Cuzick models are similar.

Bowel cancer screening

www.cancerscreening.nhs.uk/bowel

Age men and women (years)	Routine screening
<60	Not invited
60–70	Every 2 years
>70	Not invited but can opt in

It is estimated that a 10-year screening programme for bowel cancer would prevent 5000 new cases and 3000 deaths a year in the UK.

The government made clear its commitment to screening for bowel cancer in the NHS Plan (2000) and the Colorectal Screening Pilot study began looking at faecal occult bloods (FOBs) and flexible-sigmoidoscopies as options, building on original studies from Nottingham and Denmark. Screening with faecal occult blood tests (FOBt) could potentially reduce mortality from bowel cancer by 15% and this is the method that has been chosen, being done by post since 2006. Studies are starting to emerge, looking at success of pick-up of cancers and uptake (e.g. the use of pre-notification seems to increase uptake) but as yet we are only 5 years into the programme.

If the results are positive, patients will be offered a colonoscopy (this will be a separate route to the 2-week cancer referrals) through the local screening centres.

A *Lancet* study (doi: 10.1016/S0140-6736(10)60551-X) over 16 years found that a single sigmoidoscope examination in men and women aged 55–64 reduced the incidence of colorectal cancer by a third and mortality by 43%.

Prostate cancer screening

www.cancerscreening.nhs.uk/prostate/prostate-patient-info-sheet.pdf

- Prostate cancer is the second most common cause of cancer death in men.
- Around 35 000 new cases are diagnosed each year, mainly aged 70–74 years.
- Around 10 000 die from the disease.
- Around two out of three men with a raised prostate-specific antigen (PSA) level will not have prostate cancer.
- Around 20% of men with prostate cancer do not have a raised PSA level.
- Around 60% of cases have metastatic disease at the time of diagnosis.

PSA is the current tumour marker being used when investigating for prostate cancer; its use for a population-based screening programme is being evaluated. Digital rectal examination has had a lot of text time and although still included in some ongoing trials it is unlikely that this would form a significant part of a screening test. Although there is no screening programme, any man can have a PSA test if he requests one, hence screening may creep in. This doesn't satisfy the criteria, however, as evidence is lacking that screening for prostate cancer would be beneficial, whereas early detection and treatment may improve morbidity and mortality.

Arguments against screening with prostate-specific antigen

The arguments include the following:

- There is a lack of consensus on treatment for early disease and a risk of harm with diagnostic biopsy.
- Despite the widespread use of PSA testing there is lack of evidence that it reduces mortality.
- For every 100 men with a raised PSA only 30 will have a prostate cancer.
- Only a minority of cancers spread to shorten life expectancy.
- The PSA is unable to distinguish between indolent and aggressive tumours (speed of change is not an accurate reflection).
- PSA is not tumour specific and can also be raised in prostatitis, benign prostatic hypertrophy, urinary retention, instrumentation and ejaculation.
- There is no specific cut-off below which the risk of prostate cancer is zero.
- The values we currently use would be unreliable in obesity; PSA level is often lower.
- Recent genetics could mean a screening programme may be possible with no PSA.

Screening decreases prostate cancer mortality: 11-year follow-up of the 1988 Quebec prospective randomised controlled trial

Prostate 2004; 59(3): 311–18

Two studies have now found that yearly screening reduces mortality by as much as 8%. This particular study looked at 46 486 men aged 45–80 years in Quebec and found 74 deaths due to prostate cancer occurred in the unscreened group compared to 10 deaths in the screened group (mean follow up of 7.93 years). The statistics used were a Cox proportional hazards model of the age at death from prostate cancer, which showed a 62% reduction ($p < 0.002$) in screened men.

'It's a maybe test': men's experiences of prostate specific antigen testing in primary care

Br J Gen Pract 2007; 57(537): 303–10

This study was undertaken as little was known about the views of men regarding PSA testing. It found that men were uncertain about the test, the results and further interventions offered, all of which caused anxiety. The decision to have the test was based on social and media factors rather than it being patient-led.

Smoking

- Smoking is the number-one preventable cause of ill health (81 400 deaths/year in England).
- One in four adults in the UK smoke (13 million in total in the UK).
- The cost to the NHS is £1500 million/year.
- Sixty-seven per cent of smokers want to stop (National Statistics, 2010).
- Smoking cessation by someone with angina may decrease their chances of having a myocardial infarction by up to 50%.
- Quality Outcomes Framework – note targets vary each year.

NHS Stop Smoking Services were introduced in 1999 and have been shown to be effective at improving quit rates. Smoking accounts for up to a 50% difference in life expectancy between affluent and disadvantaged groups in England (*Lancet* 2006; 386(9533): 367–79).

Since 1 July 2007 there has been a ban on smoking in enclosed public places and work places (including company cars in some instances).

Some useful smoking cessation websites are:

- Smokefree Resource Centre (www.smokefree.nhs.uk/resources).
- Action on Smoking and Health (www.ash.org.uk).
- UK Centre for Tobacco Control Studies (an online training resource) (www.ukctcs.org).

1998 White Paper 'Smoking kills'

In this framework for the NHS on smoking cessation, funding was initially only guaranteed in New Health Action Zones before being rolled out nationally.

It was recommended that practitioners should:

- assess smoking 'at every opportunity'!
- advise patients to stop smoking
- provide accurate information
- recommend nicotine replacement therapy
- refer patients to specialist services as necessary
- follow up patients.

The government advocates at least a 30-second approach of AAA:

Ask: about quitting.

Advise: quit information and direction.

Act: refer or prescribe.

Obesity

- Obesity is defined as a body mass index (BMI) >30 kg/m^2.
- Over 20% of men and women are obese in the UK. It is a huge medical, public health and economic problem with genetic and environmental determinants.
- Six per cent of all deaths can be attributed to obesity (National Audit Office, 2001).

Reducing obesity is one of the six priorities of the 'Choosing health' White Paper. The strategies go beyond the recommendations of the House of Commons Select Committees Report of May 2005. The government's response to the report lays out 52 recommendations. It includes the recognition that further data collection is needed, the approach schools should take, the role of the Office for Standards in Education, Children's Services and Skills (Ofsted) in assessing these directives, a national walking strategy, the roles of healthcare professionals (pharmacological, surgical, psychological and behavioural aspects), as well as the need for a dedicated framework for obesity building on the current National Service Frameworks. One specific recommendation is that there should be a wide-ranging programme of solutions:

- health promotion
- education about food
- restriction of promotion of unhealthy foods for children
- a comprehensive care pathway on obesity.

Weight watchers and slimming world vouchers (probably more effective that GP nurse management) are being offered on the NHS in some areas.

***Obesity: guidance on the prevention, identification, assessment and management of overweight and obesity in adults and children*, December 2006**

www.nice.org.uk/nicemedia/pdf/word/CG43NICEGuideline.doc

Staying a healthy weight improves health and reduces risk of diseases associated with being overweight or obese. These recommendations focus on health promotion (in schools and in a health context) and management of lifestyle depending on co-morbidities and a willingness to change. They also grade obesity based on BMI.

Multicomponent interventions should encourage:

- increased physical activity
- improved eating behaviour (stimulus control, self-monitoring, goal setting)
- healthy eating.

Medication options looks at orlistat and sibutramine (not rimonabant/Acomplia) with the following guidelines for adults:

- Prescribe if BMI is 28.0 kg/m^2 (27 for sibutramine) with risk factors or BMI 30.0 kg/m^2 without.
- Continue at 3 months if there has been 5% weight loss (less strict for non-insulin-dependent diabetes mellitus).
- Continue at 12 months after discussion, depending on progress (for orlistat, sibutramine is not recommended for longer than 12 months).

A *Drugs and Therapeutic Bulletin* (2007; 45(6): 41) article compared drug treatments (including rimonabant) based on the evidence available and concluded that orlistat had the better efficacy and safety profile.

Medication for children was not recommended under 12 years, and for over 12 only if there are co-morbidities (prescribing should be started by a multidisciplinary team.

Prognosis in obesity (we all need to move a little more and eat a little less)

BMJ 2005; 330: 1339–40

A fantastic title that, no matter how many guidelines are produced, says it all.

This editorial touches on lots of points, most topically the 2004 White Paper 'Choosing health' and the subsequent action plan *Choosing a Better Diet*, which have both set tough targets to reduce childhood obesity. Both sides of the energy balance equation must be tackled and are well within the range of day-to-day variability in activity and diet.

Exercise

www.nice.org.uk/nicemedia/live/11000/30364/30364.pdf

Active adults live longer!

Obesity in the UK, both in children and adults, is increasing. This has numerous implications for health (non-insulin-dependent diabetes, coronary heart disease, osteoarthritis and so forth). Exercise is effective for long-term weight reduction/regulation, although you can appreciate it would be difficult to perform blinded trials. The White Paper 'Choosing health', National Service Frameworks and care pathways are some of the documents that touch on the importance of exercise.

The current advice from the National Institute for Health and Clinical Excellence obesity guidance is that 30 minutes of moderate intensity exercise five times a week (or several shorter, 10-minute sessions) should be aspired to although 45–90 minutes may be needed to maintain loss and prevent further weight gain. Even if this does not help loss of weight it should be encouraged from a cardiovascular fitness point of view.

Effects on cardiovascular disease

- Exercise reduces primary and secondary cardiovascular disease.
- Coronary heart disease can be reduced by 20%–30% in men.
- Stroke could be reduced by 30%–40%.
- Blood pressure can be reduced by up to 10 mmHg systolic and 8 mmHg diastolic.
- Exercise increases high-density lipoprotein cholesterol levels.

Musculoskeletal effects

- Exercise has been shown to increase mobility and reduce falls in the elderly.
- It can reduce the rate of hip fracture by up to 50%.
- If weight bearing it can increase bone density.

Psychiatric effects

- Exercise reduces and relieves anxiety.
- It appears to have an antidepressant effect.

Other effects

- Exercise can prevent non-insulin-dependent diabetes in 25% of cases.
- It improves glucose tolerance in non-insulin-dependent diabetes mellitus.
- People who exercise live longer.
- Graded aerobic exercise improves fatigue, functional capacity and fitness in patients with chronic fatigue syndrome.

Four commonly used methods to increase physical activity: brief interventions in primary care, exercise referral schemes, pedometers and community based exercise programmes for walking and cycling

www.nice.org.uk/nicemedia/pdf/PHYSICAL-ALS2_FINAL.pdf

This guidance looks at how effective the four methods are at encouraging people to be more active. It recommends that we opportunistically encourage people to be more active (30 minutes for 5 days a week or more), using their judgement as to when this would be appropriate, and that we could use the General Practitioners Physical Activity Questionnaire to identify inactive individuals. In giving advice we should take into account their individual needs, preferences and circumstances and supply written advice.

Healthy people: promoting health and preventing disease: questions

1 Which of the following is not found in the Wilson's criteria for screening (1966)?
   a. The condition must be common.
   b. The test must have high sensitivity and specificity.
   c. The condition must be important.
   d. Once diagnosed by screening it must be a condition that is treatable.
   e. If there is no latent period, this does not preclude screening, as long as there is treatment available.

2 Which of the statements below is correct with regard to cervical screening?
   a. Cervical cancer has two peaks in incidence, the first at 30–35 years and the second at 70–75 years.
   b. The incidence of cervical screening is 2.4 per 100 000.
   c. Around 75% of cervical cancers are squamous cell carcinoma (the majority).
   d. Cervical cancer screening prevents around 500 deaths per year.
   e. GPs are responsible for the call and recall of patients eligible.

3 With regard to ovarian cancer, which is the most correct statement?
  a. Overall 5 year survival is below 35%.
  b. Incidence is reducing with current methods for early detection.
  c. It is the most common cancer in women.
  d. All patients with a Risk of Malignancy Index I (RMI I) score >100 should be referred to a specialist multidisciplinary team.

4 Bowel cancer screening in the UK uses FOBt. Which of the following statements with regard to screening test options are correct?
  a. Flexible sigmoidoscopy has been the most extensively studied screening test for colorectal carcinoma.
  b. False positives occur with vegetables rich in peroxidase.
  c. FOB testing has a high sensitivity and specificity of 90%–95%.
  d. FOB testing can identify 99.9% of all colorectal carcinomas.
  e. If flexible sigmoidoscopy were the screening test of choice this would detect all large bowel cancers.

5 When considering the epidemiology of smoking in the UK, select the single most appropriate answer.
  a. Smoking rates are now higher in females than males (2007 as compared with 2001).
  b. Older males were found to smoke more than younger male patients.
  c. Postcode use to identify deprivation is the single more important epidemiological tool used in trials for deprivation quantification.
  d. There has been a decrease in the proportion of patients recorded as smokers in the UK from 2001 to 2007.
  e. Patients in affluent areas had twice the rate of smokers than in deprived areas because of the current costs of cigarettes.

6 Which of the following types of intervention achieves the best success for smoking cessation?
  a. One-to-one behavioural support.
  b. Brief opportunistic advice from a clinician, especially a GP.
  c. Group support with tailored prescribing of nicotine replacement or varenicline.
  d. Over-the-counter nicotine gum.
  e. Zyban prescription.

7 In reference to the familial breast cancer guidance published by the National Institute for Health and Clinical Excellence, select the single most appropriate answer with regard to MRI screening.
  a. All patients with the TP53 gene mutation should be offered annual MRI screening from birth.
  b. Patients carrying BRCA 1 or 2 should be offered 3-yearly MRI screening from the age of 30.
  c. Patients aged 30–39 who have an 8% 10-year risk of developing breast cancer should be offered annual screening.
  d. Patients aged 40–49 years with an 8% risk should be offered annual MRI screening.

8 Which of the following statements are true with regard to the taking of blood for PSA testing in men?
   a. Exercise has not been found to affect the PSA value in blood.
   b. If a patient has a urinary tract infection, PSA testing should be avoided until this is treated.
   c. It is a misnomer that digital rectal examination affects the PSA level.
   d. PSA testing should be postponed for 72 hours after a digital rectal examination (although there are some disagreements throughout professionals!).
   e. Ejaculation should be avoided for 7 days prior to PSA testing.

9 Which of the following statements with regard to management of obesity with pharmacological methods is correct?
   a. Weight loss of more than 0.5–1 kg per week should not be expected.
   b. Sibutramine has been shown to be clinically safe and effective.
   c. Orlistat should not be used for longer than 12 months.
   d. Waist measurement is done to guide purchases of new clothes rather than for any clinical reason.
   e. Orlistat is only ever able to be offered under the NHS when the BMI is $>30\,kg/m^2$.

10 Which of the following statements with regard to abdominal aortic aneurysm screening is correct?
   a. It is hoped to have been rolled out nationwide by 2020.
   b. It is being offered to men on their 70th birthday.
   c. It is being offered to men and women on their 70th birthday.
   d. Screening will cut premature death from a ruptured aortic aneurysm by up to 50%.
   e. The screening offered is computed tomography or MRI scanning, as this has been shown to increase sensitivity and specificity as compared with ultrasound.

Healthy people: promoting health and preventing disease: answers

1 **e** High sensitivity and specificity equate to a high positive predictive value. Wilson's criteria specifically mentions a latent period. Although this doesn't quite fit the breast cancer model of screening, the question specifically asks about Wilson's criteria. Wilson's criteria (1966) can be briefly summarised as follows:

- The condition must be:
  — common
  — important
  — diagnosable by acceptable methods.
- There should be a latent period where effective interventional treatment is possible.
- Screening must be:
  — cheap/cost-effective
  — continuous
  — safe

  - repeatable
  - non-invasive
  - acceptable to patients
  - the test for screening must have a high positive predictive value.
- There must be a treatment available.

2 a Cervical screening facts:

- The incidence of cervical cancer in the UK is 9.6 per 100 000.
- The mortality rate is 5 per 100 000.
- The incidence of disease peaks at 30–35 and 70–75 years of age.
- Around 95% of cervical cancers are squamous cell and 5% are adenocarcinomas.
- The most important risk factor is human papillomavirus. At least 50% of sexually active people will get human papillomavirus (type 16, 18, 31, 33 or 35). Smoking and the age at first intercourse are also important factors.
- Around 80% of women aged 25–64 years have been screened (3.8 million women).
- Cervical screening prevents around 5000 deaths per year in the UK. The incidence of cervical cancer fell by 42% between 1988 and 1996 (in England and Wales) as a direct consequence of the cervical screening programme.
- The screening programme currently costs around £157 million per year and is run by the cervical screening programme.

3 a *Ovarian Cancer* (www.nice.org.uk/nicemedia/live/13464/54268/54268.pdf). Mortality is high at >35% at 5 years, although transvaginal scanning and Ca125 are available diagnostically. Neither of these nor the currently identified proteins have (as yet) been of any help with regard to screening. It is the most common gynaecological cancer in women but the fifth most common cancer overall. An RMI I score of >250 requires urgent referral. RMI = UxMxCa125 (where U relates to an ultrasound score of 1–5 points and M relates to menopause status).

4 b Faecal occult blood (Cochrane review, 1998):

- has low sensitivity and specificity (tumour needs to be bleeding) in the range of 50%–60%
- is the most extensively studied screening test for colorectal cancer
- gives false positives with red meat and vegetables rich in peroxidase.

Flexible sigmoidoscopy:

- can detect 80% colorectal cancers
- only detects cancers up to the splenic flexure (50% of cancers are proximal).

5 d This question, although mirrored by National Statistics, was taken from the *British Journal of General Practice* (Trends in the epidemiology of smoking recorded in UK general practice (*Br J Gen Pract* 2010; 60(572): e121–7). The Townsend Score is often used for deprivation. It takes into account postcode, unemployment, car ownership and non-owner occupancy. Higher scores indicate greater levels of socio-economic deprivation. The increase in non-smokers recoded may not be the complete answer and may just reflect an increase in the use of services where smoking cessation is accessed and cessation achieved in the short term. The 30-second intervention AAA is advised (Ask, Advise, Act).

6 c *Brief Interventions and Referral for Smoking Cessation in Primary Care and Other Settings* (www.nice.org.uk/nicemedia/pdf/SMOKING-ALS2_FINAL.pdf): this guidance summarised interventions as offering opportunistic advice, discussion, negotiation and encouragement usually taking 5–10 minutes and outlines four recommendations:

- Everyone who smokes should be advised to quit except in exceptional cases.
- People should be asked how interested they are in quitting.
- We should take the opportunity to encourage people to quit at every consultation and refer to services to help them; where they are unable to do this they should be offered pharmacotherapies.
- Nurses in primary care should be recommending smoking cessation as well.

The Smoking Cessation Action in Primary Care Taskforce (SCAPE) was launched in September 2001. The aim of this initiative was to encourage GPs and practice nurses to maintain the impetus of smoking cessation services. It suggests the 30-second approach:

- Do you smoke?
- Would you like to stop?
- Would you like my help to stop?

The aim is to catch people at the right point of the cycle of change to help them engage with services. A major concern of GPs (in a survey published by SCAPE in May 2001) is workload implications. With regard to smoking cessation, 93% of GPs thought it was 'the best thing you could do for their health'. Around 91% of GPs put off advising patients to stop because of time pressures.

7 c *Familial Breast Cancer* (www.nice.org.uk/nicemedia/live/10994/30244/30244.pdf). TP53 carriers should be offered annual screening from the age of 20. BRCA 1 and 2 should be offered annual screening for ages 30–49 years. Patients aged 30–39 with a 10-year risk of >8% should be offered annual MRI screening or if aged 40–49 with a 10-year risk of >10% or >12% where mammography has shown a dense pattern.

8 b PSA testing should be avoided for 48 hours after strenuous physical exercise and ejaculation. This is increased to 7 days following a digital rectal examination and 6 weeks following prostate biopsy. Some surgeons feel the delay after digital rectal examination may be excessive, but current guidelines suggest waiting the 7 days (www.cancerscreening.nhs.uk/prostate/prostate-patient-info-sheet.pdf).

9 a Although sibutramine was clinically effective, the licence (at the time of writing) in the UK has been withdrawn because of safety concerns. Orlistat is used initially for a 6–12 month trial but can continue if sustained weight loss is seen, reinforcing lifestyle changes. Waist circumference measurement is done as this is a guide to morbidity but also because inch lost rather than weight loss can be equally important depending on the lifestyle changes being made. Orlistat can be offered where the BMI is >28 kg/m^2 if there are other risks associated. The Obesity Care Pathway 2005 (www.nationalobesityforum.org.uk) publication offers a toolkit for healthcare professionals and considers the following:

- the need for baseline patient data and investigations

- patient motivation
- healthy eating
- physical activity
- integrated weight management programmes
- the role of pharmaceuticals.

It highlights the use of waist circumference alongside BMI as an aid to stratifying risk and monitoring success.

10 d By 2013 it is hoped to be nationwide; ultrasound scanning will be offered to all men on their 65th birthday (NHS Abdominal Aortic Aneurysm Screening Programme, aaa.screening.nhs.uk/professionals).

Statement 6

Genetics in primary care

Genetics is a rapidly evolving area of medicine and is so much more directed than the exercise GPs do as part of a cardiovascular risk assessment. I would imagine most of us go into family history details in a small number of cases. It is an area that creates many ethical issues, primarily because we may know the patient's family history through our knowledge of other family members; what you won't always know is whether that is information that has been shared in the family, and so care has to be taken to not unwittingly breach confidentiality.

The genetics service would see a wide range of cases from antenatal counselling to children with problems that may be genetic in origin, through to adults for predictive testing of late-onset disorders.

Our local genetics unit is Birmingham and as well as having a useful website, they also provide guidance, advice and a downloadable form available (www.bwhct.nhs.uk/family_history_form_july_2009.pdf) for patients to be able to complete with their family history/pedigree prior to any appointments. Although this will vary across areas, the principles will be the same.

The source referenced in the Royal College of General Practitioners curriculum for a family pedigree is available online (www.clingensoc.org/Docs/Standards/CGSPedigree.pdf). Similarly, more information is available on the UK Genetic Testing Network website, with regard to the tests available (www.ukgtn.nhs.uk/gtn/Home/NHS+Professionals).

Genetics: an overview

Update January 2009 p. 46

This article is a good summary of current genetic applications. Although there is often very little that can be done with the results from genetic testing, it can help people to forward plan and make decisions in cases such as: chromosome abnormalities which could cause birth defects, learning delay or reproductive issues; single-gene disorders such as cystic fibrosis, Huntington's disease and Duchenne muscular dystrophy; family cancers; and birth defects with a genetic component such as neural tube defects and clefts.

Antenatal genetic screening tests

The integrated test identifies pregnancies at high risk of Down's syndrome, Edwards's syndrome and neural tube defects. Diagnostically, chorionic villus sampling or amniocentesis may be offered. Polymerase chain reaction tests are then used to identify aneuploidy of chromosomes 13, 18 and 21, and sometimes a full karyotype is offered.

Neonatal genetic screening tests

Neonatal screening tests and the monospot test is covered elsewhere (thalassaemia, sickle cell).

Family history cancer screening

This is specifically related to breast and bowel cancer at present, although reasons to involve a genetic team would be three or more relatives with a tumour at the same site (ovary, prostate, pancreas, melanoma, thyroid, sarcoma), or multiple primary cancers in one individual.

Other areas for referral

Although you can talk to the genetics team or refer for advice, other conditions to consider referral for would be neurodegenerative problems, Von Hippel–Lindau disease, Cowden syndrome, neurofibromatosis and learning disabilities (5% of children will be born with chromosomal abnormalities).

Genetics in primary care: questions

1 Which of the following best describes the change in chromosome structure referred to as a translocation?
   a. A chromosome breaks and the genetic material is lost.
   b. A piece of chromosome breaks off and attaches to another chromosome.
   c. A part of the chromosome is copied too many times.
   d. A chromosome breaks in two places resulting in pieces of DNA being reversed and reinserted into the chromosome.
   e. A chromosome that breaks on the long (q) arm or the short (p) arm.

2 Familial bowel cancer: which of the following would not be a reason to refer to genetics?
   a. Both parents diagnosed with colorectal cancer at any age.
   b. Three or more close relatives diagnosed with colorectal cancer, other gastrointestinal cancers, uterine or ovarian cancer at any age.
   c. One close relative under the age of 45 years diagnosed with colorectal cancer.
   d. One close relative under the age of 45 years with multiple colorectal polyps.
   e. One close relative under the age of 60 years diagnosed with colorectal cancer.

3 Fragile X: which of the following statements is true for Fragile X syndrome?
   a. No males born to fathers with fragile X syndrome will be carriers or be affected.
   b. Antenatal testing with chorionic villus sampling can be performed as early as 10 weeks.
   c. Although there are often no physical features, microcephaly is a recognised manifestation.
   d. It is not known to affect Afro-Caribbean populations.
   e. A female affected with Fragile X cannot have a child who is unaffected.

4 Familial breast cancer: which of the following is a suggested reason to seek further specialist genetics advice?
   a. Two second-degree relatives with breast cancer at any age.

b. Three first- or second-degree relatives with breast or ovarian cancer.
c. One first-degree relative aged 42 years with breast cancer.
d. One first-degree relative aged 46 years with breast cancer.
e. A first-, second- or third-degree relative with bilateral breast cancer at any age.

5 Relations: which of the following would be considered a second-degree relative?
a. Daughter
b. Parent
c. Sister
d. Brother
e. Uncle

6 Turner's syndrome: which of the following is true with regard to the effects on the cardiovascular system in Turner's syndrome?
a. There is a 54% chance of coarctation of the aorta.
b. The risk of a bicuspid aortic valve is 1%–2%.
c. Aortic dissection is known to occur without structural abnormalities.
d. There is a reduced risk of hypertension.
e. Cardiological investigation is only recommended for clinical signs and symptoms.

Cystic fibrosis: for each of the statements regarding cystic fibrosis in questions 6–10, answer true or false.

7 It is an autosomal recessive disease affecting 8000 people in the United Kingdom.
8 The gold standard test for diagnosis is now DNA analysis.
9 The neonatal screening test in the United Kingdom is done in the Guthrie heel prick test.
10 Twenty per cent of patients with cystic fibrosis have pancreatic insufficiency.

Genetics in primary care: answers

1 b In a translocation such as this the arrangement is described as balanced, as there is no overall loss or gain of genetic material. Option (a) is referring to a deletion – the ensuing chromosome imbalance usually results in learning difficulties. Option (c) is referring to duplication – this can be associated with learning difficulties with or without congenital abnormalities. Options (d) and (e) are inversions. An inversion that involves the centromere is called a pericentric inversion; one that does not involve the centromere is called a paracentric inversion.

2 e Two close/first-degree relatives under the age of 60 years diagnosed with colorectal cancer would be a reason to consider referral, although it would probably be more significant if they were under 45 years of age.

3 a Fragile X syndrome is the most commonly identified cause of inherited learning disability (Down's syndrome is the most common cause of learning disability, but this is rarely inherited). It also causes behavioural problems and developmental delay. The gene FMR1 is responsible, on the tip of the X chromosome.

Two-thirds of female carriers would be expected to have a normal IQ and one-third mild learning difficulties. Males will have female children that are carriers or males that are not (as they have passed on the Y chromosome, not the X). Although genetic testing can be performed early with chorionic villus sampling, this is not usually before 12 weeks. Although there are often no physical features, a larger (rather than smaller) head, long face, arched palate and dental crowding despite a pronounced jaw are recognised. A female can produce children of either sex who are affected by, carriers of or clear of the gene altogether. Refer to the Fragile X Society website for more information (www.fragilex.org.uk).

4 b Further genetics advice would also be wise in the following cases: two first- or second-degree relatives under the age of 60 years with breast cancer, or ovarian cancer at any age on the same side of the family; one first-degree female relative under the age of 40 years with breast cancer or one first-degree male relative diagnosed with breast cancer at any age; or a first-degree relative with bilateral breast cancer.

5 e Options (a) through to (d) are all first-degree relatives. Second-degree relatives would include grandparents, niece/nephew, aunt/uncle and half-sister/half-brother. Visit the National Genetics Education and Development Centre website for more information (www.geneticseducation.nhs.uk). Search the American Medical Association site for articles on family history (www.ama-assn.org). The National Human Genome Research Institute has online tools for drawing family history (www.genome.gov/11510372).

6 c 'Diagnosis and management of Turner's syndrome' (*MIMS Women's Health* 2011; 6(2): 26–68). Turner's affects 1 in 2500 female live births, 1.5 million women worldwide. Typically, there is short stature, congenital web neck, cubitus valgus and gonadal dysgenesis. Risk of coarctation is 11% and bicuspid aortic valve 16%.

7 True Seventy per cent of the disease gene mutations are related to Phe508del deletion.

8 False DNA testing can be used, but the gold standard is still the sweat test (raised sodium chloride is due to the cystic fibrosis transmembrane regulator being unable to absorb chlorine).

9 True This measures immunoreactive trypsinogen, the pancreatic enzyme that is elevated in the first few days of life.

10 False Eighty-five per cent of patients with cystic fibrosis have pancreatic insufficiency. It can present with signs of malabsorption, especially fat and fat-soluble vitamins (A, D, E, K). Cardiological investigations are recommended at the time of diagnosis (24-hour blood pressure (for nocturnal hypertension), heart and aorta imaging with echocardiography and electrocardiography, in older patients magnetic resonance imaging and echo).

Statement 7

Care of acutely ill people

The Royal College of General Practitioners highlights this part of the curriculum as the area where candidates often seem to do less well, possibly because we don't focus enough of our attention on it in revision (treatment would often be superficial and supportive as they are transferred to the nearest hospital) and possibly because this is an area we deal with infrequently. However, this can be said about a lot of the curriculum, and the point is to become a competent and well-rounded generalist.

You will have considered most of the issues regarding the care of acutely ill people in other statements, e.g. ectopic pregnancy in Statement 10.1 (Women's health), the use of advanced directives in Statement 12, and so forth.

Cardiopulmonary resuscitation

www.resus.org.uk

This should be something that you are better at than your trainer. It is important to have your yearly refresher course up to date for your day job. The courses often cover anaphylaxis, choking and use of automated defibrillation, as well as basic life support for adults, children and neonates.

Death certification

This could have been in many sections and is not always unexpected, but it is something that needs dealing with urgently and it is often associated with acutely ill patients, not just in a palliative setting.

Death certification provides legal evidence of the fact and cause(s) of death, which then allows the death to be registered. It has been a statutory obligation in England since the 1830s. It is important to be as accurate as possible and a mode of dying is not acceptable as a cause of death.

Terms that imply a mode of dying include:

Asphyxia	Asthenia	Brain failure
Cachexia	Cardiac arrest	Cardiac failure
Coma	Debility	Exhaustion
Hepatic failure	Renal failure	Respiratory arrest
Shock	Syncope	Uraemia

Old age can only be used as a cause of death if the person is over 70 years of age and a more specific cause of death cannot be given, although with reforms this may become less acceptable unless a patient is older.

Duties of the medical practitioner of the deceased:

- If you were in attendance in the deceased's last illness you are required to certify the cause of death, if you are able.

- You are legally responsible for the delivery of the death certificate to the registrar. This may be done personally, by post or by a relative (or other nominated person).
- You should also complete the notice to the informant (attached to the death certificate) and the counterfoil in the book for your records.

There are three kinds of certificate:

1. Medical Certificate of cause of death (Form 66) – any death after the first 28 days of life.
2. Neonatal Death Certificate (Form 65) – any live-born death within 28 days of birth.
3. Certificate of Still-Birth (Form 34) – any death of an infant after 34 weeks of pregnancy who showed no signs of life after delivery from the mother.

When to refer to the coroner

There is no statutory duty to report to the coroner (this would otherwise be done by the registrar), but voluntary reporting where suggested avoids unnecessary delay and anxiety for the relatives.

A death should be referred if:

- the cause of death is unknown
- the deceased has not been seen by the certifying doctor either after death or within 14 days before death
- the death was violent, unnatural or was suspicious
- the death may be due to an accident (whenever it occurred)
- the death may be due to self-neglect or neglect by others
- the death may be due to industrial disease or related to the deceased's employment
- the death may be due to an abortion
- the death occurred during an operation or before recovery from the effects of an anaesthetic
- the death may be suicide
- the death occurred during or shortly after detention in police or prison custody.

Death certification and doctors' dilemmas: a qualitative study of GPs' perspectives

Br J Gen Pract 2005; 55(518): 677–83

This paper gives a good introduction to the additional uses of death certification:

- to monitor trends and patterns of disease
- to guide health promotion, resource allocation and service planning
- for research and epidemiology
- for the settlement of estates, welfare and pensions entitlements.

Inaccuracies of death certification are thought to range from 20% to 65%, and when looking at determining influences on the recording of a cause of death it was found that clinical uncertainty and the role of the deceased's family were the two main themes.

The Shipman Inquiry

www.dh.gov.uk

The Shipman Inquiry was set up in January 2001 following the conviction of Harold Shipman for the murder of 15 of his patients. Its purpose was to investigate the extent of Shipman's unlawful activities, enquire into the activities of statutory authorities and other organisations involved, and to then make recommendations on steps needed to protect patients for the future.

Inquiry chair Dame Janet Smith and her team have published five reports. The first three look at the extent of Shipman's criminal activities (looking into the care of more than 800 patients), the police investigation and death certification. The fourth report (*The Regulation of Controlled Drugs in the Community*, published in July 2004) looks in detail at the prescribing, dispensing, storing and disposing of controlled drugs. The fifth report (*Safeguarding Patients: lessons from the past – proposals for the future*, published in December 2004) looks at revalidation and monitoring of GP performance, the role of the General Medical Council, disciplinary procedures, whistle-blowing and the handling of complaints.

Recommendations for death certification include the following:

- A coroner's office should be notified of all deaths.
- The officer should examine two forms before certifying the cause of death:
  - Form 1 – completed by a health professional, recording the facts surrounding death, including the persons present at the time of death.
  - Form 2 – to be completed by the doctor who last treated the patient; relevant sections of the patient's notes could be attached.

A practical method for monitoring general practice mortality in the UK: findings from a pilot study in a health board of Northern Ireland

Br J Gen Pract 2005; 55(518): 670–6

Following the Shipman cases, the Baker Report recommended monitoring mortality rates. This would pose several challenges. The data would need to be of a high quality linked to general practices. It would not be certain how easy it would be to distinguish variations in mortality and, if any variation was identified, what should be done with the information.

This pilot study looked at cross-sectional and longitudinal mortality rate variations and assigning variation reasons (e.g. nursing homes, levels of deprivation, age/sex profiles). The ultimate aim of the data collection in the pilot was to improve quality of care. There was a consensus of apprehension about the release of any such data to the public and how it may be incorrectly interpreted.

Recommendations for revalidation include:

- A mandatory knowledge-based test at least every 7 years, or every 5 years if the clinician is over 50 years of age.
- It should include a folder of mandatory evidence (e.g. prescribing data, complaints record, evidence of continuing professional development).
- Primary care trusts would be able to issue warnings and impose financial penalties to underperforming GPs.

Concerns raised about the General Medical Council include:

- There has been a failure to lay down clear policies governing fitness to practice procedures.
- There has been a failure to take into account the difficulties faced by complainants.
- There has been a failure to investigate complaints.
- There has been a tendency to lean towards preservation of a doctor's privacy and against the legitimate public interest.
- There is a concern over determination to undertake a sufficiently thorough investigation.

Learning from Tragedy, Keeping Patients Safe: overview of the government's action programme in response to the recommendations of the Shipman Inquiry

Although this report considers all aspects, the following are specific points in regard to death certification:

- Medical certificates for cause of death will be checked by an independent medical examiner attached to clinical governance teams.
- If not satisfied with the cause of death this can be referred to the coroner at any point.
- The medical examiner should have full access to the medical records and should be allowed to discuss the death with the doctor signing the certificate and with the family.
- All unexpected deaths will be treated as significant events and will be followed up by a clinical audit team.

A medical examiner would have at least 5 years of full registration. A draft bill is currently being looking into, and certification by a single doctor in burial cases will cease, as would payment for cremation certificates. Instead, a fee would be payable in all cases to the medical examiner service. There is some concern that after death a body may not be seen by a healthcare professional and the responsibility would be with the Ministry of Justice.

Care of acutely ill people: questions

1 Atrial fibrillation: which of the following would be correct in an acute presentation of atrial fibrillation?
   a. Patients should be immediately warfarinised to reduce the risk of stroke.
   b. If presenting with associated dyspnoea the patient should be started on bisoprolol.
   c. If presenting with associated bibasal crackles, they need urgent admission for cardioversion.
   d. Thyroid function test is the most important blood test required.
   e. If asymptomatic it is acceptable to do nothing for the first 7 days; if the atrial fibrillation reverts in that time, it is by definition paroxysmal atrial fibrillation.

2 What is the correct management in a non-bleeding patient with an INR of 8.3?
   a. 1 mg intravenous vitamin K given orally.
   b. 1 mg intravenous vitamin K given intravenously.

c. Omit warfarin until INR <5, then restart.
d. Reduce warfarin by 50% and repeat the INR in 48 hours.
e. Omit the warfarin for 48 hours, then restart at usual dose.

For each of the statements in questions 3–5, select the single best response. Each answer can be used once, more than once or not at all.
a. Aortic dissection.
b. Myocardial infarction.
c. Gastro-oesophageal reflux.
d. Pulmonary embolism.
e. Pancreatitis.
f. Cholecystitis.

3 This case presented with sudden sharp severe chest pain, with right arm BP of 102/70 and left arm BP of 142/70 with ST depression.

4 This case presented in a diabetic patient with shortness of breath but no other features.

5 This case can present with fever and shoulder-tip pain.

6 You review a patient who has recently had a cold and has been taking 2 × 500 mg paracetamol with Lemsip Max over the last 2–3 days. They still have their upper respiratory tract symptoms. What is your best course of action?
a. Upper respiratory tract infections are self-limiting; just reassure the patient.
b. Arrange a chest X-ray to ensure there is no underlying cause.
c. Prescribe co-codamol for use with the Lemsip Max to reduce the cough.
d. Prescribe antibiotics to resolve symptoms.
e. Immediate admission.

7 A 4-year-old child weighing 20 kg is having an acute exacerbation of asthma (viral trigger); pulse is 110/minute and respiratory rate 36/minute. There are no life-threatening features. Which of the following prednisolone regimes would be the most appropriate?
a. 40 mg for 5 days.
b. 10 mg for 3 days.
c. 10 mg for 5 days.
d. 20 mg for 3 days.
e. 20 mg for 5 days.

8 A 70-year-old woman is discharged from hospital following a routine hip replacement. She is back on her warfarin for atrial fibrillation. Her only other past medical history is an ischaemic stroke. When checked 2 days post discharge her INR is 1.4. What is the best course of action?
a. Continue at the 4 mg dose with a further INR check the next day.
b. Increase the warfarin to 5 mg daily and repeat the INR after 72 hours.
c. Increase the warfarin to 5 mg and repeat the INR after 48 hours.
d. Increase the warfarin to 6 mg and repeat the INR after 72 hours.
e. Arrange for subcutaneous low-molecular-weight heparin to be given.

Care of acutely ill people: answers

1 **c** Warfarinisation is dependent on a CHAD score >2 in the absence of contraindications. If presenting with dyspnoea the patient should be admitted for assessment of cardioversion. Bibasal crackles would be suggestive of heart failure; this as well as chest pain, syncope or neurological features should be admitted for cardioversion. Thyroid function tests may be important, but assessment for acute ischaemia in a new presentation (troponin T) may be more urgent. Paroxysmal atrial fibrillation if of fewer than 7 days' duration, but you cannot sit and wait; you need to assess properly and treat accordingly.

2 **a** This question is from the National Patient Safety Agency, *Alert 18: actions that can make anticoagulant therapy safer* (www.nrls.npsa.nhs.uk/). Risk factors for bleeding include: over 70 years of age, hypertension, previous bleeding/poor control.
- INR 4.5–6: omit warfarin, restart when INR <5.
- INR >6.0–8.0: omit warfarin and restart when INR <5.0; give vitamin K 1 mg orally if there are risk factors.
- INR >8.0: omit warfarin and 1 mg oral vitamin K.

3 **a** In dissection you may also expect carotid bruits. If untreated the mortality is 1%–2% per hour in the first 24 hours and 90% at 30 days without surgery. Survival can be 70%–90% with surgery.

4 **b** The other options would still present with pain.

5 **f** Although this can be seen in pancreatitis secondary to pancreatic head cancer, cholecystitis is the most likely cause.

6 **e** Lemsip Max also contains paracetamol, so there is a high risk of paracetamol overdose in this case. The patient needs levels, liver function tests, prothrombin time, INR and kidney function tests and electrolytes. Treatment will be difficult to work out, as the ingestion has been over 2–3 days. This question is from a *BMJ* article, 'Management of paracetamol poisoning' (*BMJ* 2011; 342: d2218).

7 **d** In children 2–5 years of age, 20 mg for 3 days; in children over 5 years of age, 30–40 mg for 3 days (from the British Thoracic Society guidelines).

8 **e** This woman has atrial fibrillation, is at high risk of a further stroke and is also at high risk given she is in the post-operative period and is still relatively immobile. Her INR is subtherapeutic, so she needs subcutaneous heparin. You would be altering her warfarin dose alongside this, but the question is about the single best response.

Statement 8

Care of children and young people

0–18 Years: guidance for all doctors

www.gmc-uk.org/

This is the first publication from the General Medical Council issuing guidance on children. It outlines roles and expectations and may help in making decisions that are in the best interest of the child/young person, assess capacity and consider consent issues.

Child health surveillance

There have been four editions of the Hall report, *Health for all Children*.

- The first set out a programme of routine reviews for all preschool children.
- The second suggested how this may be delivered.
- The third is a response to evolving professional perceptions of preventive healthcare coupled with rapid changes in the political context in which that care is provided (1996).
- The fourth report adds to the emphasis of health promotion and moves away from a medicalised model of screening.

In September 2003 the Green Paper *Every Child Matters* was published, highlighting the need to maximise opportunity, minimise risk and support children to be healthy, safe, make a positive contribution and achieve economic well-being. It sets out the strategy for child health promotion. This report was followed by *Every Child Matters: the next steps* in March 2004, which started to set out the plan for delivery, and in September 2004 the National Service Framework for Children, Young People and Maternity Services was launched (www.dh.gov.uk). It comprises 11 standards: the first five apply to all children, standards 6–10 apply to children in special circumstances and standard 11 is for maternity services.

Standard 1: Promoting health and well-being, identifying needs and intervening early.
Standard 2: Supporting parenting.
Standard 3: Child, young person and family-centred services.
Standard 4: Growing up into adulthood.
Standard 5: Safeguarding and promoting the welfare of children and young people.
Standard 6: Children and young people who are ill.
Standard 7: Children and young people in hospital.

Standard 8: Disabled children, young people and those with complex health needs.
Standard 9: The mental health and psychological well-being of children and young people.
Standard 10: Medicines for children and young people.
Standard 11: Maternity services.

The Child Health Promotion Programme replaced the Child Health Surveillance Programme and includes:
- assessment of the child's and the family's needs
- health promotion
- childhood screening
- immunisations
- early interventions to address identified needs.

This table gives an overview of health promotion services offered.

Age	Intervention
Soon after birth	General physical examination with emphasis on heart, eyes and hips Administration of vitamin K BCG and hepatitis B vaccinations in high-risk babies
5–6 days old	Blood spot test for hypothyroidism, phenylketonuria, sickle cell, cystic fibrosis and MCADD (medium-chain acyl-coenzyme A dehydrogenase deficiency)
New birth visit	This is usually around 12 days and done by the health visitor or midwife As well as assessing the family's needs parents are also given the personal child health record and the 'Birth to five' guide
6–8 weeks	Physical examination and administration of first set of immunisations: polio, diphtheria, tetanus, whooping cough, *Haemophilus influenzae* type b and meningitis C
3 months	Second set of immunisations
4 months	Third set of immunisations
By 12 months	Further developmental assessment
Around 13 months	Immunisation against measles, mumps and rubella
2–3 years	Health visitor performs further developmental assessment
3–5 years	Further immunisation against measles, mumps and rubella; polio; diphtheria; tetanus; and whooping cough
4–5 years	A review at school entry (usually school nurse) The foundation stage profile assessment by the child's teacher to look at development of physical, emotional, social and creative development as well as communication, language and literacy
10–14 years	BCG vaccination given to those who require it Tetanus, diphtheria and polio boosters (age 13–18 years)

NSF for Children, Young People and Maternity Services 2004

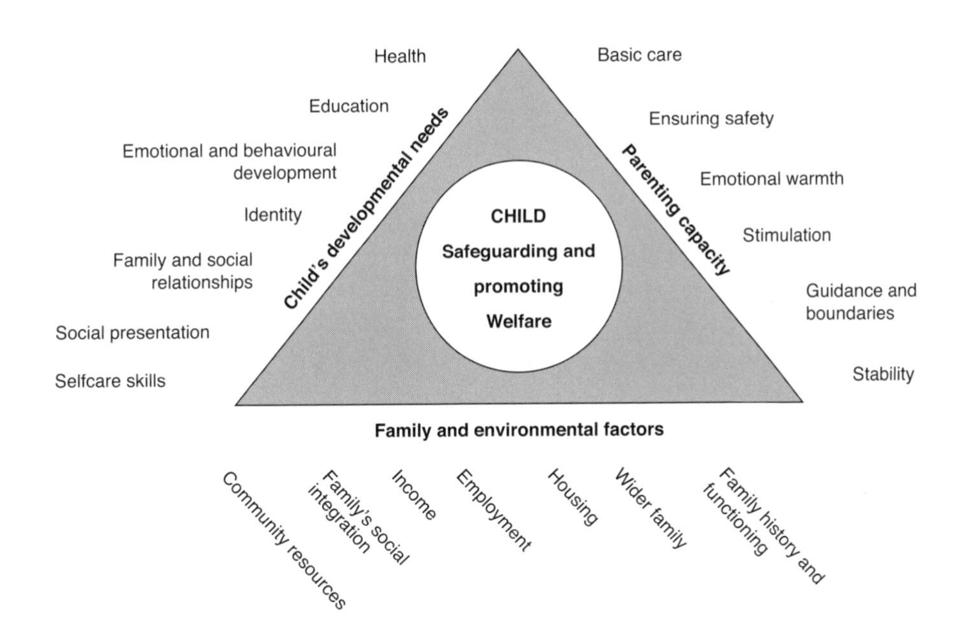

Vaccination programme

www.immunisation.nhs.uk

The immunisation schedule has saved more lives than any other public health measure (apart from the publication of the Sanitary Act in 1866 requiring provision of clean water and effective sewage disposal). The success of a vaccine is not the number of primary cases of the disease but the number of secondary cases generated from the one primary source.

Childhood immunisation

Routine childhood immunisation programme

When to immunise	Vaccine given
2 months old	Diphtheria, tetanus, pertussis (whooping cough), polio and *Haemophilus influenzae* type b (Hib) (DTaP/IPV/Hib) Pneumococcal (Pneumococcal conjugate vaccine, PCV)
3 months old	Diphtheria, tetanus, pertussis, polio and *Haemophilus influenzae* type b (Hib) (DTaP/IPV/Hib) Meningitis C (meningococcal group C) (MenC)

(*continued*)

Routine childhood immunisation programme

When to immunise	Vaccine given
4 months old	Diphtheria, tetanus, pertussis, polio and *Haemophilus influenzae* type b (Hib) (DTaP/IPV/Hib) Meningitis C (meningococcal group C) (MenC) Pneumococcal vaccination (Pneumococcal conjugate vaccine, PCV)
Around 12 months old	*Haemophilus influenzae* type b (Hib) and meningitis C (Hib/MenC)
Around 13 months old	Measles, mumps and rubella (German measles) (MMR) Pneumococcal vaccination (PCV)
3 years 4 months to 5 years old	Diphtheria, tetanus, pertussis (whooping cough) and polio (dTaP/IPV or DTaP/IPV) Measles, mumps and rubella (MMR)
13–18 years old	Diphtheria, tetanus, polio (Td/IPV)

Measles, mumps and rubella

A report from the World Health Organization (2007) included England and Wales in the seven European countries that could expect a measles epidemic in the near future. Their objectives and advice include:

- aim to maintain a high vaccine uptake
- strengthen routine vaccination programmes
- aim catch-up campaigns at susceptible age groups
- stress the safety of the vaccine
- aim for eradication of measles by 2010.

Although the ongoing surveillance has discredited the link with autism and Crohn's disease, this remains an emotive topic for all parents. The single vaccines are not licensed for use in the United Kingdom (other than rubella). If a single vaccine is requested it must be done on a named patient basis and be approved by the Medicines Control Agency. The website (www.nhs.uk/conditions/mmr) is an excellent reference site and gives direct links to other useful sites and evidence.

The MMR scare from 1998 resulted in a 4% drop in uptake, reducing immunisation to 85%. To eliminate measles there needs to be an uptake of 94%–96%. Figures from the NHS Information Centre show a small increase with current uptake running nationally at 85% for the first vaccine (still only around 75% for the booster), which is 9% lower than seen for other vaccines (94%).

The Joint Committee on Vaccination and Immunisation is an independent group that was first set up in 1963 to advise the government on matters relating to communicable disease preventable through immunisation. Their role continues today.

Chickenpox vaccine

The Joint Committee on Vaccination and Immunisation is considering whether to include varicella into the childhood immunisation schedule because of the severity and sequelae in some children and patient groups.

Thiomersal in vaccines

Thiomersal is a mercury-based antimicrobial preservative that is found in some diphtheria, tetanus and pertussis preparations (and some Hib vaccines outside the United Kingdom). This caught media attention because of suspected links with autism. Thiomersal has never been part of live vaccines (MMR and BCG). The theoretical concerns are that in combination the cumulative mercury dose could exceed recommended safety levels.

The US and Europe regulatory bodies have recommended that it is phased out. The World Health Organization has endorsed this, as well as stressing that if thiomersal-free vaccines are not available, vaccination programmes should not be compromised (i.e. children should still be vaccinated).

Three diphtheria, tetanus and pertussis vaccinations with or without Hib would give a maximum cumulative dose of 75 μg ethylmercury – less than half of the 187 μg dose that causes concern. This is cleared quickly and is not known to be cumulative.

A thiomersal and vaccine fact sheet can be found online at (www.dh.gov.uk).

Human papillomavirus vaccine

Around 95% of all cervical cancer is attributed to human papillomavirus (HPV) and development of a vaccine that prevents this is one of the most exciting developments in modern medicine. The Joint Committee for Vaccination and Immunisation has now recommended vaccinating girls aged 11–12 years. It is hoped that this will be started in the near future; similarly, there is discussion about rolling out the vaccine coverage to boys as well.

Gardasil (quadrivalent HPV (types 6, 11, 16 and 18) recombinant vaccine) has been found to prevent 100% of cases of high-grade pre-cancerous lesions as well as non-invasive cancers (CIN II and III or adenocarcinoma in situ) associated with HPV 16 and 18. This was seen after a 2-year follow-up following a three-dose regime. Cervarix (bivalent: HPV types 16 and 18) is also licensed in the United Kingdom.

The need for booster vaccines, administering the vaccine in women already infected with HPV, changes to the cervical screening programme, the therapeutic role of vaccines and cost-effectiveness (as well as whether men should be included in the vaccination programme) are all areas that will need clarification.

Screening

www.nsc.nhs.uk/ch_screen/child_ind.htm

It is important to make parents aware that screening tests are just that: screening tests. If they have any worries or concerns they need to seek advice from their GP or health visitor.

Developmental dysplasia of the hip

This is a spectrum of conditions where the head of the femur is partly or completely displaced from the acetabulum. If this is not treated it can lead to a significantly abnormal gait and to disability. Risk factors include family history, breech presentation, oligohydramnios, postural deformities of the feet, firstborn, caesarean delivery and female. It affects 1%–3% of newborns (*BMJ* 2009; 339: 1242).

Early detection and conservative treatment are often successful, avoiding the need for surgery. Routine screening with Ortolani's test and Barlow's manoeuvre (valid up to 3 months of age) misses up to 70% of cases. This is a falsely reassuring screening test for both parents and doctors. Some European countries now have a universal ultrasound screening programme. The United Kingdom targets babies with risk factors or with a positive Ortolani or Barlow result, aiming for an ultrasound scan by 8 weeks. A later sign would include asymmetrical leg creases.

Ultrasonography in screening for developmental dysplasia of the hip in newborns: systematic review

BMJ 2005; 330(7505): 1413

A total of 188 studies were selected for full assessment, of which 10 met the inclusion criteria for analysis. They made three important findings. First, there is insufficient evidence for the use of ultrasound as a screening tool. Second, ultrasound is likely to increase treatment rates, possibly unnecessarily. Third, the duration of intervention was likely to be lowered by ultrasound screening.

Screening for hearing defects

www.hearing.screening.nhs.uk/

- Around 840 children are born with permanent hearing impairment each year. This equates to around two babies in every 1000 born.
- Around 50% were previously not diagnosed until they were 18 months old.
- Around 25% were previously not diagnosed until they were 3 years old (i.e. the distraction test did not pick up some children early enough).

Permanent hearing impairment impacts on communication skills, educational attainment and quality of life. If there is intervention by 6 months the outcome for all of the above as well as the cost to society is improved.

The NHS Newborn Hearing Screening Programme screens all babies within 48 hours of birth. This is called otoacoustic emissions testing.

***Feverish Illness in Children*, NICE (May 2007)**
www.nice.org.uk/nicemedia/pdf/CG47NICEGuideline.pdf
Assessment and initial management of feverish illness in children younger than 5 years: summary of NICE guidance
***BMJ* 2007; 334(7604): 1163–4**
This problem-focused guidance was published for use in the assessment and initial management for children under 5 years of age with a feverish illness. There are no targets, just advice based on evidence and consensus opinions. It recommends that the guidelines are followed until a diagnosis is made; at that point the child should be treated according to guidelines for that condition.

Assessing the severity of fever uses a traffic light system taking into account colour, respiratory symptoms, hydration and miscellaneous factors. It also highlights that even if a child is apyrexial when you see them, it is important to take all reports of fever seriously.

Measure and record	Assess for signs of dehydration
Temperature	Prolonged capillary refill time
Heart rate	Abnormal skin turgor
Respiratory rate	Abnormal respiratory pattern
Capillary refill time	Weak pulse
	Cool extremities

The findings outlined in the table should be recorded.

The guidelines look at criteria for admission, antipyretic interventions and care at home, including advice about when to seek further advice.

Paracetamol and ibuprofen for the treatment of fever in children: the PITCH randomised controlled trial
***Health Technol Assess* 2009; 13(27): 1–163**
This trial looked at the clinical and cost-effectiveness of paracetamol plus ibuprofen as compared with paracetamol or ibuprofen alone.

For additional time without fever in the first 24 hours, combination treatment was found to be superior to individual treatment (4.4 hours less than with paracetamol alone and 2.5 hours less than with ibuprofen alone), although there was no difference in fever-related symptoms. It concluded that ibuprofen (unless contraindicated) should be used first.

Autistic spectrum disorders

Autistic spectrum disorders (a group of development disorders that include autism, Asperger's syndrome and atypical autism) are lifelong developmental disabilities affecting social and communication skills with varying degrees of severity on a somatic pragmatic scale. Onset is usually by the age of 3 years, but it can go undiagnosed. Early diagnosis enables behavioural therapy, facilitated communication and educational techniques to be introduced, hopefully improving long-term outcome.

The Scottish Intercollegiate Guidelines Network, following the National Autism

Plan for Children in England and Wales, produced evidence-based guidelines for autistic spectrum disorders in 2007. The National Institute for Health and Clinical Excellence published guidelines in September 2011 (www.nice.org.uk/nicemedia/live/13572/56431/56431.pdf) looking at recognition, assessment, diagnosis and management.

Early identification of autism by the CHecklist for Autism in Toddlers (CHAT)

J R Soc Med 2000; 93(10): 521–5

The Checklist for Autism in Toddlers is a screening tool that can be used at the 18-month check by GPs or health visitors.

The Checklist for Autism in Toddlers is frequently used; these guidelines consider various warning signs in both preschool and school-age children. Communication and social impairments are most easily recognisable but impairment in interest with lack of flexibility and recognition of other odd behaviour are also important in coming to a diagnosis.

SECTION A

1	Does your child enjoy being swung, bounced on your knee and so forth?	Yes/No
2	Does your child take an interest in other children?	Yes/No
3	Does your child like climbing on things, e.g. stairs?	Yes/No
4	Does your child enjoy playing peek-a-boo/hide-and-seek?	Yes/No
5	**Does your child ever pretend, for example, to make a cup of tea using a toy cup and teapot, or pretend other things?**	**Yes/No**
6	Does your child ever use his/her index finger to point to ASK for something?	Yes/No
7	**Does your child ever use his/her finger to point to indicate interest in something?**	**Yes/No**
8	Can your child play properly with small toys, e.g. bricks, cars, without just mouthing or fiddling with them?	Yes/No
9	Does your child ever bring objects over to show you something?	Yes/No

SECTION B

1	During the appointment has the child made eye contact with you?	Yes/No
2	**Get child's attention and then point across the room at an interesting object and say 'Oh Look! There's a – name the toy'. Does the child look across and see what you are pointing at?**	**Yes/No**
3	**Get the child's attention, then give the child a toy cup and teapot and say, 'Can you make a cup of tea?' Does the child pretend to make or drink the tea?**	**Yes/No**
4	**Say to the child, 'Where is the light?' Does the child point?**	**Yes/No**
5	Can the child build a tower of bricks? (If so, how many?)	Yes/No

If the items in bold are absent at 18 months then the child is at high risk for a social communication disorder. If no is the response to all five items then the child is at high risk.

A 12-point autism checklist is not dissimilar to this questionnaire but it is based on a scoring system.

The National Autistic Society (www.autism.org.uk) is a good source of information for both families and professionals.

Sudden infant death syndrome

The confidential enquiry into maternal and child health has an interim report dated October 2007 available to view online, but it is in the process of being reassigned to a different investigating body.

Risk factors in the infant include:

- low birthweight
- prematurity
- sex (60% of cases are boys)
- multiple births
- high birth order (parity).

Risk factors in parents for sudden infant death of their child include:

- young maternal age
- unmarried mothers
- maternal smoking in pregnancy
- smoking after birth – this increases the risk by fivefold, and is the biggest risk.

Environmental risk factors include:

- low socio-economic class
- sleeping prone (the Back to Sleep campaign was launched in 1994)
- winter
- overheating
- used cot mattresses (this is being considered in more detail)
- recent data is suggesting that babies sleeping with a dummy have a reduced risk of cot death.

Care of the Next Infant and the Foundation for the Study of Infant Deaths have been established to support parents. They provide counselling and apnoea alarms as well as many other resources.

Uncertainty in classification of repeat sudden unexpected infant deaths in Care of the Next Infant programme

BMJ 2007; 335(7611): 129–31

It is rare for a family to experience sudden infant death, and even more so to experience two such deaths. It summarised that a recent study of families with two sudden infant deaths concluded that 13% of second deaths were homicide. Review of published material shows this to be a minimum estimate, as the cause of many second deaths could not be ascertained (compare with screening for MCADD).

Child protection

Maltreatment in children is not uncommon, with over half a million referrals being made to social services. It is a sensitive subject and if you are wrong, despite having a child's best interest at heart, it can leave a family scarred and distrustful of health and social services.

In 2007 there were 27 900 children under a Child Protection Plan; these children would be on a child protection register because they were at risk of ongoing abuse. This abuse could be physical, sexual (this includes contact and non-contact), neglect and emotional ill-treatment.

Following the Victoria Climbié trial (the 8-year-old child murdered by her guardians in 2000) there have been renewed efforts to keep us all informed on child protection issues, and *Working to Safeguard Children* was published in 2006. The General Medical Council guidance *0–18 Years: guidance for doctors on child protection* followed this in 2007, and then in 2008 the National Society for the Prevention of Cruelty to Children produced a helpful toolkit with the Royal College of General Practitioners (www.rcgp.org.uk/clinical_and_research/safeguarding_children_tookit.aspx). Finally, NICE published *When to Suspect Child Maltreatment* and the British Medical Association published their toolkit.

As GPs we are not expected to be trained in forensics, but we should remain vigilant, keep good records, be prepared to set investigations in motion through the child protection agency and maintain close contact with other health professionals and the family. This is often tricky in that, although the welfare of the child must be placed above all other considerations, usually all members of the family are under our care and often at the start of an investigative process you may be reporting only suspicions. Since this there has been the high profile case of Baby P (Peter Connelly), the 17-month-old baby.

Care of children and young people: questions

1 MCADD: which of the following statements is correct?
   a. MCADD is treatable.
   b. MCADD is untreatable.
2 Developmental dysplasia of the hip: which of the following is not a risk factor of developmental dysplasia of the hip?
   a. Positive family history.
   b. Polyhydraminos.
   c. Calcaneovalgus deformity of the feet (even if unilateral).
   d. Breech presentation.
   e. Firstborn child.
3 Neonatal jaundice: which of the following would be considered a risk factor for developing significant hyperbillirubinaemia?
   a. Visible jaundice day 6–7.
   b. Gestational age at delivery term +10 days.

c. A breastfed baby who has formula top-ups.
d. A bottle-fed baby.
e. A previous sibling with neonatal jaundice.

4 Cardiac murmurs in children: which of the following would be an indication that a murmur needed referral for further investigation as it may be more than innocent?
a. A murmur noticed in a child with a temperature of 38.6°C.
b. A parasternal vibratory ejection systolic murmur.
c. A venous hum that can be abolished by head movement.
d. A soft ejection murmur heard at the left upper sternal border.
e. A thrill over the suprasternal notch.

5 pGALS (paediatric Gait, Arms, Legs, Spine): which of the following would not be considered an appropriate time to do a pGALS assessment on a child?
a. A child with joint pain.
b. A child with a fractured toe, having jumped off a sofa.
c. A child with a limp.
d. A clumsy child in the absence of neurological pathology.
e. A child with regression of their motor milestones.

6 Motor development: at what age would you expect a child to be able to run, although relatively stiffly?
a. 8 months.
b. 12 months.
c. 16 months.
d. 18 months.
e. 20 months.

7 In a 6-year-old boy, which of the following is the most likely cause of a new limp if constitutionally well?
a. Juvenile chronic arthritis.
b. Perthes's disease.
c. Developmental dysplasia of the hip.
d. Slipped upper epiphysis.
e. Septic arthritis.

For questions 8–10, which of the following could be considered safe antipyretic interventions in a feverish child? Answer each question as true or false.

8 Having a cold bath.
9 Antipyretic drugs such as paracetamol or ibuprofen.
10 Tepid sponging.

Care of children and young people: answers

1 **a** From 2009, screening for MCADD was offered to babies in the England. This is a rare, life-threatening, autosomal recessive condition making it difficult for the body to change fat into energy. It is a known cause of sudden infant death and it is treatable.

2 **b** Oligohydramnios is a risk factor. Options (a), (c) and (d) are major risk factors

alongside birthweight of >5 kg. Minor risk factors would include swaddling, prematurity and oligohydramnios.

3 e Risk factors include jaundice in the first 24 hours of life, gestational age of <38 weeks, a baby who is only breastfed and where there has been a previous sibling with jaundice. This question is taken from the *BMJ* summary of the NICE guidance ('Neonatal jaundice: summary of NICE guidance' (*BMJ* 2010; 340: c2409)).

4 e All the other options are features of a usually innocent murmur. Indications that a murmur is probably not innocent are cyanosis or clubbing, abnormal breathing, failure to thrive, absent femoral pulses (or diminished), hepatomegaly, thrill over prechordium or suprasternal notch, an ejection click, radiation through to the back, a diastolic murmur or abnormal heart sounds. This question was taken from the British Heart Foundation's *FactFile: cardiac murmurs in children* (February 2011).

5 b This is not uncommon and it is unlikely to be the cause of abuse (which would suggest you needed to do a pGALS examination. pGALS is a simple screening approach to the musculoskeletal examination. For this question I used the review in the Reports on the Rheumatic Diseases Series, *Hands On: practical advice on management of rheumatic disease* (Number 15, June 2008).

6 c

7 b In juvenile arthritis and septic arthritis you would expect the child to be unwell. Developmental dysplasia of the hip would be a longer history. Perthes's happens in children aged 4–8 years and it is a type of avascular necrosis of the femoral head. A slipped upper epiphyses happens in older children. A new limp needs urgent admission to either paediatrics or orthopaedics for X-ray/MRI/bloods.

8 False This can vasoconstrict and cause core temperature to shoot up, hence increasing the risk of fits.

9 True Recommendation is to alternate dosing.

10 False These questions are taken from the NICE guidance on management of fever in children.

Statement 9

Care of older adults

Older people

National Service Framework for Older People

www.dh.gov.uk

Although this was published in March 2001 it remains in the third edition because it is important and ageism is a political hot potato. It is an action plan to improve health and social services for older people wherever they live. It focuses on the following:

- rooting out age discrimination which is seen to happen because of society, education and resources
- patient-centred care
- promoting older people's health and independence/an active life
- management of specific clinical conditions, with timely access to specialist care.

There are eight standards:

1. Root out age discrimination, providing care on the basis of clinical need alone.
2. Person-centred care, treating patients as individuals. Planning for a single assessment process with integrated provision of services, and GPs will be mainly involved in the contact assessment.
3. Intermediate care – to enable early hospital discharge and to prevent premature or unnecessary admission to long-term residential care.
4. General hospital care – delivered through appropriate specialist care, by staff with the skills to meet their needs.
5. Stroke – the NHS will take action to prevent strokes (primary and secondary). It will provide treatment by specialist stroke services with a multidisciplinary programme of secondary prevention and rehabilitation.
6. Falls – the NHS and councils will take action to prevent falls and reduce resultant fractures or other injuries. Advice will be provided through specialised falls services.
7. Mental health in older people – there will be access to integrated mental health services (for patients and carers).
8. Promotion of health and active life in older age.

As well as these eight standards, there are five other major projects underway to drive up quality, availability and consistency of services.

1. Changes in long-term care funding including availability of NHS nursing care.
2. Expansion of intermediate care (and community equipment) services.

3 Establishment of Care Direct to provide comprehensive information and ease of access to health, housing, social care and social security.
4 Various initiatives (retirement health check, flu immunisations) to help older people stay healthy.
5 Use of Section 31 of the Health Act 1999 to promote joint working between NHS and social services.

The NHS Modernisation Board and the Older People's Taskforce will oversee progress. The Department of Health will publish the *Information Strategy for Older People*, which is due out later this year and will describe how GPs will be supported in achieving this.

Falls

- Falls are the leading cause of accidental death in people aged >75; treatment of fractures alone cost the NHS £1.7 billion per year (Department of Health, 2003).
- Every year 33%–50% of people >65 suffer a fall (the percentage increases with age) of whom 20% will need medical help and 10% will have sustained a fracture.
- The current blood pressure targets seem to be causing an increase in falls due to postural hypotension and medication.

Falls: the assessment and prevention of falls in older people

www.nice.org.uk/nicemedia/pdf/CG021NICEguideline.pdf

One of the most important things to understand in this document, at this stage, is how you would offer a multifactoral assessment of falls by assessing:

- fall history – gait, balance, mobility and muscle weakness
- osteoporosis risk
- visual and cognitive impairment
- urinary incontinence
- home hazards, including footwear and floor rugs
- cardiovascular examination and medication review.

Functional assessment in older people

BMJ 2011; 343: d4681

This recent article provides a good review of the evidence for strategies promoting health and function. It concludes that it is necessary to take PULSE into account:

P: Physical condition
U: Upper limb function
L: Lower limb function
S: Sensory
E: Environment.

Most health benefits can be gained from regular physical activity of moderate intensity. Promoting health and fitness throughout life could achieve substantial gains.

Health professionals should consider:

- activities of daily living

- comprehensive geriatric assessment
- disability
- frailty
- functional ability.

Falls assessments

There are a number of reasons why clinicians aren't doing this:

- Patients don't tell us they've fallen/slipped.
- Don't know how to do it.
- Seeing people at surgery, not home.
- Forget or run out of time.

Consider the following:

- Do they know why they fell/was there LOC?
- Are there environmental elements? If so, consider occupational therapy.
- Was the patient able to get up? If not, consider physiotherapy.
- Are the falls recurrent or unexplained? Consider specialist falls referral.
- Don't forget to review medications, blood pressure, eyesight and footwear.

Dementia

Dementia is a chronic deterioration of intellect and personality.

- Around 5% of people over 65 years of age have some form of dementia.
- Around 20% of people over 80 years of age have some form of dementia.
- 60% of cases of dementia are thought to be an Alzheimer's type, accounting for 340 000 cases in the United Kingdom.
- One in seven elderly people with dementia are in residential care.
- It is important to diagnose dementia early and to identify the type of dementia to improve care and reduce morbidity for our patients and their carers.

The Mental Health Foundation has published a report, *Tell Me the Truth*, which reveals that most people who develop dementia are not usually told what is wrong with them. It is this information that, although initially difficult to accept, helps patients to understand the changes in themselves and helps them to adapt.

The Alzheimer's Society website is comprehensive, informative and useful for professionals, patients and families (www.alzheimers.org.uk).

Dementia – National Institute for Health and Clinical Excellence and Social Care Institute for Excellence (November 2006)

www.nice.org.uk/nicemedia/pdf/CG042NICEGuideline.pdf

These guidelines consider Alzheimer's disease, dementia with Lewy bodies, frontotemporal dementia, vascular dementia and mixed dementias. The guidelines go through diagnosis, assessment, principles of care (with a view to promoting independence) treatments, end-of-life challenges and support for carers.

Risk factors and prevention

Primary prevention

General population screening is not recommended and preventive treatments such as statins, hormone replacement therapy, vitamin E and non-steroidal inflammatory drugs are not advised. In rare cases it is inherited via the AD gene, and there are also connections to the Apo-E gene but no useful diagnostic or prognostic test is yet available. The National Institute for Health and Clinical Excellence (NICE) recommends offering referral for genetic counselling of familial cases of dementia such as autosomal dominant Alzheimer's disease or frontotemporal dementia, cerebral autosomal dominant arteriopathy with subcortical infarcts and Huntington's disease.

Secondary prevention

As arteriovascular risk factors are also risk factors for dementia it is recommended that these are targeted. Smoking, alcohol excess, obesity, hypertension and raised cholesterol levels would all be important.

Diagnosis and assessment

The clinical cognitive assessments recommended are the Mini-Mental State Examination (MMSE), General Practitioner Assessment of Cognition, six-item Cognitive Impairment and the 7-minute screen.

Blood tests would routinely include biochemistry, haematology, thyroid function tests as well as vitamin B_{12} and folate levels.

If imaging were required this would be requested through the specialist service, and referral at an early stage is recommended (this is also recommended in the National Service Framework for Older People).

A protein called clusterin is being looked at as it has been found to be raised in patients with Alzheimer's; it may be that this could indicate severity of disease although as yet doesn't have a place in clinical practice.

Treatment of dementia

Non-pharmacological

In the initial stages this is geared towards support for patients and their families.

Pharmacological

Three cholinesterase inhibitors have been licensed in the United Kingdom for mild to moderate Alzheimer's disease: donepezil, rivastigmine and galantamine. It is recommended that these are started if the MMSE is 10–20/30 (i.e. for moderate dementia). Although the drugs costs can amount to around £1000/year it is thought the costs may ultimately be offset by delaying the need for residential care. (Of interest, in the initial draft of the guidance it was recommended that these treatments should no longer be available on the NHS because of lack of effectiveness. This met with a great deal of resistance and the final guidance was revised).

The specialist team starting care should review the effects of the medication.

Interventions for non-cognitive symptoms and behaviour

Non-pharmacological

Following early assessment to identify potential causes, holistic therapies such as aromatherapy, massage and animal-assisted therapies are suggested.

Pharmacological

It is suggested that antipsychotics (contraindicated in dementia with Lewy bodies, and be aware of the increased risk of cardiovascular events) and acetylcholinesterase inhibitors are only used if there is severe distress or risk of harm to the patient or others.

Palliative and end-of-life care in dementia

Information on end-of-life care is available on the National End of Life Care Programme website (www.endoflifecareforadults.nhs.uk). It is recommended that this approach is adopted from diagnosis until death to enable patients to die with dignity.

Support for carers

Assessments of carers should seek to identify psychological distress and impact on the carer. Care plans and support as well as psychological therapy should be offered.

Effectiveness of acetylcholinesterase inhibitors: diagnosis and severity as predictors of response in routine practice

Int J Geriatr Psychiatry 2006; 21(8): 755–60

This Oxfordshire-based 4-year study looked at the monitoring of cholinesterase inhibitor prescribing and an MMSE improvement of 2 or more points was defined as a 'cognitive response'. Medication was prescribed for 1322 patients and outcome data were available on 1250. Subsequently, 939 patients were reassessed after a mean of 120 days. The finding that cognitive, but not clinical, response was more likely in those with moderate dementia than in those with mild dementia accords with the findings from randomised studies in the January 2006 revision of the NICE *Appraisal Consultation* document.

Dementia: still muddling along?

Br J Gen Pract 2007; 57(541): 606–7

Professors Lliffe and Manthorpe wrote an insightful article about the industry that is guideline production and then focused on the reasons why we should use these guidelines. The first reason is that incidence is increasing; the estimated annual cost of dementia in the United Kingdom (1998) was £5.5 billion. The second reason is that dementia is now included in the Quality and Outcomes Framework. The third reason is that public expectations about dementia, and treatments, are changing so we may have more people presenting early. The fourth, because when it comes to implementing new treatments and moving medicine forward, we are a fundamental part of the NHS.

The same authors also wrote a review article for *GP Clinical* in July 2007, bringing attention to the PAID acronym for the management of problems related to dementia:

P: Physical problems, like pain, may trigger behavioural change.
A: Activities of others are annoying or frightening for the patient.
I: Intrinsic features of dementia are appearing, like wandering.
D: Depression underlies the behaviour change, or there are delusions/psychotic symptoms.

Miscellaneous factors and Alzheimer's disease

Other treatments for Alzheimer's disease

Selegiline and vitamin E

Treatment with either was found to slow progression of the disease. A Cochrane review in 2000 found selegiline was better than placebo at improving cognitive function, behavioural disturbance and mood.

Vitamin C and vitamin E for Alzheimer's disease

Ann Parmacother 2005; Oct 14

This article concluded that vitamin C and E supplements do not have the supporting evidence to be recommended for use in Alzheimer's disease.

Ginkgo biloba (40 mg three times daily)

One systematic review (of eight randomised trials) reported that ginkgo biloba improved cognitive function and was well tolerated in patients with Alzheimer's disease (*Clin Drug Invest* 1999; 17: 301–8). A more recent study (*JAMA* 2008; 300: 2253–62) has found that it made no great difference.

Reality orientation

This involves presenting information designed to reorientate a person in time, place and person. It may be a noticeboard giving the day, date and time or a member of staff reorienting patients at each contact.

Clinical evidence found one systematic review of small randomised controlled trials that showed improvement in cognitive function and behaviour compared with no treatment.

Vaccine

The bapineuzumab vaccination is a monoclonal antibody that has been shown to reduce the build-up of beta-amyloid plaques. This is still in development and has no clinical application at present.

None of the treatments listed in this section as other treatments for Alzheimer's disease are recommended by NICE.

Leisure-time physical activity at midlife and the risk of dementia and Alzheimer's disease

Lancet 2005; 4(11): 705–11

This was a study of 1239 people aged 65–79 years of age. The study found that exercising at least twice a week was associated with a 50% lower relative risk of dementia and 60% lower risk of Alzheimer's disease. This was especially so (once adjusted for other factors) in carriers of the APOE gene.

Diet

This is a difficult topic, as good nutrition is interlinked with so many other lifestyle issues and attitudes. Most recently the Italian paper 'Lifestyle-related factors in predementia and dementia syndromes' looked at observational studies. It is hard not to think that a healthy diet is good for you; it certainly wouldn't be harmful, and the social interaction of meal times similarly so.

Lifestyle-related factors in predementia and dementia syndromes

Expert Rev Neurother 2008; 8(1): 133–58

In older subjects, healthy diets, antioxidant supplements, the prevention of nutritional deficiencies, and moderate physical activity could be considered the first line of defence against the development and progression of predementia and dementia syndromes. However, in most cases, these were only observational studies, and results are awaited from large multicentre randomised clinical trials.

Driving and dementia

www.dft.gov.uk/dvla/medical/ataglance.aspx

Having dementia doesn't mean that a patient is unsafe to drive; the loss of this ability affects independence, especially in rural parts of the country. It is not our role to formally assess fitness to drive – that is the responsibility of the Driver and Vehicle Licensing Agency (DVLA) and patients can often continue to drive subject to a yearly review. However, we do have to do the following:

- Inform the patient that they must contact the DVLA and their insurance company.
- If there is consent complete the medical report requested by the DVLA.
- Consider whether a patient is fit to drive while awaiting assessment.
- Inform the DVLA if we consider there is a danger to themselves or others.

How to assess capacity to make a will

BMJ 2007; 335(7811): 155–7

This is written with legal input because due to an increasing number of wills that are contested after a testator's death solicitors are asking doctors to certify testamentary capacity in certain cases (capacity for making a will). There is a useful summary box on tests for capacity.

What the testator must be capable of understanding:

- the nature and effect of making a will
- the extent of his/her estate

- the claims of those who might expect to benefit from the will (both those who have been included and excluded).

What the testator should not have:
- a mental illness that influences the testator to make bequests that he/she would otherwise not have made.

Our role as doctors is about satisfying ourselves of the testator's capacity and understanding, and recording these findings (known as the 'golden rule'). The solicitor will detail the legal tests, we assess (writing answers verbatim) and then check the extent of the estate and previous wills with the solicitors.

Care of older adults: questions

1 Dementia: chose the single most appropriate answer for a patient with early dementia.
   a. Donepezil would be the best pharmacological option to reduce cognitive decline.
   b. Rivastigmine would be the best pharmacological option to reduce cognitive decline.
   c. Galantamine would be the best pharmacological option to reduce cognitive decline.
   d. Memantine would be the best pharmacological option to reduce cognitive decline.
   e. The focus should not involve pharmacological treatments.
2 With regard to behavioural problems in severe dementia, chose the best answer from the following.
   a. Consider referral to secondary care for memantine.
   b. Haloperidol regularly would be in everyone's best interest.
   c. Risperidone would be the best medication to use on a regular basis.
   d. Zopiclone would be helpful to aid night-time rest.
   e. A group directive for nursing home staff to be able to administer intramuscular midazolam would be the most helpful.
3 When using the six-item cognitive impairment test for assessment of dementia, which of the following is correct?
   a. A score of 5/28 would be indicative of severe dementia.
   b. A patient is allowed to make two errors when counting backwards from 20 without being penalised.
   c. A patient is allowed one error when saying the months of the year in reverse order without being penalised.
   d. The memory recall test is based on remembering an address phrase.
   e. A patient can have 10 points deducted for incorrect recall on the memory test.

For questions 4–6 regarding xerostomia, determine whether each statement is true or false.

4 Patients can present with a burning mouth.

5 Extractable nuclear antigen antibodies are useful blood tests.

6 Pilocarpine should be avoided, as it can make symptoms worse.

7 Which of the following activities would be considered abnormal in the 'get up and go test'?

a. Being unable to walk heel to toe for ≥3 metres.
b. Turning en bloc.
c. Being unable to stand still with their eyes closed.
d. Being unable to touch their nose.
e. Being unable to lie flat without feeling light-headed/dizzy.

8 Which of the following is the correct answer regarding dabigatran for anticoagulation?

a. Dabigatran should be monitored using INR on a regular basis.
b. Dabigatran is currently licensed as an alternative anti-thrombotic for prevention of venous thromboembolism in joint replacement.
c. Dabigatran has no risk of haemorrhage.
d. Dabigatran is known to be more effective than warfarin in preventing stroke in a patient with atrial fibrillation.
e. If used post-DVT (first occurrence) it is advisable to use as lifelong prophylaxsis.

Care of older adults: answers

1 e The focus should not be pharmacological but defining a positive strategy approach.

Memantine is an N-methyl-D-aspartate receptor antagonist that is thought to reduce oxidative stress. It is used for moderate to severe Alzheimer's disease for agitation or aggression and prescribed by secondary care. Donepezil, rivastigmine and galantamine are used in moderate dementia with shared care arrangements.

2 a Antipsychotics such as haloperidol and risperidone increase the risk of stroke and patients are more likely to die if these types of medication are used (although there genuinely may not be a better alternative) (*MeRec* Extra Issue 39 'Antipsychotics increase mortality in elderly patients with dementia'). Sleeping tablets potentially increase the risk of falls and fracture, and while the group directive sounds ideal this isn't quite the done thing in primary care!

3 d Health professionals are allowed to use Six-Item Cognitive Impairment Test freely. A score of 0–7/28 is regarded as normal, and >8/28 is significant (this cut-off having a 90% specificity and 100% sensitivity).

Six-Item Cognitive Impairment Test (6CIT) (the Kingshill version, 2000)		
1 What year is it?	Correct	0 points
	Incorrect	4 points
2 What month is it?	Correct	0 points
	Incorrect	3 points
3 Give the patient an address phrase with five components to remember (e.g. John, Smith, 42, High Street, Bedford)		
4 About what time is it (within 1 hour)?	Correct	0 points
	Incorrect	3 points
5 Count backwards from 20 to one	Correct	0 points
	One error	2 points
	More than one error	4 points
6 Recite the months of the year in reverse	Correct	0 points
	One error	2 points
	More than one error	4 points
7 Repeat the address phrase	Correct	0 points
	One error	2 points
	Two errors	4 points
	Three errors	6 points
	Four errors	8 points
	All wrong	10 points
	6CIT score	/28

4 True

5 True These are useful for identifying Sjögren's syndrome.

6 False It is used for treatment alongside replacement saliva, sips of water and so forth. It works parasympathetically to increase production of saliva.

7 b Although all of the above symptoms may point to cerebellar, ENT or cervical spondylosis-type problems, only turning en bloc would be considered abnormal in the specifics of the test. For functional assessment in older people see *BMJ* 2011; 343: 469–73. When the patient is in their normal footwear and using their customary walking aid, ask the patient to:

- rise independently from an armless chair, or with arms folded
- stand still
- then walk 3 m (10 feet)
- turn 180°
- return to chair
- sit down.

Abnormalities that may be seen include unsteadiness, need for external support, apraxia (short steps, shuffling and en bloc turning), lack of arm swinging, hesitancy, antalgic gait).

8 b A licence for stroke prevention is expected soon. One of the positives of this drug is that no monitoring is needed (RE-LY trial, *Lancet* 2010; 376: 975–83).

Statement 10.1

Women's health

Breast cancer

Breast cancer accounted for 27% of all female cancers in 1995. It is the most common female cancer and it is the cause of 18% of all female deaths.

- Around 5% of all breast cancers are linked to specific single-gene defects.
- Between 50% and 80% of breast cancers are due to BRCA (breast cancer genes) 1 or 2.
- BRCA 1 and 2 are linked with colon cancer and possibly prostate cancer.
- Women with dense breasts on mammography are more likely to develop breast cancer (*N Engl J Med* 2007; 356: 227–36).

See Statement 5 for breast, cervical and ovarian cancer screening information.

Cervical cancer

www.cancerresearchuk.org

- The incidence of cervical cancer in the UK is 9.6 per 100 000.
- The mortality rate is 5 per 100 000.
- The incidence of disease peaks at 30–35 and 70–75 years of age.
- Around 95% of cervical cancers are squamous cell, 5% are adenocarcinomas.
- Most important risk factor is human papillomavirus: at least 50% of sexually active people will get human papillomavirus (type 16, 18, 31, 33 or 35). Smoking and the age at first intercourse are also important factors.

Ovarian cancer

www.nice.org.uk/nicemedia/live/13464/54268/54268.pdf

- Ovarian cancer is the fourth most common female cancer in the UK.
- The incidence in the UK is 20 per 100 000 (and it appears to be increasing).
- Each year there are 6900 new cases.
- Women with BRCA 1 gene have 50% lifetime risk and those with BRCA 2 have a 30% lifetime risk (the same risk as if two first-degree relatives have ovarian cancer).

Menopause

Herein lies a dilemma: is this a medical problem or a social problem? The answer in some cases is both. About 10%–20% of women have distressing menopausal symptoms, and as a GP your role is very much to help patients with health promotion (the calcium effect), empowerment and symptom management.

Managing the menopause – British Menopause Society Council Consensus Statement on hormone replacement therapy (10 June 2005)

This statement concludes that results from recent papers have thus far given no reason to make any changes in current clinical practice. The following is a brief summary of the statement.

Benefits

- **Vasomotor symptoms** – there is good evidence from randomised controlled trials (RCTs) with improvement usually noted within 4 weeks.
- **Urogenital symptoms and sexuality symptoms** – respond well to oestrogens (topically or systemically), long-term treatment is often needed.
- **Osteoporosis** – there is evidence from RCTs (including the Women's Health Initiative (WHI) and the Million Women Study) that hormone replacement therapy (HRT) reduces hip as well as other osteoporotic fractures. It is not advised that HRT be used as first-line treatment for prevention of osteoporosis. Benefit wears off rapidly after cessation of use.
- **Colorectal cancer** – results from the oestrogen progestogen arm (WHI) only shows that HRT reduces the risk of colorectal cancer, it is not advised that HRT be used for prevention.

Risks

- **Breast cancer** – mammographic density is increased in about 25% of women.
  - HRT appears to confer a similar degree of risk as that associated with a late natural menopause (2.3% compared with 2.8% per year, respectively). The lifetime risk is significantly increased with current long-term use when started over 50 years (relative risk (RR), 1.35; 95% confidence interval (CI) 1.2–1.49). Such effect is not seen in women who start HRT for a premature menopause, indicating that it is the duration of lifetime hormone exposure that is relevant.
  - Progesterone addition increases the risk of breast cancer and has to be balanced against the fact that if not used the risk of endometrial cancer will increase.
  - Breast cancer risk falls after cessation of use, being no greater than if never been exposed by 5 years.
- **Endometrial cancer** – unopposed oestrogen increases endometrial cancer; sequential progesterone does not eliminate this risk.
- **Venous thromboembolism** – HRT increases the risk twofold, the highest risk being in the first year of use. Absolute risk is small, at 1.7 per 1000 in women over 50 years of age.
- **Gallbladder disease** – HRT increases the risk (confirmed in WHI).

Uncertainties

- **Cardiovascular disease** – the role of HRT for primary and secondary prevention remains uncertain. WHI showed a transient increase in coronary heart disease, absolute risk at 50–59 years was 5, and at 60–69 years was 1.

- **Dementia and cognition** – while oestrogen may delay or reduce the risk of Alzheimer's, it does not seem to improve established disease.
- **Ovarian cancer** – with oestrogen only after more than 10 years of use there seems to be an increase in the risk; in continuous combined therapy this does not seem to be the case.
- **Quality of life** – difficult to evaluate, there is no conclusion as yet.

Hormone replacement therapy

HRT is a collective term to encompass a variety of sex steroids, oestrogens and progesterones given in various forms. Treatment with HRT is a curious ethical problem and is always topical.

Menopause in the UK is around 51 years of age and our current target population of women who should be given the opportunity to make an informed decision on whether to take HRT or not includes the following:

- Women with menopausal symptoms affecting quality of life (usually short-term use).
- Women who have had a premature menopause (under the age of 45 years).
- Women who have had a surgical menopause (hysterectomy and oophorectomy) under 40 years of age. Use of HRT in this group is usually until the age of 52.

Managing the menopause

BMJ 2007; 334(796): 736–41

Helen Roberts wrote this clinical review that, although it discussed most issues, provided detail using the type of simple table I find most helpful when explaining risk to patients: a table of absolute risk. The table shows the number of extra women who would suffer an event if they took HRT for 1 year (aged 50–79). Where there is a negative number this means there is a risk reduction.

Difference in absolute event rates for hormone replacement therapies compared with placebo/10 000 women/year

Event	Oestrogen and progestogen versus placebo	Oestrogen only versus placebo
Breast disease	8	≤7
Heart disease	7	≤5
Pulmonary embolus	8	7
Stroke	8	12
Hip fracture	≤5	≤6
Colorectal cancer	≤6	1

Alternatives to HRT

For hot flushes

The research base for these products is limited, although undoubtedly some women get very real relief from these products. Some of these may contain oestrogenic properties and women need to be aware of the implications of this if they have a history of oestrogen-sensitive tumours.

- Phyto-oestrogens – chickpeas, lentils, soya products, red clover. There have been several small RCTs comparing, for example, soy flour to wheat flour and they have found no significant reduction in hot flushes.
- Black cohosh – a recent study in *Maturitas* (2005; 16: 134–46) found that it offered no significant benefit.
- Dong quai (*Angelica sinensis*).
- Evening primrose oil (*Oenothera biennis*).
- Ginkgo biloba.
- Agnus castus (also suggested for premenstrual tension).
- Clonidine (an alpha adrenoceptor agonist available on prescription).
- Selective serotonin reuptake inhibitors (SSRIs).
- Acupuncture (usually a small tack left in at the ankle that can be massaged).

For osteoporosis

HRT is no longer used as a first-line treatment for osteoporosis

- bisphosphonates (e.g. aledronate, etidronate, residronate)
- strontium ranelate.

For mood disturbances

- St John's wort
- antidepressant medication.

Heavy Menstrual Bleeding

www.nice.org.uk/nicemedia/live/11002/30403/30403.pdf

Heavy menstrual bleeding (menorrhagia) is a loss of >80 mL of blood per cycle (with either regular or irregular cycles). It is important to assess the condition properly for primary and secondary causes.

- Around 28% of women feel menstruation is excessive and 5% consult their GP.
- One in 20 women aged 30–49 years consult their GP each year with menorrhagia.
- One in five women will have a hysterectomy before the age of 60 years.
- GPs should focus on quality-of-life issues.

These National Institute for Health and Clinical Excellence (NICE) guidelines consider important factors in the history, necessary initial investigations (full blood count is the only routine test advocated). Further investigations should be directed, depending upon the history. For example, high vaginal and chlamydia swabs if there is a suspicion of infection; clotting studies should be considered if there is a significant family history. Ultrasound scan should be considered where there is a pelvic mass or the uterus is palpable abdominally, or where there is treatment failure.

Referral for endometrial biopsy should be considered:

- in women over 45 years
- where there is persistent intermenstrual bleeding
- where treatment has failed.

Premenstrual syndrome

www.rcog.org.uk/womens-health/clinical-guidance/management-premenstrual-syndrome-green-top-48

This is a distinct disorder (of emotional and physical symptoms) that affects 5% of women. It occurs in the luteal phase of the cycle, due to release of progesterone triggered by ovulation, and continuing until menstruation. There is no evidence of a specific hormonal imbalance. Meta-analyses have confirmed that treatment with progesterone products is no more effective than with placebo.

There is no diagnostic test. The best way to diagnose premenstrual syndrome (PMS) is by asking the patient to keep a two-cycle diary, which should show cyclical premenstrual deterioration with postmenstrual cure.

Premenstrual Dysphoric Disorder Symptoms **(DSM-IV, 1994)**

- depressed mood and interest
- marked anxiety, tension, difficulty concentrating
- marked affective lability, lethargy with either hypersomnia or insomnia
- marked anger, irritability or increased interpersonal conflicts.

This is an extreme part of the PMS spectrum. Patients can be treated in two broad ways: suppressing ovulation or changing ovulation status.

First-line treatment

- Exercise, cognitive behavioural therapy, vitamin B_6 (maximum of 100 mg, as there is a risk of neuropathy).
- Combined oral contraceptive pill has a variable response, newer pills (e.g. Yasmin) may have a better effect.
- Continuous or luteal phase (days 15–28) SSRIs.

Second-line treatment

- Oestrogen patches or implants – progestogenic endometrial protection (e.g. mirena) is needed as well as assessment of the endometrium at the outset of treatment so as not to risk falsely reassuring women that bleeding is normal when she may indeed have endometrial cancer.
- Higher-dose SSRIs (continuous or luteal phase).

Third-line treatment

- Gonadotrophin-releasing hormones (pharmacological menopause – time limited unless add-back HRT or tibolone is used).

Fourth-line treatment

- Oophrectomy and hysterectomy (rarely justified).

Other treatment options

- Agnus castus fruit extract: this fruit from the Chast tree has been a traditional remedy for PMS. The article 'Treatment for PMS with agnus castus fruit extract:

prospective, randomised, placebo-controlled trial' (*BMJ* 2001; 322(7279): 134–7) reports on 178 German women who were randomised for three cycles. Agnus castus fruit was found to be significantly more effective than placebo, and it appears to be safe.
- St John's wort: initial studies have shown a possible benefit. It does help depressive features, irrespective of other symptoms.
- Dietary changes such as increasing soy isoflavins and magnesium supplementation have been seen to give some improvement.
- Complementary therapies: acupuncture has been shown to help features of dysmenorrhoea. Homeopathy has been found in a pilot study of 20 women to have a 90% improvement compared with placebo. Qi therapy, aromatherapy, reflexology, photic stimulation and magnetic therapy all have some supporting anecdotal evidence.

Antenatal care

***Antenatal Care: routine care for healthy pregnant women* (2010)**
www.nice.org.uk/nicemedia/live/11947/40115/40115.pdf

The National Services Framework for Children, Young People and Maternity services was published in 2004 and is another useful tool as part of your revision. This looks at all areas of antenatal care (pre-conception, pre-birth, birth and postnatal community care).

Down's syndrome screening

Down's syndrome is the most common chromosomal abnormality at birth. The incidence is related to maternal age and the Down's syndrome screening programme is part of routine antenatal care.

In the 2010 guidance, NICE advises that pregnant women should be offered the following tests (which would provide detection rates above 75%):
- From 11 weeks 0 days to 13 weeks 6 days – the combined test (nuchal translucency, beta-human chorionic gonadotrophin (β-hCG) and pregnancy associated plasma protein A.
- From 15 to 20 weeks (in patients who book late) the triple or quadruple test (the quadruple test includes β-hCG, AFP, uE3, inhibin A).

Human immunodeficiency virus testing

- If a human immunodeficiency virus (HIV)-infected woman is unaware of her infection status her baby has around a one in four chance of being infected.
- Around 300 babies per year are born with HIV (mainly in London).
- Up to 80% of babies infected by vertical transmission could be prevented with the use of antivirals (antenatally, during delivery and for the infant), lower segment caesarean section and avoiding breastfeeding.

Women are now being offered HIV screening at booking to reduce the risk of transmission (national targets were adopted in 1999). Although screening is offered, there is not always counselling to fully explain the implications of not having the test or a positive test. HIV testing antenatally is becoming a more acceptable, routine test given the scope of treatment for the neonate and the mother.

Group B *Streptococcus*

www.rcog.org.uk/files/rcog-corp/uploaded-files/GT36SummaryGroupBStrep.pdf

The United States, Canada and Australia encourage routine screening for Group B *Streptococcus* antenatally (vaginal and rectal swabs at 35–37 weeks) as it is known to cause severe early onset of infection in neonates. The incidence of early onset Group B *Streptococcus* disease in the UK is 0.5 per 1000 births. Screening is not advocated in the UK, as it is still not clear whether screening may cause more problems that it would solve.

Pre-eclampsia

This condition complicates 2%–8% of pregnancies, and 6% of maternal deaths are due to eclampsia (as reported in the Confidential Enquiry into Maternal Deaths). There are many theories on reasons for development of pre-eclampsia: genetics (maternal, paternal and foetal), raised homocysteine levels in initially normotensive women and Leiden factor V gene are all being given consideration in current journals; as yet there are no useful screening tests. UK research is looking into a saliva test to detect raised urate levels and determine whether there is a clinical application.

The Royal College of Obstetricians and Gynaecologists Guideline 10(A) consider severe pre-eclampsia and eclampsia in more detail (www.rcog.org.uk/files/rcog-corp/GTG10a230611.pdf).

The Confidential Enquiry into Maternal Deaths 2003–05 reported 18 deaths from eclampsia, and detailed the incidence as 26.8 cases per 100 000 pregnancies (95% CI 23.3–30.7), which was a significant decrease from 1992.

Risk factors for pre-eclampsia at antenatal booking: systematic review of controlled studies

BMJ 2005; 330(7491): 565

The authors looked at studies published from 1966 to 2002 and found an increased risk in the following cohorts:

- a previous history of pre-eclampsia (RR, 7.19; 95% CI 5.85–8.83)
- the presence of antiphospholipid antibodies (RR, 9.72; 95% CI 4.34–21.75)
- pre-existing diabetes (RR, 3.56; 95% CI 2.54–4.99)
- twin pregnancies (RR, 2.93; 95% CI 2.04–4.21)
- nulliparity (RR, 2.91; 95% CI 1.28–6.61).

Family history, raised blood pressure (> 80 mmHg diastolic) at booking, maternal age over 40 years, raised body mass index before pregnancy and multiparous women were also shown to increase the risk.

Aspirin and pre-eclampsia

There is the theoretical belief that anti-platelets may have a role in prophylaxis but there is a lot of conflicting evidence. The CLASP (collaborative low dose aspirin study in pregnancy) trial and subsequent meta-analyses showed no benefit.

Low dose aspirin in pregnancy and early childhood development: follow up of the collaborative low dose aspirin study in pregnancy

***Br J Obstet Gynaecol* 1995; 102(11): 861–8**

This was the 12- and 18-month follow-up of children born to women who had been at high risk of complications from pre-eclampsia. The findings were reassuring about the safety of aspirin but they showed no clear evidence of benefit.

A protein VEGF165b has been associated with women who have pre-eclampsia; at 12 weeks the levels have been found to be lower than in normal pregnancies.

Postnatal depression

- One in 10 women become depressed after childbirth (70 000 women every year).
- Around 50% are still having problems 6 months postnatally.
- This is different from 'baby blues', which are common day 3–5 (up to day 10) and which do not require treatment, and it is less severe than puerperal psychosis.
- Postnatal depression tends to start around 4–6 weeks after delivery.
- It is important to diagnose and treat early to minimise problems with bonding within the family.

NICE published guidance, *Antenatal and Postnatal Mental Health*, in February 2007 (www.nice.org.uk/nicemedia/live/11004/30432/30432.pdf). The guidance considers our role as GPs in detecting problems, referring to psychiatric services and prescribing based on a risk benefit assessment.

Edinburgh Postnatal Depression Scale

***Br J Psych* 1987; 150: 782–876**

This scale was developed in primary care to improve detection through screening. It is used at 6–8 weeks postnatally and is scored by a health professional (GP, health visitor or midwife).

1 I have been able to laugh and see the funny side of things	
As much as I always could	0
Not quite so much now	1
Definitely not so much now	2
Not at all	3
2 I have looked forward with enjoyment to things	
As much as I ever did	0
Rather less than I used to	1
Definitely less than I used to	2
Hardly at all	3
3 I have blamed myself unnecessarily when thing went wrong	
Yes, most of the time	3
Yes, some of the time	2

	Not very often	1
	No, never	0
4	I have been anxious or worried for no good reason	
	No, not at all	0
	Hardly ever	1
	Yes, sometimes	2
	Yes, very often	3
5	I have felt scared or panicky for no good reason	
	Yes, quite a lot	3
	Yes, sometimes	2
	No, not much	1
	No, not at all	0
6	Things have been getting on top of me	
	Yes, most of the time I haven't been able to cope at all	3
	Yes, sometimes I haven't been coping as well as usual	2
	No, most of the time I have coped quite well	1
	No, I have been coping as well as ever	0
7	I have been so unhappy that I have had difficulty sleeping	
	Yes, most of the time	3
	Yes, sometimes	2
	Not very often	1
	No, not at all	0
8	I have felt sad or miserable	
	Yes, most of the time	3
	Yes, quite often	2
	Not very often	1
	No, not at all	0
9	I have been so unhappy that I have been crying	
	Yes, most of the time	3
	Yes, quite often	2
	Only occasionally	1
	No, never	0
10	The thought of harming myself has occurred to me	
	Yes, quite often	3
	Sometimes	2
	Hardly ever	1
	Never	0

If the calculated total score is >13 then there is a 92.3% chance that the woman is suffering from a depressive illness. The score should not override clinical judgement.

Treatment of postnatal depression

Treatment of proven benefit includes cognitive behavioural therapy and counselling by a health visitor. SSRIs and tricyclic antidepressants appear to be safe in pregnant and breastfeeding women, guidance is to use the lowest effective dose and drugs in the group with the most data (fluoxetine, amitryptyline and imipramine).

Teenage pregnancy

www.bpas.org

The age of consent (from a legal perspective) to any form of sexual activity is 16 for both men and women. In children aged 13–16 years, there are series of laws to help protect them from abuse, and in children under 13 years there is a maximum life imprisonment for rape – there is no defence of mistaken belief about age as there is in 13- to 15-year-olds.

Teenage sexual health, pregnancy and termination is always topical. Teenage Pregnancy Unit statistics have found the following:

- In England there are 41 325 conceptions per year to women under 18 (2008).
- Almost half of these lead to termination.
- Nationally the rate is starting to fall (London remained stable from 1998 to 2003) but we still have the highest teenage pregnancy rate in Western Europe.
- Forty in 100 girls aged 15–17 years will become pregnant.
- Approximately 12.4% of all terminations are to women under 18 years, following either a previous birth (5%) or a previous termination (7.4%).

It is well recognised that teenage pregnancies:

- are seen at higher rates in deprived areas
- mean that teenage mothers are less likely to finish their education or find a job
- mean teenage mothers are more likely to bring their children up in poverty
- generally lead to poorer antenatal health and low-birthweight babies
- when resulting in a birth, the infants have twice the mortality rate seen in the population.

National teenage pregnancy strategy

www.education.gov.uk/consultations/downloadableDocs/4287_Teenage%20pregnancy%20strategy_aw8.pdf

This link gives you the information on the teenage pregnancy strategy beyond 2010.

The original aims were:

- Halve under-18 conception rates in England by 2010.
- Increase the participation of teenage mothers in education, training or work by 60% by 2010, to reduce the risk of long-term social exclusion.

Progress so far:

- There has been an 11.8% decline in under-18 conception rates (lowest rate for 20 years).
- There has been a 12.1% decline in under-16 conception rates (lowest rate for 20 years).

- Approximately 46% of conceptions still end in abortion (this has been fairly static since 1998).

Issues relating to teenage pregnancies

Provision of health and sex education

Teenagers are often unaware how to obtain contraceptive advice and believe they have to be over 16 years to obtain treatment. Teenagers are often willing to run the risk of sexually transmitted infections and pregnancy as they think their parents will find out if they see their GP (confidentiality is needed at all levels).

Contraceptive services need to be accessible

This includes GPs, family planning services, school nurses, youth clinics and so forth.

Role of schools

This includes sex education/behavioural interventions as well as the need to develop communication skills and sustain the truth that virginity is still in the majority (apparently).

Women's health: questions

1 Varicella zoster infection in pregnancy can cause foetal varicella syndrome and maternal mortality. Which of the following cases below would be eligible for varicella zoster immunoglobulin?
   a. A seronegative woman who has stood in a supermarket queue for 1–2 minutes next to a person whom, because of facial dry scabs, she believes to have had a chickenpox rash.
   b. A seropositive woman who looked after her nephew who went on to develop classical chickenpox rash 24 hours later.
   c. A seronegative woman who develops a vesicular chickenpox rash.
   d. A seropostitive woman who develops a purpuric rash that starts behind the ears.
   e. A seronegative woman who attended an antenatal clinic and was in the waiting room for 20 minutes with a woman who 24 hours later went on to develop chickenpox.

2 In young women with menorrhagia and a regular menstrual cycle, which of the following investigations is the most appropriate?
   a. Thyroid function tests.
   b. Full blood count.
   c. Endometrial biopsy.
   d. Clotting studies.
   e. Full blood count and thyroid function tests.

3 In a 50-year-old menopausal woman starting on HRT for systemic symptoms of flushing, mood changes and vaginal dryness, which of the following statements is the most appropriate?
   a. Topical vaginal oestrogen preparation, such as Vagifem.

b. Where the woman is still having a regular menstrual cycle, an unopposed oestrogen patch to be changed every third and fourth day.
c. Where the woman has a Mirena coil for contraception (fitted 2 years previously), unopposed oestrogen patch to be changed twice a week.
d. Replens vaginal moisturiser with Sylk as additional lubrication for intercourse.
e. Where the lady stopped her periods 6 months ago, a continuous combined preparation of HRT so as not to inconvenience her by causing regular withdrawal bleeds again.

4 Which of the following would be an indication to screen a pregnant woman for gestational diabetes?
a. A previous macrosomic baby weighing 3.5 kg or more.
b. A patient with a booking BMI of 27 kg/m^2.
c. A patient at 30 weeks with a BMI of 30 kg/m^2.
d. A previous baby with shoulder dystocia.
e. A patient of South Asian descent.

5 Which of the following is contraindicated in pregnancy?
a. Ferrous fumarate.
b. Folic acid 5 mg.
c. Vitamin D.
d. Vitamin A.
e. Ferrous sulphate.

6 With regard to ectopic pregnancy, which of the following statements is correct?
a. There is a 50% chance of recurrence.
b. If β-hCG is <1000 IU/L then no ultrasound scan is necessary.
c. If β-hCG is >1000 IU/L a single dose of intramuscular methotrexate would be expected to cause miscarriage in 86%–90% of ectopic pregnancies.
d. If β-hCG is >5000 IU/L intramuscular methotrexate would be appropriate treatment.
e. A dose of methotrexate should never be repeated if initially unsuccessful.

7 Although no longer recommended as a way of assessing foetal well-being, foetal movements would normally be considered within normal limits if:
a. Ten movements were felt within a 12-hour period.
b. Ten movements were felt by lunch time.
c. Ten movements were felt within a 24-hour period.
d. Ten movements were felt over a 2-hour period.
e. Ten movements were felt while on bed rest over a 12-hour period.

8 Which of the following tests is not included in routine antenatal care in the UK?
a. Blood group with rhesus status.
b. HIV test.
c. Rubella test.
d. Syphilis (treponema pallidum) test.
e. Hepatitis B test.
f. Varicella zoster test.

9 Which of the following are symptoms of pre-eclampsia?
a. Epigastric pain.

b. Double vision.
c. Dysuria.
d. Low platelets.
e. Raised alkaline phosphatase.

10 Galactorrhoea: what is the most likely diagnosis in a 22-year-old woman (pregnancy test negative) with milky nipple discharge?
a. Sebaceous cyst.
b. Apocrine breast cyst.
c. Ductal ectasia.
d. Fibroadenosis.
e. Prolactinoma.

Women's health: answers

1 e Significant contact is 15 minutes' face-to-face contact. Once the lesions are dry they are unlikely to shed any virus. A person can transmit the virus 2 days prior to the rash developing. Varicella immunoglobulin has no therapeutic effect once the rash has developed; oral acyclovir may be appropriate (www.rcog.org.uk/files/rcog-corp/uploaded-files/GT13ChickenpoxinPregnancy2007.pdf).

2 b This question is taken from the NICE guidance on heavy menstrual bleeding (www.nice.org.uk/nicemedia/live/11002/30403/30403.pdf). Out of the above options full blood count is all that is suggested. The guidance does not advocate thyroid function testing (we often do this in practice and pick up to three new cases of hypothyroidism a year where menorrhagia has been the only symptom). Endometrial biopsy may be advocated if the woman is having irregular and prolonged bleeding, especially if over 45 years.

3 c This question is about knowing the difference between local and systemic symptoms as well as the types of HRT. MIMs has excellent tables in the back pages. In this case there are different scenarios, the Mirena coil gives the progestogen protection to the endometrium so unopposed oestrogen is absolutely fine. In options (b) and (d) the treatment suggested does not give the correct progestogenic protection so would further increase the overall risk of endometrial carcinoma.

4 e Patients that should be offered screening for gestational diabetes would be those at booking with a BMI of 30 kg/m^2, a previous macrosomic baby (4.5 kg or more), a first degree relative with diabetes or family origin with high prevalence of diabetes (South Asian, black Caribbean or Middle Eastern ethnicities).

5 d Vitamin A, especially >700 μg, may be teratogenic. Although folic acid is usually used at 400 μg, 5 mg may be used in certain circumstances. Vitamin D isn't regularly used but can be in patients with no sunlight exposure or inadequate intake. Iron is not used routinely but can be depending on routine blood results.

6 c There is a 15% chance of recurrence of an ectopic. If the β-hCG is <100 IU/L an ultrasound scan is needed, if no sac is detected then expectant management is acceptable. Methotrexate in not indicated where the β-hCG is greater than 5000, the patient is in a collapsed state, an adnexal mass is greater than 4 cm or the patient is in severe pain. Follow-up after methotrexate would usually be days 4, 7 and 14 for serum β-hCG levels and LFTs; if the β-hCG drops less than 15% then a further dose of methotrexate may be needed. Liver function tests may rise but the changes are usually reversible.

Methotrexate is prescribed at an intramuscular dose of 1 mg/kg; it is teratogenic, so contraception is needed.

7 d Movements can be felt from between 18 and 20 weeks (often from week 16), usually there are 4–100 movements per hour but women could usually expect to feel 10 movements over a 2-hour period (*Antenatal Care*, www.nice.org.uk/nicemedia/live/11947/40145/40145.pdf).

8 f

9 a Epigastric pain – pre-eclampsia until proven otherwise (beware the Gaviscon request without a blood pressure check) (*Hypertension in Pregnancy* (August 2010), www.nice.org.uk/nicemedia/live/13098/50416/50416.pdf). Vision could be blurred, not doubled. Headaches, vomiting and oedema of the face, hands and feet would all be recognised symptoms. You can get protein in the urine but not dysuria. The other options are not symptoms.

10 e

Statement 10.2

Men's health

Several studies have shown that men seek help for a given illness later than women. Although they do care about health issues, men find it more difficult to express their fears.

Erectile dysfunction

www.bssm.org.uk/downloads/BSSM_ED_Management_Guidelines_2007.pdf

- Around 50% of men aged 40–70 years experience some degree of erectile dysfunction (ED).
- ED is frequently a manifestation of underlying vascular disease and men should be screened for risk factors and signs of vascular disease as part of the assessment.
- The incidence is doubled in hypertensives, tripled in diabetics and quadrupled in men with coronary heart disease.
- Cigarette smoking increases the prevalence of all of the above twofold.
- Lipids and glucose should be measured in all patients.

If there is a normal libido and secondary sexual characteristics, it is unusual to find a low testosterone level (if measuring, the sample should be taken between the hours of 8 a.m. and 11 a.m.). If sex hormone binding globulin and testosterone are requested, a ratio can then be determined (i.e. the availability of testosterone), which may help management. Also, consider whether testing for thyroid hormone and prolactin are needed.

Treatment

Involve the partner as well as the patient, where possible. Patients who received an NHS prescription before 14 September 1998 can continue to receive ED treatment (not just the first method they were prescribed) on the NHS (the script should be endorsed 'SLS'). Otherwise treatment is only available on the NHS for patients with certain medical problems, e.g. prostate cancer, diabetes, spinal cord injury, Parkinson's disease, multiple sclerosis and so forth (twelve in total). Private scripts can be written for those not eligible for NHS treatment.

Lifestyle

Reducing alcohol intake if excessive, stopping smoking and losing weight if overweight are all recommended. These factors should also help reduce cardiovascular risks (treatment of cardiovascular risk should be as per guidelines).

Phosphodiesterase type 5 inhibitors (sildenafil, tadalafil and vardenafil)

These are selective inhibitors of phosphodiesterase type 5 and are currently the favoured option, but are contraindicated in patients taking nitrates. The best responders are those with psychogenic symptoms and are mainly effective in arousal because they prolong the production of nitric oxide (a vasodilator). The response seen may be less marked after around 2 years of use. There is an understanding that if the treatment is used regularly the response is better than if used infrequently. A study recently found that in men with a history of ischaemic heart disease and hypertension, using sildenafil and tadalafil increased the risk of non-arteritic anterior ischaemic optic neuropathy and blindness (*Br J Ophthalmol* 2006; 90(2): 154–7). Use is not contraindicated, but it would be prudent to warn patients.

Apomorphine (Uprima) (dopamine receptor agonist)

This drug has been licensed for ED. Currently there are no prescribing restrictions. There is a 1 in 500 risk of syncope due to vasovagal response, so care is needed with the first dose and when increasing from 2 to 3 mg.

Intra-cavernosal prostaglandin E1 (alprostadil)

Around 80% of men have a satisfactory erection with this method. There is a greater need for education on how to self-inject.

Intra-urethral prostaglandin E1

The MUSE (medicated urethral system for erections) system of pellets gives around 30% of men some discomfort after use, which causes discontinued use of treatment. One randomised controlled trial showed a satisfactory effect in 40% of men.

Yohimbine (alpha blocker)

This drug is not yet licensed. It has been found to be effective in some placebo controlled trials, but its effectiveness is probably inadequate for treatment of most.

Benign prostatic hypertrophy/lower urinary tract symptoms

www.gpnotebook.co.uk

- Approximately 3.3 million men in the United Kingdom have benign prostatic hyperplasia (BPH).
- One in three men over the age of 50 will have symptoms.
- The prime concern in management, besides symptom control, is to ensure that those men with outflow obstruction do not go on to develop renal failure.

The International Prostate Symptom Score

www.gp-training.net/protocol/docs/ipss.doc

This is a way of assessing symptoms over time with treatment, and the BPH Impact Index is a way of assessing how troublesome symptoms are.

Management

Alpha blockers

Alpha blockers (e.g. prazosin, indoramin) relax the smooth muscle of the prostate; they haven proven more effective than placebo in randomised controlled trials. They usually show an improvement within 2–3 weeks. If there is no improvement within 3–4 months then an alternative should be tried.

5-alpha-reductase inhibitors

These (e.g. finasteride) inhibit 5-alpha-reductase, which converts testosterone to dihydroxytestosterone, and is known to influence prostate growth. Randomised controlled trials have confirmed that they are more effective than placebo. They cause hyperplasia to regress over 3–6 months (allow 12 months for maximum effect), so are especially suitable if the prostate is enlarged. These may reduce the prostate-specific antigen by up to 50%.

Impact of baseline symptom severity on future risk of benign prostatic hyperplasia-related outcomes and long-term response to finasteride. The PLESS study group

Urology 2000; 56(4): 610–16

The Proscar long-term efficacy and safety study have published several outcome studies.

A total of 3040 men with BPH were treated for 4 years with either finasteride or placebo. Finasteride reduced the risk of surgery and acute urinary retention in all groups ($p < 0.001$).

Dutasteride

Dutasteride has been shown to reduce symptoms scored, reduce retention, reduce prostate volume, improve flow rates and reduce the need for surgery.

Plant extracts

- Saw palmetto (*Serenoa repens*) (Permixon): this is an extract from a cactus-like plant. It has had some success (although the trial did not use a placebo arm) and is thought to work in a similar way to finasteride.
- Beta-sitosterol: trials have shown that this is more effective than placebo in short term. The side effects include gastrointestinal symptoms and impotence.
- Rye grass pollen extract: it has been suggested that this is beneficial, but trials as yet are inconclusive.

Botulinum A toxin

When this is injected into the prostate it has been shown to improve symptoms of BPH.

Prostate cancer

There is no formal screening (see Statement 5) or prevention available at the time of writing, but the use of finasteride and the potential vaccine development may become more topical over the next few years.

The Influence of finasteride on the development of prostate cancer

N Eng J Med 2003; 349(3): 215–24

This was a study of 18 882 men aged 55 years and older who had a normal digital rectal examination and a prostate-specific antigen level of less than 3 ng/mL. The subjects were randomised to either treatment with finasteride or placebo for 7 years. Finasteride was found to have a reduction of 24.8% of prostate cancer, although tumours of Gleason grades 7–10 were more common in this group, as were sexual side effects.

PSA testing is the main current blood test that we have to detect prostate cancer, although there is research into the use of antibody-based blood tests (specifically to protasomes) which is ongoing and may prove to be more specific.

Prostate cancer vaccine

Prostate-specific membrane antigen has been a target for vaccines, as has radioactively labelled monoclonal antibodies against prostate-specific membrane antigen. Although certain vaccines are in the clinical trial phase, as yet there are no conclusive results on efficacy.

Men's health: questions

1 ED: which of the following is considered permissible for an NHS prescription of cialis for ED?
   a. A patient with ischaemic heart disease.
   b. Diet-controlled diabetic.
   c. A patient who had a fall resulting in a back fracture.
   d. A patient with ED following a prostate biopsy, biopsy reported as normal.
   e. A patient who had already been receiving treatment under the NHS for ED (outside the current guidance in the British National Formulary) prior to 14 September 2006.
2 Haematospermia: which of the following would not be considered a cause for haematospermia?
   a. BPH.
   b. Prostate cancer.
   c. Testicular cancer.
   d. Human papilloma virus.
   e. Seminal vesicle calculi.
3 Vasectomy: when counselling a patient with regard to chronic pain following vasectomy, which of the following statistics is correct?
   a. Chronic scrotal pain occurs in 1% of men post-vasectomy.
   b. Chronic scrotal pain occurs in 5% of men post-vasectomy.
   c. Chronic scrotal pain occurs in 1%–5% of men post-vasectomy.

d. Chronic scrotal pain occurs in 1%–15% of men post-vasectomy.
e. Chronic scrotal pain occurs in 15% of men post-vasectomy.

4 ED: when would a PDE5 inhibitor (phosphodiesterase 5) be least successful as treatment for ED?
a. In a type 1 diabetic patient with an HbA1c of 8.2%.
b. Following a prostatectomy.
c. In a patient where the testosterone level was found to be <8 nmol/L.
d. In a patient where the testosterone level was found to be >12 nmol/L.
e. In a patient with a prostate-specific antigen level of 10.2.

5 Infertility: when considering causes of infertility in a couple, what percentage of cases are usually due to male factors?
a. 50%
b. 30%
c. 10%
d. 5%
e. 3%

6 This may present in a 17-year-old male with no history of trauma but sudden severe scrotal pain associated with swelling. Select the single most appropriate answer.
a. Retrograde ejaculation.
b. Scrotal varicocoele.
c. Testicular cancer.
d. Epididymo-orchitis.
e. Testicular torsion.

7 Renal stones: which of the following treatments have been found to be helpful in reducing the time taken to pass a renal stone once the decision has been made not to intervene surgically?
a. Furosemide
b. Bendroflumethazide
c. Ramipril
d. Diclofenac
e. Alfuzosin

Questions 8–10 are differential diagnoses of gynacomastia (breast tissue growth in males). Answer each number as true or false.

8 Chronic liver disease.
9 Treatment with frusemide.
10 Zoladex treatment for prostate cancer.

Men's health: answers

1 b Patients who are entitled to NHS prescription are listed in the British National Formulary (general guidance, although this may vary across the United Kingdom, is a total of four tablets per month – there are safe and sensible ways around this if it is important). Ischaemic heart disease is not included. Diabetes, renal failure on dialysis, Parkinson's disease, single-gene neurological disease (note this is disease, not disorder), multiple sclerosis and spina bifida are all included. A fractured back would not be included unless this had resulted in severe pelvic injury or a spinal cord injury. All patients who were being treated with ED medication prior to 14 September 1998 would be entitled to continue with their medication or an alternative if this became ineffective (as may happen after a couple of years' use).

2 d Although sexually transmitted infections can be responsible (often due to prostatitis as well as superficial lesions), human papilloma virus affects the squamous epithelium, so it would not be responsible for a true haematospermia. Other causes include simple cysts of the seminal vesicles and trauma. If the patient is over 40 years of age then the likelihood that there is a more serious cause underlying the problem is increased. This question was based on a clinical review article published in *General Practice* (15 October 2010).

3 d This question was written using the clinical review article 'Investigating and managing chronic scrotal pain' (*BMJ* 2010; 341: c6716). Chronic scrotal pain is seen in 1%–15% of men post vasectomy, and severe scrotal pain is seen in 1%–6% of men (10-year follow-up in the study).

4 c In this instance increasing the testosterone is more likely to be helpful. The testosterone may be reduced in obesity because of the action of aromatase (the enzyme that metabolises testosterone to oestradiol), which causes a further increase in the abdominal fat deposition and further lowering of the testosterone level. This is adapted from the article, 'Erectile dysfunction in association with co-morbid conditions' (*Guidelines in Practice* 2009; 12(7): 25–30).

5 b Thirty per cent male, 25% ovulatory, 25% unexplained, 20% tubal, 5% endometriosis, 5% coital problems, 3% cervical problems, <1% uterine causes. In 15% of cases there is more than one cause.

6 e Testicular cancer wouldn't usually present with sudden pain. This can occur in men aged 20–40 years. Epididymo-orchitis can be difficult to distinguish from torsion, although the pain is usually of a more gradual onset. Torsion most commonly occurs between ages 13 and 17, but it can happen under the age of 30 years.

7 e The distal ureter has many alpha-1 receptors, so blockade increases relaxation and expulsion rate. Diclofenac helps pain and reduces the spasm around the stone.

8 True

9 False With spironolactone.

10 True All gonadorelin analogues.

Statement 11

Sexual health

Contraception

www.fsrh.org/pages/clinical_guidance.asp

The global population is estimated to reach 8.9 billion by 2050 and with it are significant risks of overpopulation. The goals of contraception are ultimately to reduce the number of unplanned and unwanted pregnancies by safe, well-tolerated and reversible methods.

Combined oral contraception

In the UK 25% of women aged 16–49 years and 50% of women in their twenties are on the combined oral contraceptive pill (COCP). Currently all pharmacological methods of contraception are reversible and made from synthetic steroids, containing no natural oestrogens or progesterones.

There are three generations of combined pill:

1. First generation (e.g. Norinyl-1, Ovran):
   - first produced in the 1960s and no longer used
   - high dose of oestrogen (increased venous thromboembolism (VTE) risk).
2. Second generation:
   - lower oestrogen
   - similar progestagen to first-generation pills.
3. Third generation:
   - produced in the 1980s
   - lower dose of oestrogen
   - new form of progestagen (less androgenic than second-generation products).

Risk assessment

The UK Medical Eligibility Criteria (UKMEC) for the COCP is printed in summary in the guidance of the Royal College of General Practitioners' Faculty of Sexual and Reproductive Healthcare on prescribing the combined contraceptive pill.

It is important to assess risk before initiating treatment and at each review.

- Venous thromboembolic (VTE) risk increases with age.
- A body mass index (BMI) >35 kg/m^2 quadruples the risk of VTE – there are other alternatives so use them if you possibly can.
- Smoking doubles the risk of VTE.
- Family history – if patients have a first-degree relative under 45 years of age with VTE/primary thrombotic tendency, then combined pills should not be used.
- Ask about migraines (focal), breast cancer, pregnancy, undiagnosed vaginal bleed and diabetes.

- Measure blood pressure.

Venous thromboembolism

In 1 year:

- Five per 100 000 women years will develop VTE (not pregnant and not using a COCP).
- Fifteen in 100 000 if taking second-generation pill (levonorgestrel/norethisterone).
- Twenty-five in 100 000 if taking third-generation pill (gestodene/desogestrel).
- Sixty in 100 000 in pregnancy.

The absolute risk, as opposed to the relative risk, is small.

If a woman has not experienced a clot after 1 year of pill use, it is thought that the subsequent risk will then be much lower.

Since the 1980s, the accepted risk for VTE due to COCPs was 30 in 100 000. Therefore, studies did not necessarily suggest an increased risk in third-generation pills but, rather, a reduced risk, and an increased risk with second-generation pills compared with what was originally thought.

Long-Acting Reversible Contraception, National Institute for Health and Clinical Excellence (October 2005)

The following recommendations have been identified as priorities:

- Contraceptive provision:
  - Information and choice of all methods of contraception should be offered.
  - Contraceptive service providers should be aware that all currently available long-acting reversible contraceptive methods (intrauterine devices (IUDs), intrauterine systems (IUSs), injectables and implants) are more cost-effective than the pill at 1 year. IUDs, IUSs and implants are more cost-effective than injectables, and increasing the use of long-acting reversible contraceptives will reduce the risk of pregnancy.
- Counselling and provision of information:
  - This should be both written and verbal and include: efficacy of method, duration of use, risk and possible side effects, non-contraceptive benefits, procedure for initiation and discontinuation, and when to seek help while using the method.
  - Should include advice on safer sex.

Nexplanon

www.fsrh.org/pdfs/CEUGuidanceProgestogenOnlyInjectables09.pdf

This was launched as Implanon in September 1999 (following withdrawal of Norplant relating to the insertion and removal of six rods many years ago now). It consists of a single semi-rigid rod with dimensions of 40 × 2 mm, and insertion should be subdermal. It releases etonogestrel 30–40 μg per day. The device lasts for a total of 3 years and has a failure rate of <4 in 1000 over 2 years if used in licence.

Amenorrhoea is reported in around 21% of women, and irregular bleeding can be problematic (as expected with progesterone methods) in around 17% of women, although by 6 months this has often settled.

Enzyme inducers such as antiretrovirals and probably St John's wort can reduce effectiveness (antibiotics are still thought to be safe). There is no need to replace the rod early in obesity although you may do so if there is an early return of bleeding.

Coils

www.fsrh.org/pdfs/CEUGuidanceIntrauterineContraceptionNov07.pdf

1 Copper coils (380 mm copper) are relatively easy to insert, even in nulliparous women. The licence is usually from 8 to 10 years, depending upon the type of coil and the time of insertion related to the menopause. The failure rate is around 2% at 5 years (mostly due to expulsion). At least 300 mm of copper is needed for contraception to be effective.
2 Mirena is licensed for 5 years (7 years if fitted over the age of 45 years) for contraception and 4 years for endometrial protection in hormone replacement therapy. The National Institute for Health and Clincical Excellence guidelines state that if the woman is ammenorrhoeic it is fine to keep the IUS in situ until it is no longer needed for contraception (not as straightforward as it may seem, given the need for contraception is usually based on having stopped menses with no hormonal influence). Failure rate is around 1% at 5 years.
3 Gynaefix is a frameless IUD consisting of six copper tubes (total of 330 mm^2 copper) on a nylon thread, knotted at one end, that anchors into the uterine fundus. The failure rate is <1% in up to 5 years of use, and the expulsion rate is low.

Current contraception issues

1 Depot medroxyprogesterone: there has been a drive to limit the use of depo in younger women and women approaching the menopause, as well as to limit the duration of use to 2 years, following a better understanding that this affects the bone mineral density.
2 Evra patch (norelgestromin and ethinyloestradiol) was licensed in the United Kingdom in 2003. It is worn for 3 weeks of a 4-week cycle and the patch needs to be changed weekly.
3 YAZ is a new combined pill, not yet licensed in the United Kingdom, with ethinyloestradiol and drosperidone. It has 24 active pills, with a 4-day pill-free interval.
4 Immunocontraception is a novel new approach that is receiving a considerable degree of attention. Sperm have unique proteins and targeting antibodies to these gamete-specific antigens could be successful. Currently vaccines targeting the HCG molecule are undergoing phase I and II trials on humans.
5 Folic acid-supplemented contraception is being given consideration. As there are still some preventable foetal abnormalities occurring, this may help, for example, in women who miss or stop the pill to conceive but forget to take folic acid.

Emergency contraception

www.fsrh.org/pdfs/CEUguidanceEmergencyContraception.pdf

A MORI survey has indicated that 43% of 15- to 24-year-olds reported having casual sex in the last 10 years, and 40% of these had failed to use a condom. Around 12% of patients who require emergency contraception are under 16 years of age. Emergency contraception is available free of charge on prescription from GPs, family planning clinics, youth clinics, walk-in centres, genitourinary clinics, some A&E departments and some pharmacists.

In 1983 the Attorney General ruled that emergency contraception is not a form of abortion, as there is no pregnancy to terminate. This was further supported by another test case in 2002 where it was judged that life legally begins at implantation (in the UK).

Levonelle is now first line (ulipristal acetate, ellaOne, is new to the market) and has been shown to be effective with a stat dose of 1.5 mg. For women on enzyme-inducing drugs, the advice for Levonelle is that patients take two 1.5 mg tablets as soon as possible after unprotected sexual intercourse. This is also considered sensible if women are over 70 kg in weight. Women should be warned of the greater risk of ectopic pregnancy following emergency contraception.

Other options for emergency contraception

- Copper coil can be used up to 5 days after unprotected intercourse (i.e. up to day 19 of a regular 28-day cycle, but should be based on the shortest cycle if periods are irregular). Medicolegally, this is not procuring an abortion (having been tested in the courts).
- Ulipristal (EllaOne) can be taken up to 5 days after unprotected intercourse.

Young people: sex, contraception, consent and the law

The age of consent for heterosexual sex is 16 years for both men and women. In England, Scotland and Wales the age of consent for sex between men is also 16 years.

The Sexual Offences Act 2003 updated offenses chargeable and a significant proportion was aimed at protecting children under the age of 13 years, as at this age it is not thought that one is able to consent (this applies even if involving two 12-year-olds; indeed, this would be rape even if the children were of the same age). The act does not prevent us providing confidential sexual health advice, information and treatment.

Working to Safeguard Children is a document written as part of the new child protection guidelines. In its draft phase there was a move to make it mandatory for all healthcare professionals to report all children under 16 years of age who were sexually active; this was contested and is not necessary. We should report any concerns of abuse or exploitation against anyone under 18 years of age using the Child Protection Procedures.

Working Together (2006) lists a concerns checklist (listed in part):

- Is the young person competent to understand and consent to the sexual activity in which they are involved?
- Nature of the relationship – consider age and power imbalances.

- Whether aggression, coercion or bribery was involved (including drug or alcohol use).
- Whether a young person's behaviour places them at risk.
- Whether there have been any attempts to secure secrecy by the sexual partner.

Action in children under 13 years of age who have disclosed sexual activity:
- Consult the child protection lead.
- Always refer, except in exceptional circumstances (keep full records of the reasons why not referred).

Gillick test and Fraser competence

The Gillick test is used to judge whether a child under 16 years of age is mature enough to understand what treatment involves, including the risks, and it shows that a child is competent to consent to treatment (such as contraception and vaccinations). In issues such as contraception where an adult with parental responsibility would not necessarily be involved, then you can apply the Fraser guidelines on competence:
- They understand the doctor's advice.
- The doctor cannot persuade them to involve their parents that they are seeking contraceptive advice.
- They are likely to begin or continue having sex whether or not you prescribe contraception.
- Unless they receive contraception their physical or mental health is likely to suffer.

Gillick or Fraser? A plea for consistency over competence in children

BMJ 2006; 332(7545): 807

This is an excellent editorial by Robert Wheeler. He explains the original case brought by Victoria Gillick, who challenged the health service guidance that would have allowed her daughters, under 16, to receive confidential contraceptive advice without her knowledge. Wheeler then explains Lord Fraser's concern over the dilemma of providing contraceptive advice to girls where their welfare may depend on it.

Gillick competence provides an objective test of competence whereas Fraser guidelines are more narrow, relating only to contraception.

Standards for the Management of Sexually Transmitted Infections (STIs)

medfash.org.uk/Projects/BASHH_standards/Final_pdfs/Standards_for_the_management_of_STIs.pdf

This was published in January 2010 and covers the ethos behind provision of sexual health services (relevant to commissioning). Although this is a thorough document, useful for case-based discussions and thinking about service provision, I doubt any Applied Knowledge Test questions will be based around this.

National Strategy for Sexual Health and HIV **(2001)**
www.dh.gov.uk/prod_consum_dh/groups/dh_digitalassets/@dh/@en/documents/digitalasset/dh_4058945.pdf

In July 2001 a consultation document was published that outlined the government's proposed strategy for sexual health and human immunodeficiency virus (HIV). The main aim of the strategy is to prevent sexual causes of premature deaths and ill health, as well as to ensure that services are available for those patients who need them. Local networks of providers will be based on three service levels.

Level 1: to be provided by GPs

- sexual history and risk assessment
- contraceptive information and services
- pregnancy testing and referral
- cervical cytology screening and referral
- sexually transmitted disease testing for women
- assessment and referral for men
- HIV testing and counselling
- hepatitis B immunisation.

Level 2: intermediate care to be provided by primary care teams with a special interest (e.g. an enhanced service), genitourinary medicine or family planning clinics

- IUDs and contraceptive implants
- testing and treatment of sexually transmitted diseases (STDs)
- invasive STD testing for men
- partner notification and contact tracing
- vasectomy.

Level 3: specialist clinical teams across more than one primary care group

- outreach contraceptive services
- outreach STD prevention
- specialised infection management, including contact tracing
- specialised HIV treatment and care.

A large proportion of GPs already provide level 1 services (the exception being HIV testing).

The additional services of the current GP contract cover contraceptive services, while the enhanced service would allow a greater role of sexual health provision, as per the strategy.

Chlamydia

www.ons.gov.uk/ons/search/index.html?newquery=chlamydia

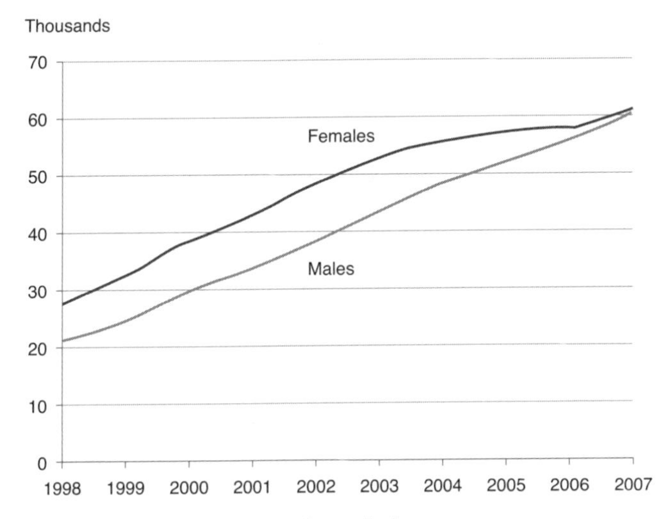

New episodes of genital chlamydia (uncomplicated): by sex, UK

- There were 121 986 cases of chlamydia in 2007.
- Sixy-eight per cent of these cases were in the under-25 age group.
- Around 70% of women and 50% of men are asymptomatic; there may be non-specific symptoms.
- It is the most common curable sexually transmitted disease in Europe.
- It can cause ectopic pregnancy, pelvic inflammatory disease (in 10%–30% of cases), infertility, perihepatitis (Fitz-Hugh-Curtis's syndrome) and there can be neonatal transmission.
- National postal chlamydia screening is available for those under 25 online (www.b-clear.org.uk).

High-risk groups are 16- to 25-year-olds and women undergoing a termination of pregnancy. Behavioural risk factors include teenagers leaving school at a young age, women with multiple partners, being single and people from ethnic minorities.

Screening for chlamydia

www.chlamydiascreening.nhs.uk/

www.b-clear.org.uk

It is important not to confuse opportunistic screening of asymptomatic men and women with the need for a full complement of swabs and blood tests in high-risk individuals where it is important to consider all sexually transmitted infections.

National Chlamydia Screening Programme

This was launched in 2003 with the following aims:

- controlling chlamydia through early detection and treatment of asymptomatic infection

- reducing onward transmission
- prevention of the consequences of untreated infection.

Opportunistic genital chlamydia screening will be offered to sexually active individuals:
- under 25 years of age
- under 16 years of age who are deemed Fraser competent
- whenever there is a change in sexual partner.

In men, a first pass urine has 75%–100% sensitivity; in women, a self-taken vulvovaginal swab has over 80% sensitivity, with 99% specificity (urine in women has been shown to be less sensitive but is now used as part of the screening, as it is more acceptable). Endocervical swabs at the time of a cervical smear may also be used.

Although the screening is initiated in primary care (general practice, antenatal clinics, family planning, colposcopy clinics and so forth), the chlamydia screening office then coordinates the result notification, treatment if needed (azithromycin 1 gm stat is first line, taking 1 week to work) and contact tracing.

The person undergoing the test has the option of receiving the results by telephone (text messaging is offered in some regions) or in person. Further pilots are in place with the chemist Boots looking at their role in offering screening.

Screening implications for general practitioners

1. Extra time is needed by clinical staff for:
   - taking samples from at-risk patients or explaining how to do a self-test
   - training for practice staff
   - sexual history from all patients under 25 years of age
   - pre-test counselling
   - counselling for patients who test positive; although the office will coordinate things, it is inevitable that there will be some fallout
   - partner notification and treatment
   - ensuring compliance and follow-up to treatment.
2. Extra resources needed:
   - staff training
   - laboratory tests.
3. Issues:
   - compliance – requires sexual abstinence for 1 week
   - contact tracing (6-month history from patients)
   - consider a test of cure
   - genitourinary referral – confidentiality issue/insurance forms and so forth.

Sexual health: questions

1. If a patient using the COCP has post-coital bleeding, what is the most appropriate cause of action?

   a. A pregnancy test.

   b. A urine chlamydia test.

c. A low vaginal self-swab for chlamydia.
d. A speculum examination with vaginal and cervical swabs.
e. Colposcopy.

2 Contraception: which of the following is an absolute contraindication (UKMEC Category 4) for combined contraceptive pill use?
a. Diabetic neuropathy.
b. Immobility.
c. Migrainous headaches with a past history of aura at any age.
d. Highly active antiretroviral treatment.
e. Obesity with a BMI >35 kg/m^2.

3 Chlamydia: which of the following is more commonly associated with chlamydia trachomatis infection?
a. Behçet's syndrome.
b. Seropositive polyarthropathy.
c. Reiter's syndrome.
d. Genital ulceration.
e. Wegener's granulomatosis.

4 HIV: which of the following skin conditions is not associated with HIV?
a. Kaposi's sarcoma.
b. Severe psoriasis.
c. Seborrhoeic dermatitis.
d. Multidermatomal herpes zoster.
e. Koebnerisation.

For questions 5–10, answer true or false. The following are requirements when a person dies of hepatitis C.

5 By law you must inform the undertakers.
6 The body must remain in a sealed body bag in the coffin.
7 You must complete a notification of disease form for the Communicable Disease Surveillance Centre.
8 Body bags should be labelled biohazard with tape or tags.
9 All bodies must be cremated (burial is not permissible by law).
10 Coffins must be hermetically sealed (e.g. lid soldered shut).

Sexual health: answers

1 d This question is taken from the Faculty of Sexual Health and reproductive Healthcare guidance on unscheduled bleeding (www.rcog.org.uk/files/rcog-corp/UnscheduledBleeding23092009.pdf). You can't rely on just testing for chlamydia in this case; although risk may be low, you need to look at the cervix. Obviously, if cervical screening is needed this could be done at the same time.

2 a See *Faculty of Family Planning and Reproductive Health Care Clinical Guidance: first prescription of combined oral contraception* (www.fsrh.org/pdfs/FirstPrescCombOralContJan06.pdf). Diabetes with neuropathy, nephropathy, associated vascular disease or duration of >20 years is UK Medical Eligibility Criteria (UKMEC) categories 3 and 4. Immobility is UKMEC 3. Migraine with aura (currently) is UKMEC 4, but past history of aura at any age is UKMEC 3 (note migraine without aura comes under UKMEC 2 and 3). Highly active antiretroviral treatment comes under UKMEC 2. Obesity with a BMI 35–39 35 kg/m^2 is UKMEC 3, whereas BMI >40 kg/m^2 is UKMEC 4.

3 c Reiter's is a triad of seronegative arthritis, urethrits and conjunctivitis caused by *Chlamydia* infection.

4 e Koebnerisation is the tendancy of scar tissue to be a focal point for certain skin pathology or for trauma to the skin to provoke the skin lesion, e.g. psoriasis, lichen planus and so forth.

5 True The body cannot be embalmed.

6 True There are implications on viewing the body – no clothes or make-up for burial.

7 False This should have already been done.

8 True

9 False

10 True

Statement 12

Care of people with cancer and palliative care

The NHS Cancer Plan

www.dh.gov.uk

The NHS Cancer Plan was introduced in September 2000, following a series of cancer guidelines, with the aim of improving cancer care and outcome in the NHS. A multidisciplinary team developed the plan, but for it to have any impact it needed 'local leadership and support'. Each primary care trust will have a cancer lead.

The government will play its part by investing in the workforce and tackling shortages. There were 1000 new cancer specialists planned; histopathology and radiography were also targeted.

It is hoped that the plan is going to be achieved by increasing capacity through new ways of working and developing opportunities as well as education, recruitment and retention planning. Needless to say, there are various opinions in editorials and in the letters pages of medical journals, ranging from 'excellent, simple, clear, GP and patient centred' to 'a waste of money, politically motivated and barely enough investment to keep up with the increasing incidence of cancer'.

The plan has four main aims.

1 Save more lives.
2 Ensure people with cancer get professional support and care as well as the best treatment.
3 Tackle inequalities in health that mean unskilled workers are twice as likely to die from cancer than professionals.
4 Build a future through cancer research and preparation for a genetic revolution.

There were three planned commitments:

1 Reduce smoking in manual workers from 32% (in 1998) to 26% by 2010.
2 Reduce waiting times for diagnosis and treatment to 1 month from an urgent cancer referral to starting treatment by 2005.
3 Investing an extra £50 million in hospices and specialist palliative care.

Also discussed is the role of promoting a healthier diet, the five-a-day programme. As well as raising public awareness, children aged 4–6 will be able to have a piece of fruit every day if they want (currently this works with fruit being offered at school instead of dessert and tuck and having dedicated fruit tuck days).

There were plans to extend cancer screening in the following ways:

- Breast cancer screening will be extended to women aged 65–70 years by 2004 and available on request to those over 70 years of age.
- Cervical screening programmes will be upgraded and unnecessary repeats reduced.
- With regard to prostate cancer, prostate specific antigen tests will be available to empower men to make their own choices (no formal programme planned, as there are too many questions currently unanswered, although trials are in progress).
- Ovarian cancer screening trials are in progress.

Finally, there was planned investment in research, in particular the National Cancer Research Institute. Advances in genetics will lead to a greater understanding of inherited susceptibility in the future. As things stand the cancer genetics service needs a strategic framework to develop further. The Harper report recommended that primary care should be the principle focus for clinical cancer genetics. This in turn came from the Calman–Hine report, which recommended networks of cancer care in research, assessment, diagnosis and treatments.

Advance directives (living wills)

In medieval times a good death was a prepared death. Advance directives are statements (usually written and formally witnessed) made by a person about medical care they would and would not want if they were to become incompetent in the future. This is as opposed to an advance statement, which would explain your general wishes and views.

Is there such a thing as a life not worth living?

BMJ 2001; 322(7300): 1481–3

This article debates the practical difficulties of measurement of and ethical issues associated with determining quality of life in situations where a life has been judged to have no quality. Patients who are dying may find some quality in life even when assessed by current measures as abysmal. The use of proxies is touched on as a problem for similar reasons – namely, the disparity between an observer's assessment and the patient's own evaluation.

Legally the whole subject of advance directives is complicated. At present there are six types of advance statements:

1. A requesting statement reflecting an individual's aspirations and preferences.
2. A statement of general beliefs and aspects of life that the individual values.
3. A statement naming proxy.
4. A directive giving clear instructions relating to some or all of treatment.
5. A statement specifying a degree or irreversible deterioration after which no life-sustaining treatment should be given.
6. A combination of all of the above.

An advance directive should not preclude the provision of basic care, defined as maintenance of bodily cleanliness, relief of sustained pain and provision of oral nutrition and hydration.

The current legal situation in the UK

- A person must be competent at the time of declaration (Mental Capacity Act 2005).
- The person must be informed in broad terms about the nature and effect of treatments and procedures.
- The person must have anticipated and intended the refusal to apply to the circumstances that subsequently arise.
- The person must be free from undue influence when issuing the declaration.

Adherence to advance directives in critical care decision-making: vignette study

BMJ 2003; 327(7422): 1011

This article raises the point that advance directives are open to widely varying interpretation, partly because of ambiguity of a directive's terminology and partly because of willingness of health professionals to make value judgements concerning quality of life.

A GP is likely to be involved with advance directives in one of two ways:

1. Advising patients when advance directives may be appropriate and of the phrasing of the directive (Age UK [www.ageuk.org.uk] provides access to information and a pack to help in drawing up a directive).
2. As a repository of the advance directive, which could be forwarded to the appropriate department on request.

An advance directive has been legally binding on a doctor in common law since 1994 and has been endorsed by the medical (British Medical Association since 1995) and legal professions. Most experts believe that directives should be reviewed periodically (e.g. every 5 years). Formatted versions are available from either the Terrence Higgins Trust (tel +44 (0)171 831 0330) or Dignity in Dying (tel +44 (0)20 7479 7730).

MedicAlert is allowed to engrave bracelets advising that the patient has a living will. They can also keep a copy and fax it to the appropriate department or read it to the paramedics over the telephone.

Treatment and care towards the end of life: good practice in decision-making, General Medical Council, July 2012

www.gmc-uk.org

This publication looks at guiding principles and a doctor's ethical obligations to show respect for human life, dilemmas of starting and stopping treatment, a framework of good practice and areas of special consideration.

Assisted dying and euthanasia

Both assisted dying and euthanasia involve medical assistance. Providing a patient with the means to end life (e.g. medication) is termed 'physician-assisted suicide', while ending the life if a patient who is physically unable to do so is termed 'voluntary euthanasia'. Both are illegal in the United Kingdom, and a World Medical Association resolution has condemned the practice as unethical.

On the sanctity of life

Br J Gen Pract 2007; 57(537): 332–3

Weingarten writes an interesting article about duration versus quality, the difficulties doctors and religious people have and the perception that this would be a killing. In both doctrines there are circumstances where the duty to save life is not absolute, e.g. when it is no longer possible to use life for its God-given purpose it loses its state of holiness. The final thought is that the term 'sanctity of life' confuses the debate.

Moral dimensions

BMJ 2005; 331(7518): 689–91

Tännsjö considers the following three moral outlooks:

1. Deontology – the view that some kinds of actions are unconditionally prohibited, the sanctity of life doctrine is often the argument against euthanasia.
2. Basic (negative) moral rights – meaning that individuals are free to do as they see fit with themselves. With this view we have no positive right to receive help when we are in distress.
3. Utilitarianism – an action is wrong if, and only if, an alternative is available with better consequences.

Although many doctors and politicians oppose legalised euthanasia, this article concludes that in limited circumstances it may be beneficial.

Taking the final step: changing the law on euthanasia and physician assisted suicide

BMJ 2005; 331: 681–3

This is written from a legal perspective and opens with a profound statement: doctors in the UK can accompany their patients every step of the way, up until the last. The law stops them helping their patients take the final step.

The proposed legislation under the Assisted Dying for the Terminally Ill Bill, would allow a competent adult (who has lived in the UK for at least 1 year), who is suffering unbearably as a result of a terminal illness, to receive medical assistance to die at his or her request. The bill includes various safeguards to protect both the patient and the physician. Current public opinion is 82% in favour of allowing assisted dying.

There are many concerns that are discussed following this *BMJ* paper. The authors look at the Oregon model of assisted suicide, legalisation in Sweden, the need for our own patients to travel when they are at one of the most vulnerable points in life (for themselves and their family), often in pain. Similarly, the worries doctors have if they were to consider undertaking such a role and the impact on their own personal and religious beliefs. Although the bill may go some way to addressing these concerns and providing a legal framework, the issues will continue to be debated at length.

Recently, the House of Lords Select Committee has been asked to consider the Assisted Dying for the Terminally Ill Bill, and the US courts have recently concluded that doctors could lawfully withdraw hydration and nutrition from a patient in a vegetative state. Both of these, and the fact that life expectancy has increased (through public health and improved medical care), increased knowledge of human rights and the limitations of modern technologies mean that interest in assisted dying, in the media and society, has increased.

Care of people with cancer and palliative care: questions

1 Breast cancer: which of the following is contraindicated when a patient is taking tamoxifen?
   a. Paroxetine
   b. Replens
   c. Sylk
   d. Clonidine
   e. Paracetamol

2 Breast cancer: in women who are oestrogen receptor positive, being treated with an aromatase inhibitor, and found to have a T-score of less than −1.0 to −2.0, which of the following would be considered the most appropriate action?
   a. Lifestyle advice.
   b. Stop the aromatase inhibitor, as the risk of fracture is too great.
   c. Change the aromatase inhibitor to tamoxifen.
   d. Calcium and vitamin D supplementation.
   e. Start bisphosphonate treatment.

3 In a case of persistent hiccups in an otherwise well patient, which of the following statements is the most correct?
   a. They would usually be benign, ultimately self-limiting and the patient can be reassured.
   b. They should be investigated to determine whether there is an underlying malignancy.
   c. They can be cured by Butekyo breathing exercises.
   d. They can be cured by sipping iced water.
   e. They can be cured by taking antiemetics that stimulate gastric motility.

4 Which of the following would be the least likely to indicate a brain tumour?
   a. Headache worse on waking.
   b. Headache that wakes someone in the night.
   c. Headache that is worse with sneezing.
   d. Headache that is worse with bending over.
   e. Headache that is worse at the occiput having come on suddenly.

Staging of prostate cancer helps categorise the disease to allow individualised discussions on treatment, as there is no clear consensus on optimum management at different stages. Consider the following statements in questions 5–9 and answer each one either true or false.

5 A Gleason score is extrapolated from a biopsy and looks at glandular differentiation, relationship of glands to stroma and differentiation (Grade 1 = well differentiated; Grade 5 = poorly differentiated).

6 In localised disease, high risk would be classified as Gleason grade 8 or more.

7 In advanced metastatic disease, from prostate cancer, radical prostatectomy would be an effective first-line treatment.

8 Low-dose rate brachytherapy is as effective as external beam radiotherapy for patients with localised disease.

9 Active surveillance with yearly prostate-specific antigen testing may be suitable for some men with low-risk localised disease.

10 The risk of colorectal cancer can be reduced in many ways. From the following options, select the answer where there is known evidence of a reduction in mortality.

a. Hormone replacement therapy for the menopause.
b. Aspirin 75 mg daily.
c. Screening using faecal occult bloods.
d. Screening using flexible sigmoidoscopy.
e. Proton pump inhibitors.

Care of people with cancer and palliative care: answers

1 a Interaction of serotonin reuptake inhibitors with tamoxifen (*BMJ* 2010; 340: 324–5). The risk of death from breast cancer increased with the length of concomitant treatment with paroxetine (but not other selective serotonin reuptake inhibitors). The authors go through a clever explanation that it is due to the strong CYP2D6 inhibiting properties of paroxetine.

2 d A DEXA (dual energy X-ray absorptiometry) scan of this score would be osteopenic. Lifestyle advice would not be adequate, although it would be additionally to the calcium and vitamin D supplement. Changing to tamoxifen would not be appropriate – patients on aromatase inhibitors will often have already completed 5 years on tamoxifen. If a repeat DEXA scan at 24 months shows a T-score of less than −2.0 or an annual rate of bone loss >4% at the lumbar spine or hip, then you could add a bisphosphonate (*Guidelines in Practice* 2011; 14(5): 11–22).

3 b It is important to assess hiccups properly – looking at renal and liver function and considering underlying malignancy. Although there are tricks to ease the hiccups, be a little cautious.

4 e This is suggestive of a subarachnoid haemorrhage; all the other options are suggestive of raised intracranial pressure.

5 True These answers are taken from the CancerBackup site.

6 True Maximum would be grade 10.

7 False In advanced disease, hormone therapy to cause androgen deprivation (usually with a luteinising hormone-releasing hormone analogue) would be first line.

8 **True** Shown to be as effective as external beam radiation therapy and radical prostatectomy up to T2a.

9 **False** Active surveillance may be suitable but would involve 3-monthly prostate-specific antigen testing, re-imaging and biopsy at 12–18 months.

10 **c** This question on colorectal cancer is taken from the *Drugs and Therapeutics Bulletin* (2006; 44(9)) and the NHS screening information, and updated from ongoing papers and reviews. Hormone replacement therapy is known to reduce the risk of colorectal cancer but not yet mortality; aspirin 300 mg daily is known to prevent and reduce recurrence of adenocarcinomas, not mortality. Neither flexible sigmoidoscopy nor colonoscopy is known to reduce mortality, although they are excellent methods for investigation and screening.

Statement 13

Care of people with mental health problems

The Mental Capacity Act 2005

www.opsi.gov.uk/ACTS/acts2005/ukpga_20050009_en_1

The Mental Capacity Act 2005 was revised from 1983 and came fully into force on 1 October 2007. The act defines 'mental disorder' as 'any disability or disorder of the mind or brain whether permanent or temporary which results in an impairment or disturbance of mental functioning'. Not only is the definition broad but also it is an emotive subject, where patients and public have preconceived ideas, especially with regard to loss of rights. The reformed act goes some way towards addressing difficult issues but it is important to remember there is a distinct difference in treating mental disorders and in exercising social control.

A New Mental Health (and Public Protection) Act was first published in 1959, the main issues being that decisions on involuntary treatment for mental disorders became primarily a matter for doctors. Limits to medical discretion were set out in 1983.

The key issues with regard to mental health are:

- Risk of patients to themselves and others:
  - Care and treatment provided should reflect the best interests of the patient.
- Simpler template for formal assessment:
  - Assessment will be conducted by two doctors and an approved social worker.
  - The template will be set out in a formal care plan, which must be of 'direct therapeutic benefit' or address the management of 'behaviours arising from the disorder'.
  - After 28 days compulsory treatment would have to be re-authorised by the Mental Health Tribunal (a new independent body).
  - It will be followed by a care and treatment order applicable in both civil and criminal justice, which would be made by the Mental Health Tribunal or by a court.
- Care and treatment in the community:
  - Care and treatment orders may apply to patients outside hospital.
  - There will be contingency plans if patients refuse to take their medication in the community to prevent patients becoming a risk to themselves and others.
- Safeguards:
  - There is entitlement to free legal service.
  - There is a statutory obligation for care plans.
  - The Mental Health Tribunal is an independent body taking advice from the

clinical team, patients, independent experts and other agencies. It is also concerned with long-term use of compulsory powers. It may exceptionally reserve the right not to accept the clinical supervisor's decision to discharge a patient if there is serious risk of harm to others.
- The New Commission for Mental Health has responsibilities for maintaining formal powers and looking after people subject to care and treatment orders.

Assessing lack of capacity is a fundamental part of the act. A person is regarded as lacking in capacity if they are unable to:
- understand and retain information to enable them to make a decision
- consider the information
- communicate their decision.

This is in keeping with the General Medical Council guidance on consent in that, for it to be valid (i.e. a decision to consent), it must be informed, competent, uncoerced and continuing. The government website (www.justice.gov.uk/about/opg.htm) has information and forms for lasting power of attorney.

Admission under compulsion

This is only to be used where the patient is suffering from a mental disorder and cannot be persuaded to enter hospital voluntarily. Never use this lightly and always keep comprehensive notes. Acceptance by the receiving hospital is necessary.

Section 2: Assessment

- Should be used where possible (Section 4 may be more appropriate in general practice).
- Applied for by an approved social worker or nearest relative.
- Supported by two doctors (one of whom must be section 12 approved and one with knowledge of the patient). The two doctors need to examine the patient within 5 days of each other.
- The maximum length of stay is 28 days.

Section 3: Admission and treatment

- Application is based on two medical recommendations.
- Length of stay is 6 months initially, typically following on from Section 2.

Section 4: Emergency in the community

- The maximum duration of admission is 72 hours.
- It is applied for by an approved social worker or nearest relative.
- It is supported by one doctor, who should have previous knowledge of the patient if possible. Both individuals must have seen the patient within 24 hours.

Depression

- The annual incidence of depression is 8%–12%.
- The economic cost in the United Kingdom is £8 billion each year (*BMJ*, 2006).

- The rate of depression in nursing/residential homes is 22%–33% (*New Generalist*, 2005).

Diagnostic and Statistical Manual of Mental Disorders, fourth edition, diagnostic scale

Five of the following options should be present over a 2-week period for the diagnosis of major depression (a score of 5–6 is moderate depression):

- At least one of the following:
  - depressed mood or irritability
  - loss of interest or pleasure.
- Plus three or four of the following (to make a total of five options):
  - appetite or weight loss
  - sleep loss/change in sleep pattern
  - psychomotor agitation or retardation
  - fatigue/loss of energy
  - worthlessness or guilt
  - poor concentration
  - recurrent suicidal thoughts/thoughts of death.

These criteria are useful in differentiating between low mood and clinical depression. In chronic depressive illness (dysthymia), be aware that patients may not meet these criteria but they could still benefit from drug treatment in the short term. GPs can improve identification of depression (it is estimated that we miss up to 50% of cases) by asking open questions, having good eye contact and not interrupting our patients.

Depression: the treatment and management of depression in adults

www.nice.org.uk/nicemedia/live/12329/45888/45888.pdf

The recommendations are presented in a practical stepped care (steps 1–4) starting with recognition of depression and going through treatment options based on severity of symptoms. The key priorities for implementation build upon the National Service Framework for Mental Health.

Screening questionnaires

These are useful to aid diagnosis and monitor progress. Although there are some data about reliability in certain age groups, less is known about the sensitivity and specificity cross-culturally.

- **Patient Health Questionnaire (PHQ-9)** – not ideal for older patients.
- **Hamilton Depression Rating Scale** – not ideal for older people, as it includes a number of somatic items that may be positive in older people who are not depressed.
- **Geriatric Depression Scale** – designed for elderly people, it avoids somatic items.
- **Beck Depression Inventory** – designed for patients with more severe depression, it tackles suicidal thinking.

- **Edinburgh Postnatal Depression Scale** – more sensitive than other scales in post-natal women.
- **Abbreviated Mental Test Score** – can be used as a guide to dementia.

Geriatric Depression Scale

1	Are you basically satisfied with your life?	Yes/**No**
2	Have you dropped many of your activities or interests?	**Yes**/No
3	Do you feel that your life is empty?	**Yes**/No
4	Do you often get bored?	**Yes**/No
5	Are you in good spirits most of the time?	Yes/**No**
6	Are you afraid that something bad is going to happen to you?	**Yes**/No
7	Do you feel happy most of the time?	Yes/**No**
8	Do you feel helpless?	**Yes**/No
9	Do you prefer to stay at home rather than going out and doing new things?	**Yes**/No
10	Do you feel you have more problems with memory than most?	**Yes**/No
11	Do you think it is wonderful to be alive now?	Yes/**No**
12	Do you feel pretty worthless the way you are now?	**Yes**/No
13	Do you feel full of energy?	Yes/**No**
14	Do you feel your situation is hopeless?	**Yes**/No
15	Do you think that most people are better off than you are?	**Yes**/No

Scoring: answers indicating depression are in bold type. Each answer given indicating depression receives 1 point. The patient should not see this scoring guidance. A score >5 indicates probable depression.

Psychometric comparison of PHQ-9 and HADS for measuring depression severity in primary care

Br J Gen Pract 2008; 58(546): 32–6

In satisfying the Quality and Outcomes Framework it is now important to detain a depression scale score. Both of these scales (the PHQ-9 and the HADS, advocated by the British Medical Association) were shown to be highly consistent and equally reliable. They differed in how they categorised severity (which may have an impact on treatment decisions), PHQ-9 categorising a greater severity than HADS.

Should we screen for depression?

BMJ 2006; 332: 1027–30

Screening for depression would be in keeping with the National Screening Committee criteria; however, screening alone cannot improve management and outcome of depression and the cost would be significant (currently we see case findings as part of the chronic disease Quality and Outcomes Framework criteria; see questions later in the chapter). On review of the literature, this article summarises that screening is unlikely to improve the well-being of the population.

Drug treatment in depression

You need to ask yourself what you are trying to achieve:

- improvement in mood, social and occupational function, quality of life
- reduction in morbidity and mortality
- prevention of a recurrence
- minimisation of adverse effects of treatment.

Antidepressants

Systematic reviews have shown that there is no clinically significant difference in effectiveness between different classes of drugs. All have an improvement of 50%–60%. On average people on selective serotonin reuptake inhibitors are less likely to stop treatment because of side effects. The selective serotonin reuptake inhibitors are now prescribed first line because of this. It is important to be aware of potential drug interactions, and to use recognised side effects to benefit the patient. If there are no side effects the drug should be used for 6 weeks before changing class or increasing dose. When stopping the drug, tail off over 4 weeks (depending upon the patient and symptoms).

St John's wort (*Hypericum perforatum*)

This is a low-grade monoamine oxidase inhibitor that is widely dispensed over the counter for low mood and depression. A systematic review of 27 studies (Cochrane Library, 1999) concluded that it was more effective than placebo. However, various different preparations of hypericum were used in each study.

It is worth noting that hypericum can induce liver enzymes and may interact with digoxin, theophylline, warfarin and the combined oral contraceptive pill (consult the British National Formulary). Also, hypericum products widely differ in composition.

Acute treatment of moderate to severe depression with hypericum extract WS 5570 (St John's wort: randomised controlled double blind non-inferiority trial versus paroxetine

BMJ 2005; 330(7490): 503

This study found that 90 mg/day of hypericum extract (WS5570) three times a day (increased if no response after 6 weeks) was at least as effective after 42 days (assessed with the Hamilton Depression Scale) as paroxetine 20 mg (or 40 mg if the dose had to be increased).

Non-drug treatments

Cognitive behavioural therapy

Cognitive behavioural therapy (CBT) is a structured treatment aimed at changing dysfunctional beliefs and negative automatic thoughts that contribute to patient's problems. This form of treatment requires the therapist to have a high level of training based on the original Beck and Ellis models. Typically there would be 16–20 sessions offered. The simple understanding is that CBT and problem-solving are successful, whereas counselling, although less successful, does have a higher patient satisfaction. More recent studies looking at long-term outcomes report, on the whole, no difference between groups.

Chocolate craving when depressed: a personality marker

Br J Psychiatry 2007; 191: 351–2

We all know that chocolate isn't all bad and we probably subscribe to the fact that it probably increases serotonin levels, albeit temporarily, in the brain. It has also been shown to reduce blood pressure. This study looked at 2692 people over the age of 18 and found 45% craved chocolate when depressed, a significant association between craving and severe depression.

Counselling in general practice

Around 51% of general practices have an on-site counsellor. Counselling is designed to help people work on their problems and become more skilled in helping themselves. It is a disciplined psychological intervention that requires specialist training in the different styles (e.g. directive, informative, confrontational, supportive and so forth). There is documented evidence that if selected appropriately then it is effective. Counsellors have their own professional code of ethics and practice. They must hold a current membership of a professional body, the British Association of Counselling. Appropriate referral and assessment is essential for cost-effective intervention. Most counsellors offer 6–12 sessions.

Suitable candidates for brief focal counselling, include those who:

- are able to express feelings and thoughts
- are able to trust the counsellor
- have mild to moderate difficulties (e.g. depression, relationship problems, anxiety, bereavement, emotional or psychological difficulties)
- are able to bear disturbing or conflicting feelings.

Unsuitable candidates include those who:

- have moderate to severe difficulties (e.g. schizophrenia, dementia, substance abuse, personality disorders, risk of suicide)
- are silent or withdrawn
- are prone to over intellectualisation
- have no close relationships
- lack of ability to think about self.

The Royal College of Psychiatrists (www.rcpsych.ac.uk) has a useful site with access to information on CBT and psychotherapy in the section providing mental health information. Increasingly, neurolinguistic programming is being used either alongside CBT or as an alternative approach, but practitioners are not reliably available on the NHS.

Mindfulness-based cognitive behavioural therapy

This is a CBT technique based on meditation that patients can use protectively to identify their own thoughts and recognise the impact they can have on their feelings and emotions. It seems to be able to reduce relapse rates for depression. At the moment it is available on a private basis (www.bemindful.co.uk).

Schizophrenia

www.nice.org.uk/nicemedia/live/11786/43610/43610.pdf
www.rcpsych.ac.uk/mentalhealthinformation.aspx

Schizophrenia was first described in the eighteenth century. There is a 1% lifetime prevalence (mainly seen in 20- to 30-year-olds), with 25% of patients being cared for by their GP. The diagnosis is made based on the World Health Organization's International Classification of Disease (ICD-10), which looks for clear evidence of past or present psychosis, absence of prominent affective symptoms and a minimum duration of illness. We also need to look for negative symptoms such as blunted affect or poor motivation.

Schneider's first-rank symptoms are:

- auditory hallucinations
- thought withdrawal or insertion
- thought broadcasting
- somatic passivity
- feelings or actions perceived as being under external control
- delusional perceptions.

Schizophrenia: core interventions in the treatment and management of schizophrenia in primary and secondary care (2009)

www.nice.org.uk/nicemedia/live/11786/43610/43610.pdf

These guidelines are relevant to adults over 18 years of age and to those diagnosed with schizophrenia below the age of 60 years. There are three phases:

1 Initiation of treatment (first episode)

- Early referral to secondary care and involvement of other services.
- Early treatment – suggests discussion with psychiatrist and urgent referral; consider atypicals first line, e.g. olanzepine.

2 Treatment of acute episode

- Single drug – administer in British National Formulary dose range for minimum of 6 weeks and monitor response.
- May need rapid tranquillisation.
- Be aware of side effects, e.g. risk of diabetes and weight gain with some atypicals.
- Address other needs: psychological, social, occupational and so forth.

There is a high risk of relapse. If treating a relapse you need to continue treatment for 1–2 years and slowly withdraw treatment thereafter, monitoring for 2 years after the last acute episode.

3 Promoting recovery (primary care)

- Care register (essential).

- Monitor mental health and treatment alongside secondary care.
- Consider referral in the following circumstances:
  - problem with compliance
  - poor response to treatment
  - suspected co-morbid substance misuse
  - increased risk to self or others
  - new to practice list – for assessment and care programme
  - where service users prefer not to receive care from GP.

DOCUMENT EVERYTHING CLEARLY

The following are essential across all phases:

- optimism
- get help early
- assessment
- working in partnership
- consent and accurate information
- addressing language and culture
- addressing the issue of advance directives (although limited in schizophrenia).

Eating disorders

www.nice.org.uk/nicemedia/live/10932/29218/29218.pdf

Anorexia nervosa

BMJ 2007; 334(7599): 894–8

The prevalence for anorexia is 0.3% (there is an even distribution across all social classes), and 80%–90% are young females, with the average age of onset being 15 years. It is the most common cause of weight loss in women. Up to 20% of those with anorexia nervosa will die as a result of their illness, death being more likely if weight fluctuates rapidly.

Many people do not ask for help, so as GPs we can play a vital role in detection of these illnesses, looking for presenting features such as depression, obsessive behaviour, infertility and amenorrhoea. All five IDC-10 criteria must be met before a diagnosis is made (the American Psychiatric Association stated in 1994 that if the diagnostic criteria for both bulimia and anorexia are met, the diagnosis of anorexia takes precedence).

Recognised risk factors include genetic factors (we don't know what is inherited, possibly a vulnerable personality type), cultural values, childhood obesity, early onset of puberty, adverse life experiences, extreme shyness, bullying, family functional style and low self-esteem. You will notice that a lot of clues boil down to personality traits.

Early diagnosis and intervention gives better outcome. CBT and selective serotonin receptor inhibitors have both been shown to improve short-term outcome compared with placebo. It is not yet clear if remission rates are reduced (Cochrane Library).

Standards 2 and 3 of the Mental Health National Services Framework outline the need to improve healthcare for patients with anorexia nervosa and bulimia nervosa.

Attention deficit disorder

***Attention Deficit Hyperactivity Disorder: diagnosis and management of ADHD in children, young people and adults*, NICE (2008)**

www.nice.org.uk/nicemedia/live/12061/42107/42107.pdf

This guidance gives an overview of diagnosis (based on ICD10 or DSM IV hyperkinetic disorder) looking at management options, side effects and involvements of other agencies such as schools.

Hyperactivity affects 1%–2% of children. Prescribing in attention deficit disorder has gradually increased over the last few years. Although these treatments are licensed it is recommended that they are only prescribed following specialist input.

- Methylphenidate is a sympathomimetic amine that works on dopamine receptors.
- It is used as part of the comprehensive treatment programme (paediatric and psychiatric).
- It is not licensed for children under 6 years, or in cases of thyrotoxicosis or tics.
- Continued prescribing and monitoring may be performed by GPs under a shared care agreement.

Benefits can be obtained with medication, behavioural therapy and educational support. Dietary supplements such as flax oil, vitamin C and omega 3 are receiving a lot of attention and there is anecdotal evidence for excluding some colourings and preservatives.

Both the parents and the GP influence access to treatment. It can lead to conflict, misunderstanding and dissatisfaction if a parent's concerns are not taken seriously.

Current research is focusing on cognitive processing, genetic factors, brain function abnormalities and the significance of co-morbidity factors.

Attention-deficit hyperactivity disorder

Lancet 2005; 366(9481): 237–48

This review estimates that this disorder of inattention and impulsivity and hyperactivity can affect up to 12% of children worldwide and that at least half of the children affected will have impairing symptoms into adulthood. It also considers treatment with methylphenidate and amphetamine effective, as well as targeted psychosocial treatments.

Care of people with mental health problems: questions

1 Admission under compulsion: which of the following would be the most appropriate section to use for a patient who, despite treatment, is suffering from severe depression and has a high risk of injuring themselves or another person? They need to be detained urgently, so it is not appropriate to delay detainment in order to get a second medical opinion.

a. Section 2

b. Section 3

c. Section 4
d. Section 5
e. Section 17

2 Generalised anxiety: in Step 3, the point at which pharmacological treatment is introduced, which of the following is the suggested treatment for generalised anxiety disorder?
a. Escitalopram
b. Citalopram
c. Fluoxetine
d. Diazepam
e. Sertraline

3 Cognitive behavioural therapy: the process of CBT helps develop new behaviours by modifying unhelpful thinking styles, which in turn reduces anxiety-linked behaviour. Which of the following conditions has the least sound evidence in a base for success with CBT?
a. Depression.
b. Borderline personality disorders.
c. Sexual dysfunction.
d. Acute psychoses.
e. Chronic fatigue.

4 Suicide: which of the following is a risk factor for suicide?
a. Female.
b. Living in a household of four or more people.
c. Smokers.
d. Aged over 42 years.
e. Schizophrenia.

5 Eating disorders: which of the following is not a recognised stem in the SCOFF questionnaire?
a. Do you believe yourself to be fat when others say you are too thin?
b. Have you recently lost more than 1 kg in a 3-month period?
c. Would you say that food dominates your life?
d. Do you make yourself sick because you feel uncomfortably full?
e. Do you worry you have lost control over how much you eat?

6 Schizophrenia: which of the following would form your differential when diagnosing schizophrenia?
a. Persistent delusional disorder.
b. Hypokalaemia.
c. Hyponatraemia.
d. Menopause.
e. Ischaemic cerebrovascular accident.

7 Obsessive-compulsive disorder: which of the following has not been reliably shown to help treatment of obsessive-compulsive disorder?
a. Counselling.
b. CBT.
c. Fluoxetine.

d. Seroxat.
e. Clomipramine.

Care of people with mental health problems: answers

1 c Section 2 is based on two medical recommendations and would allow detainment for 28 days to allow assessment. Section 3 is based on two medical recommendations to allow detainment for up to 6 months for treatment; this cannot be enforced if the nearest relative objects. Section 4 is the correct answer, allowing emergency detainment for 72 hours; only one medical recommendation is needed. Section 5 allows a patient who is already voluntarily in hospital to be detained. Section 17 allows authorised leave of a patient who is detained under the act.

2 e Sertraline is thought to be the most effective, although will not suit all patients. Diazepam is only used for short courses in times of crisis.

3 d CBT is the treatment of choice for depression, phobias, anxiety, post-traumatic stress disorders and habit disorders. There is evidence for effectiveness in chronic fatigue, psychoses, anger, stress and personality and eating disorders. In an acute psychotic episode there is little ability to rationalise thought processes, meaning that CBT would not be a treatment of choice.

4 e Suicide is the most common cause of death in men younger than 35 years, and 5000 people take their own lives each year. Risk factors include the following: male, living alone, unemployed, alcohol and drug misuse, mental illness.

5 b See 'The SCOFF questionnaire: assessment of a new screening tool for eating disorders' (*BMJ* 1999; 319(7223): 1467–8). Dr J Morgan and colleagues at George's Hospital, London, designed the SCOFF questionnaire in order to give specialists a simple screening tool with which to identify eating disorders. It comprises five questions. Score 1 point for each 'yes' answered. A score >2 indicates a likely problem.

- Do you make yourself **Sick** because you feel uncomfortably full?
- Do you worry you have lost **Control** over how much you eat?
- Have you recently lost more than **One** stone in a 3-month period?
- Do you believe yourself to be **Fat** when others say you are too thin?
- Would you say that **Food** dominates your life?

The researchers compared this tool with more lengthy questionnaires and had excellent results of 100% sensitivity and 87.5% specificity (12.5% false positive rate).

6 a See 'Clinical review on schizophrenia' in *GP* (14 May 2010). Differential diagnosis would include:

- Organic psychoses: drug use or withdrawal, epilepsy, tumours, human immunodeficiency virus, neurosyphilis, thyroid disorders, heavy metal or carbon monoxide poisoning.
- Drug induced: cannabis, amphetamines, cocaine.
- Functional psychoses: affective disorders, persistent delusional disorders.

- Dementia.
- Post-traumatic stress disorder and schizotypal personality disorder.

7 a CBT is specifically the type of therapy found to be helpful in obsessive-compulsive disorder. Although clomipramine is a tricyclic antidepressant it is also a potent serotonin reuptake inhibitor. This question is based on a *Pulse* article written by David Veale (20 April 2011).

Statement 14

Care of people with learning disabilities

There are many stakeholders within the term 'care of people with learning disabilities': the patients, families and caregivers, social care, medical care, psychiatric care and the role of charitable organisations.

The Royal College of General Practitioners recently published *A Step by Step Guide for GP practices: annual health checks for people with learning disabilities* (www.rcgp.org.uk/pdf/CIRC_A%20Step%20by%20Step%20Guide%20for%20Practices%20(October%2010).pdf). This goes hand in hand with the Enhances Services, as part of the General Medical Services contract, and both seem to have developed from the 2007 Mencap 'Death by indifference' campaign.

The step-by-step guide begins with principles from the 2006 Canadian guidelines:

- The dignity of people with learning disability, based on their intrinsic value as human beings, requires respect and does not diminish with the absence or reduction in any ability.
- People with learning disability are nurtured throughout life by human relationships.
- Primary care providers need to take into account health issues particular to adults with learning disabilities, with or without a specific cause.

The health checks should be offered annually, as it is recognised that people with learning disabilities have poorer health than the general population, and it is recommended that there is a 30-minute nurse appointment followed by a 30-minute doctor appointment.

The aims of these health checks are:

- To improve health outcomes for people with learning disabilities.
- To help identify and treat medical conditions early.
- To screen for health issues particular to people with learning difficulties and specific conditions.
- To improve access to generic health promotion in people with learning difficulties.
- To develop relationships with GPs, practice nurses and primary care staff, particularly after the comprehensive paediatric care finishes at the age of 18.

The guide provides templates for suggested letters to use when inviting patients for health checks. These letters are created using a pictorial format, which may increase uptake. The guide also provides templates for clinical use in the assessment/health check.

Consent and capacity are important to understand (as discussed in other statements of the curriculum), although 'best interest' considerations may apply.

The specific syndrome checklists are for Down's, Fragile X, Rett's and Williams's syndromes. Checklists for Angelman's, Kabuki and Noonan's syndromes are also available.

Care of people with learning disabilities: questions

1 Which of the following sets of blood tests should be requested prior to an annual health check of a patient with a learning disability?
   a. FBC, U&E, LFT, fasting glucose, bone profile.
   b. FBC, U&E, LFT, HbA1c, random glucose, TFT, CRP.
   c. FBC, U&E, LFT, HbA1c, PSA (for men)/FSH (for women).
   d. FBC, U&E, LFT, fasting glucose, ESR.
   e. FBC, U&E, LFT, calcium and phosphate, ESR, CRP, fasting glucose and lipids.

2 Which of the following is the most common problem seen in people with learning difficulties present within the community?
   a. Coeliac disease.
   b. Angina/ischaemic heart disease.
   c. Asthma.
   d. Chronic obstructive pulmonary disease.
   e. Skin infections.

3 Which of the following would be an appropriate scale to use when assessing depression in a patient with a learning disability?
   a. GDS
   b. PHQ-9
   c. HAD
   d. GDS-LD
   e. GDS-CS

For questions 4–7, select the most correct syndrome from the following list. Each answer can be used once, more than once or not at all.
   a. Down's syndrome
   b. Fragile X syndrome
   c. Rett's syndrome
   d. Williams's syndrome
   e. Noonan's syndrome
   f. Kabuki syndrome
   g. Angelman's syndrome

4 Which syndrome is the most common cause of inherited learning difficulty?

5 Which syndrome is typified by a long face, large jaw, prominent ears and enlarged testicles (post puberty)?

6 What condition has associated opthalmic problems that include cataracts, glaucoma, keratoconus and refractive errors?

7 Which syndrome has similar clinical features to Turner's syndrome, with additional characteristics of a broad forehead, downward-slanting eyes, flat nasal bridge and congential heart problems affecting the right side of the heart (as compared with the left in Turner's)?

Care of people with learning disabilities: answers

1 b Follicle-stimulating hormone test is recommended for women who haven't had a period for 6 months. Prostate-specific antigen test is recommended for men over the age of 50. Calcium and vitamin D levels are recommended if on antiepileptic drugs, if there is poor sun exposure or if the patient is from a black or ethnic minority. Lithium and antiepileptic drug levels before the morning dose ('trough' level if patients are on this type of medication).

2 e Coeliac disease is seen at increased incidence in Down's syndrome (dermatitis herpetiformis may be the presentation). A Dutch study in 2007 found that epilepsy and skin infections were the most common presenting problems in primary care.

3 d The GDS is the Geriatric Depression Scale. The GDS-LD is the Glasgow Depression Score for People with a Learning Disability (http://bjp.rcpsych.org/content/182/4/347.full). The GDS-CS is the Carer Supplement to the GDS-LD. The PHQ-9 is the Patient Health Questionnaire, and the HAD is the **HA**milton **D**epression Rating Scale.

4 b

5 b

6 a

7 e Prognosis in Noonan's is dependent on the cardiac problems experienced.

Statement 15.1

Cardiovascular problems

This section will go through some of the conditions that come under the broad heading of cardiovascular problems. The National Institute for Health and Clinical Excellence (NICE) have a comprehensive selection of guidelines that will take your revision nicely through this area (http://guidance.nice.org.uk/Topic/Cardiovascular). It is extensive, so allow a reasonable amount of time for this.

Cardiovascular disease risk assessments

This is bread-and-butter general practice. Know the difference between primary and secondary prevention!

Individuals are at increased risk of developing cardiovascular disease (CVD) if they are smokers, hypertensive, diabetic or have dyslipidaemias. It is also known that obesity, increased waist-to-hip ratio, increased alcohol consumption, family history and ethnicity all increase an individual's risk. It can be argued that preventing CVD is one of the most important tasks for GPs, and cardiovascular risk assessments have been introduced for all patients over the age of 40 in England.

Absolute risk is the probability of developing coronary heart disease (non-fatal myocardial infarction or coronary death) over a defined period of time and this can be estimated using risk assessment charts. These help us to explain risks to the patients, which in turn empowers them to make informed choices on available options. The information from the charts should not replace clinical judgement.

Problems with risk assessment tables

Risk assessment tables are valuable in primary prevention: they have given us a place to start, and they have helped us work out levels of treatment and communicate risk to patients. However, no system is perfect. You need to be aware which risk assessment tool your computer is using/what has been included in the templates. Some of the main concerns with the use of risk assessment tables are as follows:

- Tables usually calculate a 10-year risk and this becomes inaccurate with blood pressure and lifestyle changes over time, so you need to reassess periodically. JBS is considering a lifetime risk assessment, which we would be able to apply to patients under 50 years of age.
- They can be time-consuming to include opportunistically in a consultation (despite IT facilities) if done properly.
- They do not always take into account ethnicity (which can increase the risk by around 1.5, for example in the Framingham risk scores).
- They underestimate the risk if there is a strong family history of coronary heart disease below 65 years of age, or hyperlipidaemia (in these cases it is thought you need to increase the risk estimate by a factor of 1.5).

- They are dependent on you assessing variables correctly.
- How often do you assess/reassess risk?

Hypertension

You will be dealing with hypertension every day of your working life. While there are clinically grey areas that are open for debate, the guidelines are sound and easy to understand and put into practice.

British Hypertension Society guidelines, 2004

J Hum Hypertens 2004; 18(3): 139–85 and *BMJ* 2004; 328(7440): 634–40 (summary)

The British Hypertension Society published a 2004 update of previous guidelines (1989, 1993 and 1999). The guidelines state that the main determinant of benefit from blood pressure–lowering drugs is the achieved blood pressure rather than the choice of therapy.

They can be summarised as follows:

- Start antihypertensive treatment in patients with:
  - a sustained systolic blood pressure (BP) >160 mmHg
  - a sustained diastolic BP >100 mmHg.
- Start antihypertensive treatment in diabetic patients who have:
  - systolic BP >140 mmHg
  - diastolic BP >90 mmHg.
- Treat borderline BP (140–159/90–99 mmHg) if there is target organ damage, CVD, diabetes or a 10-year CVD risk >20% (this is equivalent to the coronary heart disease risk of around 15%).
- Optimal BP targets, in non-diabetics are:
  - systolic BP <140 mmHg
  - diastolic BP <85 mmHg.

The minimum acceptable control for audit purposes is 150/90 mmHg, and for patients with diabetes, chronic renal disease and established CVD it is 130/80 mmHg.

- Give non-pharmacological advice to all hypertensives (and borderline hypertensives).
- Consider statins to reduce cardiovascular risk in:
  - primary prevention, where the 10-year cardiovascular risk factor is >20%
  - secondary prevention, where high BP is complicated by CVD (irrespective of the baseline total cholesterol).

Optimal cholesterol lowering should reduce the total cholesterol by 25% (or low-density lipoprotein-cholesterol by 30%), or achieve a cholesterol <4.0 mmol/L (or low-density lipoprotein-cholesterol <2.0 mmol/L) – whichever is the greater reduction.

- Consider aspirin (75 mg/day), when the BP is controlled (<150/90 mmHg) in:
  - primary prevention if over 50 years of age with a 10-year CVD risk >20%
  - secondary prevention of ischaemic CVD.

Hypertension: clinical management of primary hypertension in adults **(2011)**
www.nice.org.uk/nicemedia/live/13561/56015/56015.pdf

- If clinic BP is >140/90 mmHg, offer ambulatory monitoring to diagnose hypertension (use average value of at least 14 measurements).
- If home readings used – three readings a minute apart, with the patient seated, done in the morning and evening preferably for 7 days (although 4 days would do), assess target organ damage: albumin-to-creatinine ratio, blood, ECG and fundoscopy.
- Medication is as shown in the table, where A is an angiotensin-converting enzyme (ACE) inhibitor or an angiotensin receptor blocker (ARB), C is a calcium channel blocker and D is a diuretic.

	Age <55 years	Age >55 years, or black person of Afro-Caribbean origin at any age
Step 1	A	C
Step 2	A + C	
Step 3	A + C + D	
Step 4	A + C + D + other diuretic, alpha blocker or beta blocker Consider referral	

Do remember that there may be certain instances where it may be sensible to not follow the order of the guidelines.

Myocardial infarction

For us in primary care the question we ask is along the lines of: 'Is this history suggestive of a myocardial infarction and do I need a blue light?'

Classification is now working towards types 1–5 based on the 2007 'universal definition' which considers history, ECG, troponin I or T levels (above the 99th percentile, with a coefficient variation of <10%). This in turn determines not only inpatient management but also the need for cardiovascular risk modification that we will need to address in our management of these patients.

Type 1: Spontaneous myocardial infarction (MI) related to ischaemia caused by a primary coronary event, such as plaque fissuring or rupture.
Type 2: MI secondary to ischaemia resulting from an imbalance between oxygen supply and demand, such as coronary spasm.
Type 3: Sudden death from cardiac disease, with symptoms of MI, accompanied by new ST elevation or left bundle branch block, in this type of MI death occurs before blood samples can be taken.
Type 4: MI associated with primary percutaneous intervention.
Type 5: MI associated with coronary artery bypass graft.

New definition of myocardial infarction (*BMJ* 2008; 337: a3078).

***MI: secondary prevention* (2007)**
www.nice.org.uk/nicemedia/pdf/CG48NICEGuidance.pdf

- Lifestyle:
  - Dietary advice should include advice to have 7 g omega-3 oil a week (not beta-carotene or antioxidant supplements) and encourage a Mediterranean-style diet.
  - Alcohol consumption should be within the current recommended limits (14 units a week for women and 21 units a week for men).
  - Encourage physical activity and smoking cessation advice.
  - Encourage to achieve and maintain a healthy weight.
- Cardiac rehabilitation – should be offered to all patients who are stable.
- Drug therapy – after an MI in the last 12 months:
  - All patients should be offered a combination of ACE inhibitor, aspirin (and clopidogrel for 12 months if non-ST-segments elevation acute coronary syndrome), beta blocker and statin.
- Drug therapy – after an MI >12 months ago:
  - ACE inhibitors, statins and aspirin should be continued if tolerated.
  - Beta blockers if started post-MI should be continued, otherwise do not start unless they are at increased risk of a further cardiovascular event.

Heart failure

Wilson described heart failure in 1997 as a complex clinical syndrome characterised by 'abnormalities in left ventricular function, neurohormonal regulation, exercise intolerance, shortness of breath, fluid retention and reduced longevity'.

- Prevalence is 3–20 per 1000 among the general population.
- Prevalence is 100 per 1000 if over 65 years of age.
- Afro-Caribbean people aged over 65 years are at 2.5 times greater risk than the general population.

Standard 11 of the NSF has targeted heart failure, as it is known that heart failure is underdiagnosed and undertreated. It highlights the need for correct diagnosis and appropriate investigation.

Heart failure is not a diagnosis. It can include features of impaired left ventricular function or reduced cardiac output, seen in a number of conditions. You need to consider causes such as ischaemic heart disease, hypertension, arrhythmias, cardiomyopathy, valvular heart disease and so on, as this will help you deliver the correct management plan. There is poor correlation between symptoms and signs when comparing the echocardiographic findings with the degree of impairment.

Atrial fibrillation

Atrial fibrillation (AF) is the most common tachydysrhythmia diagnosed. It is important to diagnose, as it may be the first sign of heart disease and is an important risk factor for strokes. There is no known cause in 20%–30% of cases; however, the majority of cases are associated with hypertension or structural valvular disease. It is seen in up to 50% of patients with heart failure secondary to ischaemic heart disease.

Overall incidence is 11.5 in men and 8.9 in women. The overall risk increases with age. Management is directed at rate and rhythm control, anticoagulation to reduce stroke and underlying pathology.

Screening

Screening is currently being considered as an option in an attempt to reduce the risk of strokes. Almost without realising, we selectively screen patients with every blood pressure we take, pulse we feel, heart we listen to and ECG we perform.

Anticoagulation

The CHADS scoring system has been used to assess risk of stroke and thromboembolism in patients with AF. More recently, the CHA_2DS_2-VAS_c has been validated against $CHADS_2$ and been found to be better at predicting high-risk patients (*BMJ* 2011; 342: d124). Ongoing studies are questioning whether this is a good enough tool to determine between high- and low-risk patients.

$CHADS_2$	Score	CHA_2DS_2-VAS_c	Score
Congestive heart failure	1	Congestive heart failure	1
History of hypertension	1	History of hypertension	1
Age >75 years	1	Age > 75 years	2
Diabetes	1	Diabetes	1
Stroke or previous transient ischaemic attack	2	Stroke or previous transient ischaemic attack	2
		Vascular disease (including peripheral vascular disease or plaque)	1
		Age >65 years	1
		Sex (female)	1

A score of 2 and above indicates warfarin would be beneficial; a score less than 2 indicates aspirin would be more appropriate.

Cardiovascular problems: questions

1 Which of the following is not used to assess cardiovascular risk in the QRISK assessment tool?
   a. Total cholesterol: high-density lipoprotein ratio.
   b. Family history of heart disease in a first-degree relative <65 years of age.
   c. Being on blood pressure treatment.
   d. Postcode.
   e. Body mass index.

2 The following would indicate treatment is needed to reduce cardiovascular risk.
   a. A QRISK score of 24% but Framingham score of 16%.
   b. A persistent systolic BP of >144 mmHg.
   c. A Framingham-based risk score of 12% in a 68-year-old man whose father died at the age of 69 years from a heart attack.

d. A total cholesterol of 5.6.
e. Left ventricular strain on an ECG done as part of a CVD risk assessment.

3 Other risk factors for CVD: which of the following is thought to have a future role as an indicator for CVD?
a. Erythrocyte sedimentation rate.
b. Calcium level.
c. Fasting magnesium level.
d. Homocysteine.
e. C-reactive protein.

4 In the NICE guidance on hypertension 2011, which of the following statements is correct?
a. All patients should have their blood pressure readings assessed over 3–4 weeks prior to a diagnosis of hypertension being made.
b. Plasma renin should be part of your initial work-up, to allow a baseline to be determined.
c. Natriuretic peptide precursor B gene is helpful in determining prognosis in individual cases of hypertension.
d. Twenty-four-hour ambulatory monitoring should be offered to all patients with two blood pressure readings of >140/90 mmHg.
e. Unless contraindicated all patients should be offered an ACE inhibitor first-line treatment for renal protection.

5 Which of the following is not a rare contributory cause of myocardial infarction?
a. Cocaine use.
b. Vessel occlusion secondary to plaque rupture.
c. Antiphospholipid syndrome.
d. Protein C and factor V Leiden deficiency.
e. Coronary artery dissection.

6 In the acute presentation of a non-ST elevated MI, which of the following antiplatelet regimens is recognised as best current management?
a. Dispersible aspirin 300 mg or dipyridamole 200 mg twice a day if known hypersensitivity to aspirin.
b. Clopidogrel 600 mg should be offered to patients where they will not need angiography in the following 24 hours.
c. A loading dose of 2 × clopidogrel 75 mg followed by maintenance dose for a minimum of 2 years.
d. Dispersible aspirin 900 mg with diamorphine 2.5 mg.
e. A loading dose of 300 mg of clopidogrel followed by 12 months of 75 mg where 6-month mortality is >1.5%.

7 When considering the use of omega-3 in current medical practice, which of the following answers is correct?
a. All patients should be encouraged to eat oily fish on a daily basis.
b. If a patient is not managing to eat 7 g omega-3 a week 6 months post MI, they should be prescribed 1 gm omega-3 ethyl esters.
c. Patients should be encouraged to eat 7 g omega-3 in the form of oily fish a week.

d. If a patient is not managing to eat 7 gm omega-3 a day 6 months post MI, they should be prescribed 1 gm omega-3 ethyl esters.
e. A patient post MI should, as with statins, be offered lifelong treatment with 1 gm a day of omega-3 ethyl esters if they are not achieving 7 gm a day in their diet.

8 Heart failure: which of the following investigations is not considered to be necessary in the diagnosis of heart failure?
a. B-type natriuretic peptide.
b. Two-dimensional echocardiography.
c. N-terminal pro-B-type natriuretic peptide.
d. Chest X-ray.

9 Heart failure: which of the following is a reasonable treatment option in heart failure with left ventricular systolic dysfunction secondary to ischaemic heart disease?
a. First-line treatment of diltiazem started alongside bisoprolol (or other cardioselective beta blocker).
b. First-line angiotensin receptor blocker in patients who are known to have chronic cough and sputum production due to chronic obstructive pulmonary disease, as opposed to ACE inhibitors.
c. Combination of ACE inhibitor and ARB in patients with severe heart failure.
d. Hydralazine in combination with verapamil in patients intolerant of ACE inhibitors and ARBs.
e. First-line beta blockers alongside ACE inhibitors in patients with peripheral vascular disease.

10 AF: a CHADS2 score of 4 would increase the annual risk by which of the following?
a. 1.9%
b. 8.5%
c. 18.2%
d. 31.7%
e. 37.6%

Cardiovascular problems: answers

1 b QRISK is felt to be more reliable than Framingham for the UK population. The original Framingham study (named after a town in Massachusetts) was published in 1971. The main concerns surrounding the use of the Framingham model are that it is based on affluent white patients and that there is no consideration of ethnicity, family history or socio-economic groupings. QRISK was devised using data collated across 531 English and Welsh general practices from 1993 to 2008 (>16 million person-years). It includes ethnicity, age, sex, smoking status, systolic BP, cholesterol, BMI, family history of heart disease <60 years old, treated hypertension and a deprivation score based on postcode. It wasn't included in the NICE 2008 *Lipid Modification* guideline (www.nice.org.uk/nicemedia/live/11982/40675/40675.pdf) because of concerns around validation. Since then the guidance has been amended, leaving the choice of risk assessment tool essentially to us (they also include ASSIGN as being similar to NICE and more predictive of risk than Framingham). 'An independent and external validation of QRISK2 cardiovascular disease risk score: a prospective open cohort study' (*BMJ* 2010; 340: c2442) found that QRISK was better than Framingham at assessing risk over CVD at the 20% threshold.

2 a A BP of 144 is not necessarily indicative of the need to treat. It would depend on the outcome of the CVD risk assessment percentages, whether they are over 20%. The Framingham score of 12%, when multiplied by the suggested 1.5, equates to 18%. Left ventricular strain is important to assess further to determine whether there is left ventricular hypertrophy.

3 d The British Heart Foundation (February 2007) looked at novel risk factors (homocysteine, C-reactive protein and fibrinogen). To be clinically valuable they must be reliably quantifiable and they must help predict more accurately the risk of developing coronary heart disease. At present there is insufficient evidence to use any of these methods, but homocysteine seems to be the most promising. In 2002, the British Cardiac Society presented research showing that elevated homocysteine levels (>12 mmol/L) doubled the risk of a second coronary event but high levels in the UK population are probably due to lack of folate and vitamin B. C-reactive protein, fibrinogen, nitric oxide and vitamin D all have some following in this area, but to a lesser degree than homocysteine. Calcium supplementation risks discussed recently do not correlate with calcium levels and are not applicable to this question.

4 d Plasma renin may be useful in patients on three antihypertensives who still have uncontrolled blood pressure. There is currently a trial (PATHWAY) underway to determine the clinical role of this. Recently, genes NPPA and NPPB have been identified – they influence hypertension due to their effect on stress markers atrial and B-type natriuretic peptides. They have no clinical application at present.

5 b This question is taken from a British Heart Foundation FactFile (May 2011). Plaque rupture in atherosclerotic disease is one of the most common causes of MI. Coronary dissection and procoagulant states are causes of a type 1 MI. Most cases of dissection occur in younger women, often in this group in pregnancy or post partum. Cocaine use is a powerful vasoconstrictor, as well as being thrombogenic and atherogenic.

6 e A loading dose of 300 mg of aspirin (dissolvable or chewable) to then be continued at 75 mg daily indefinitely (unless contraindicated). A loading dose of 300 mg of clopidogrel (600 pre-angiography is not licensed but thought sensible) followed by 75 mg daily, if there are no further events stopping after 12 months. See *Unstable Angina and NSTEMI* (NICE 2010) (www.nice.org.uk/nicemedia/live/12949/47924/47924.pdf).

7 c Omega-3 fish oils have been known to protect against coronary heart disease since the 1970s. The mechanism of action is not fully understood. NICE (*MI: secondary prevention*, 2007 (www.nice.org.uk/nicemedia/live/11008/30493/30493.pdf)) currently recommends that patients eat 7 g of omega-3 per week in

2–4 portions of oily fish. If they are not achieving this and have had an MI in 3 months you should consider prescribing omega-3 ethyl esters for 4 years.

8 d Chest X-ray and ECG are no longer considered to be necessary, other than for the consideration of other diagnoses. Similarly, bloods such as urea and electrolytes and estimated glomerular filtration rate are not diagnostic, but a low estimated glomerular filtration rate could cause raised levels of B-type natriuretic peptide without heart failure being present. Cardiac MRI scan and transoesophageal echocardiography are only considered necessary if there is poor imaging with two-dimensional echocardiography. All of these tools are necessary, as based on history and examination alone our accuracy is less than 50% (GPs and cardiologists alike – Finland and ECHOES study, and more recently the article 'Echocardiography in chronic heart failure in the community' (*Q J Med* 1993; 86(1): 17–23). See *Chronic Heart Failure* (August 2010) (www.nice.org.uk/nicemedia/live/13099/50526/50526.pdf).

9 e See *Chronic Heart Failure* (August 2010) (www.nice.org.uk/nicemedia/live/13099/50526/50526.pdf). ACE inhibitors and beta blockers are first-line treatment for heart failure even in peripheral vascular disease, diabetes, erectile dysfunction and chronic obstructive pulmonary disease. If these aren't tolerated, an ARB is a sensible option, followed by hydralazine and nitrate combination. Verapamil and diltiazem are not the best option of calcium channel blockers. ARB and ACE inhibitors in combination can be considered, but they are rarely used in combination, especially in elderly patients, because of the effects on renal function. Digoxin and spironolactone are both recognised in reducing mortality in heart failure but, especially in the case of spironolactone, they are often underused.

10 b

0 points = 1.9%
1 point = 2.8%
2 points = 4.0%
3 points = 5.9%
4 points = 8.5%
5 points = 12.5%
6 points = 18.2%

Statement 15.2

Digestive problems

Dyspepsia

Dyspepsia is defined as 'chronic or recurrent pain, or discomfort, centred in the upper abdomen'; it is a symptom, not a diagnosis. Gastro-oesophageal reflux disease (GORD) is the term used to describe reflux of gastric contents into the oesophagus causing symptoms such as dyspepsia.

- Annually, 40% of adults will have dyspepsia.
- Five per cent will consult their GP.
- One per cent will be referred for endoscopy.
- Of those having endoscopy, 40% will have a non-ulcer dyspepsia, 40% will have GORD, 13% will have an ulcer and 3% will have a gastric carcinoma.

There is a huge amount of literature published on gastro-oesophageal reflux, *Helicobacter pylori*, ulcer and non-ulcer dyspepsia. I suggest referencing the following for the most up-to-date information:

- National Institute for Health and Clinical Excellence (NICE) guidance
- eGuidelines – summarising guidelines for primary care (www.eguidelines.co.uk)
- Clinical Evidence (www.clinicalevidence.com).

Dyspepsia: management of dyspepsia in adults in primary care

www.nice.org.uk/nicemedia/live/10950/29460/29460.pdf

An important part of our initial assessment in primary care is determining if there are any ALARM features (**A**naemia, weight **L**oss, **A**norexia, **R**efractory problems, **M**elaena or swallowing problems) or an acute gastrointestinal bleed that warrants urgent investigation.

The following have been identified as priorities:

- referral for endoscopy
- interventions for uninvestigated dyspepsia
- interventions for GORD
- interventions for peptic ulcer disease
- interventions for non-ulcer dyspepsia
- reviewing patient care
- *H. pylori* testing and eradication.

Helicobacter pylori

H. pylori is a Gram-negative bacterium that colonises the stomach. It seems to have an aetiological role in gastric and duodenal ulceration, gastric lymphoma, gastric cancer (by anything up to seven times) and colorectal adenoma (*J Gastroenterol*

2005; 40(9): 887–93). Its exact role in these conditions (and in coronary heart disease) is unclear.

- It affects 20% of people under 40 years of age and 50% of people over 60 years.
- Re-infection in adults is rare (<1% per year), so eradication is almost curative.

Management

In cases of confirmed ulcers, eradication speeds healing and reduces recurrence (the number needed to treat = 2). This is not the case in GORD (the number needed to treat = 17). Most guidelines suggest that it is not necessary to test for *H. pylori* if there is a known duodenal ulcer, but, rather, to treat empirically and investigate if there are ALARM symptoms or symptoms do not improve. Triple regimen is more successful than the double; there is no difference between the different triple regimens. One week of treatment is as successful as 2 weeks' treatment.

Non-invasive tests for *H. pylori*

Stool antigen detection tests

These have superseded all other tests and are usually monoclonal tests (polyclonal tests are less sensitive). The specificity and sensitivity are up to 95%, positive predictive value is 84% and you now only need a pea-sized piece of stool. It is not known whether positive tests should ultimately lead to endoscopy to look for secondary pathology. Stool antigen tests should not be performed within 2 weeks of taking proton pump inhibitors or antibiotics.

Serology

Serology does not distinguish between old and active infection (IgG antibodies can remain in the circulation for up to 9 months after eradication), i.e. 50% of positives could be false positives. At present this is a suboptimal test and is not recommended. Its sensitivity is 60%–85%, and specificity is 80%, depending upon which paper you read.

Carbon-13 urea breath test

Urea is hydrolysed by *H. pylori* urease to carbon dioxide and ammonia. The specificity and sensitivity are 95% and positive predictive value is 88%. It is easy to use in primary care (but it does still have to be sent to the lab for analysis). It should not be used while taking antacids/proton pump inhibitors, because this causes false-negative results in some cases. The test becomes negative once *H. pylori* is eradicated. It is more expensive than serology, but it reduces the need for endoscopy so it is more cost-effective in the long run.

Invasive test/endoscopy

Histology

Histology has a sensitivity and specificity >90%. Although it is more invasive and expensive, it is preferable to empirical treatment. It decreases drug consumption, the number of visits to the doctor, and sick leave for 2 years after endoscopy compared with the year before, and patients are generally more satisfied with the treatment. The symptomatic outcome (endoscopy versus empirical treatment) is seen to be similar in the two groups.

Coeliac disease

www.pcsg.org.uk/

Coeliac disease is a gluten-sensitive enteropathy, histologically an inflammatory picture, which affects the small bowel. As part of the baseline investigation, antibodies can be looked for: IgA anti-endomysial antibody (sensitivity 90%, specificity 99%) and IgA anti-transglutaminase antibody (sensitivity 89%, specificity 98%). These are better choices than antigliadin antibody (*JAMA* 2010; 303(17): 1738–46).

Adult coeliac disease

BMJ 2007; 335(7619): 558–62

This is a clinical review of interest. It tabulates conditions known to be associated with ceoliac disease: dermatitis herpetiformis, recurrent aphthous ulcers, iron deficiency anaemia, irritable bowel and so forth. Prevalence is 0.5%–1% internationally and delay to diagnosis can be 4.5–9 years.

Banbury Coeliac Study (January 1999 *BMJ*)

This study was set up to determine the underdiagnosis of coeliac disease, and the principles are still important. In the study 1000 patients were tested for endomysial antibody (other antibody tests could include gliadin and reticulin). Thirty of these patients were positive with a positive biopsy result, 15 out of the 30 presented with anaemia and 25 out of the 30 presented with non-gastrointestinal symptoms. It found only around 20% of patients with coeliac disease are currently being diagnosed.

GPs can prescribe gluten-free foods to patients with coeliac disease or dermatitis herpetiformis but must endorse the prescription 'ACBS' (According to Borderline Substance Act), otherwise the script may be queried or rejected – these prescriptions are not meant to be luxury items. Coeliac UK produces an annual food list of gluten-free products that is available to members (www.coeliac.org.uk).

Compliance to a gluten-free diet has been shown to improve with medical follow-up. The British Society of Gastroenterology suggests that this is done yearly.

Long-term complications include small bowel lymphoma and osteoporosis (up to 50%). The Primary Care Society for Gastroenterology guidelines suggest that a DEXA scan at the time of diagnosis and a repeat after the menopause for women, or at 55 years of age for men. If a fragility fracture occurs at any age then a scan should be done, over and above current guidance for fragility fracture.

The Department of Health advises prophylactic immunisation against pneumococcus in coeliac disease patients over 2 years of age because of the risk of hyposplenism.

Enzyme treatment

Prolyl endonuclease is the enzyme identified that has been found to degrade proteins and the amino acid proline (of which gluten contains around 20%), even at low pH. Although this is purely experimental at the moment, it is thought that in the future it may allow coeliac patients to eat gluten foods.

Colorectal cancer

- Lifetime incidence of colorectal cancer is 5%.
- In the United Kingdom, 16 000 people die each year from colorectal cancer, the second most common cause of cancer death.
- Five per cent of people with bowel cancer have more than one cancer.
- Eighty-five per cent of colorectal cancers occur over the age of 60.
- Around 90% of cases are diet related and 10% genetic (*Gut* 2000; 46(6): 746–8).

Role of the GP

- Identify high-risk patients – early detection improves the 5-year survival.
- Provide detailed counselling and information about causes of colorectal cancer.
- Promote lifestyle issues that may prevent colorectal cancer (over five portions of fruit and vegetables a day, 30-minute brisk exercise daily, stopping smoking and maintaining a BMI 18.5–25 kg/m^2 throughout life).
- See Statement 5 for bowel cancer screening information.

Role of aspirin

There is increasing evidence that aspirin protects against development of colorectal cancer, but its use as a chemoprotective agent is not yet advocated for the general population. High levels of vitamin D (above 100 nmol/L) have also been mentioned in medical journals as being accountable for reducing the risk of colorectal cancer by 40% (*BMJ* 2010; 340: b5500).

Long-term effect of aspirin on colorectal cancer incidence and mortality: 20-year follow-up of five randomised trials

***Lancet* 2010; 376(9754): 1741–50**

In summary, this article found that aspirin of 75 mg taken daily for several years reduced both long-term incidence and mortality due to colorectal cancer, especially so in relation to proximal colon involvement.

Digestive problems: questions

For questions 1–4, chose the single most appropriate answer from the following options for each question/statement. Each answer can be used once, more than once or not at all.

a. Irritable bowel syndrome.
b. Adenocarcinoma.
c. Crohn's disease.
d. Ulcerative colitis.
e. Familial polyposis coli.
f. Barrett's oesophagus.

1 Which option is most likely to be linked with ankylosing spondylosis?

2 Endoscopic surveillance should take place every 2 years in this case.

3 Rome criteria can be applied for this diagnosis.
4 Cigarette smoking reduces susceptibility.

5 Which of the following skin conditions would not usually have a link to inflammatory bowel disease?
   a. Erythema multiforme.
   b. Erythema nodosum.
   c. Pemphigus vulgaris.
   d. Pyoderma gangrenosum.
   e. Urticaria.
6 Which of the following has a high negative predictive value in ruling out inflammatory bowel disease?
   a. Anaemia with a raised mean corpuscular volume.
   b. A raised stool calprotectin level.
   c. Anaemia with a low mean corpuscular volume.
   d. A raised blood calprotectin level.
   e. A negative faecal occult blood test.
7 Hepatitis B: which of the following statements with regard to hepatitis B is correct?
   a. Infection in adults is likely to lead to a chronic infection in 30% of cases.
   b. The United Kingdom is now considered an area of high prevalence.
   c. Vaccinated health professionals who do not mount an immune response to the vaccine are not permitted to work in high-risk fields.
   d. The screening test of choice for infection is hepatitis B surface antigen.
   e. Patients with previous hepatitis B infection should not receive chemotherapy or immunosuppressants because of the risk of reactivation.
8 *Clostridium difficile*: which of the following statements with regard to *C. difficile* is correct?
   a. Amoxicillin is as likely as ciprofloxacillin to cause *C. difficile*.
   b. The Health Protection Agency recommends that all stool in patients over the age of 65 with diarrhoea is tested for *C. difficile*.
   c. If diagnosed and treated promptly there is no risk of toxic megacolon.
   d. Loperamide 2 mg after each loose stool, up to maximum daily dose, is recommended to reduce the risk of hypokalaemia.
   e. There is nothing you can offer, other than supportive treatment, for *C. difficile*.
9 Non-alcoholic fatty liver (NAFLD): although there is no proven therapy for NAFLD, which of the following statements is considered correct?
   a. Weight loss is advised, but it is important not to loose weight too quickly.
   b. Statins are contraindicated.
   c. There is no additional risk of hepatocellular carcinoma.
   d. Although out of licence, metformin is recommended as part of treatment in normoglycaemic patients.
   e. Patients with NAFLD are considered eligible for the seasonal influenza vaccination.

10 Faecal incontinence: with reference to the National Institute for Health and Clinical Excellence guidance, which of the following statements is considered correct?

a. Faecal incontinence may be reversible if secondary to a rectal prolapse.
b. Dietary interventions include adequate hydration with 2–3 L of water per day.
c. Pelvic floor exercises have little effect in faecal incontinence.
d. Patients with cognitive impairment do not respond to initial management focusing on diet, bowel habit, toilet access, medication and coping strategies.
e. Rectal irrigation and stimulation should be considered as first line treatment for faecal incontinence.

Digestive problems: answers

1 d

2 f Barrett's used to be 4 years, but it is now more consistently referenced at 2 years because of the high risk of metaplastic change to oesophageal adenocarcinoma. Barrett's affects 2% of the population; the lifetime risk of change is 5% for men and 3% for women. Familial polyposis coli screening depends on the number of adenomas found and their size; it could be needed on a yearly basis.

3 a Currently, irritable bowel syndrome based on Rome criteria is recurrent abdominal pain or discomfort (meaning an uncomfortable sensation not described as pain) at least 3 days/month in the last 3 months associated with two or more of the following:

- improvement with defaecation
- onset associated with a change in frequency of stool
- onset associated with a change in form (appearance) of stool.

Criteria to have been fulfilled for the last 3 months with symptom onset at least 6 months prior to diagnosis (www.theromefoundation.org/assets/pdf/19_RomeIII_apA_885-898.pdf).

4 a As compared with Crohn's disease, where the risk is increased with smoking.

5 c

6 b Calprotectin is a marker of neutrophil influx into the bowel lumen, and hence it is a sensitive marker of inflammation. It is seemingly a better predictor of relapse than standard markers (ESR and C-reactive protein).

7 d Chronic infection occurs in <5% of cases and is defined as the presence of hepatitis B surface antigen for more than 6 months. The United Kingdom is still considered as having low prevalence (<2%); high prevalence would be >8%. Health professionals can work in these areas but if exposed (e.g. a needle stick injury from a hepatitis B patient) they would need hepatitis B immunoglobulin. If on immunosuppressant treatment or chemotherapy it is recommended that patients with previous infection have antiretroviral treatment for the course of the therapy and for 12 months afterwards.

8 b Broad-spectrum antibiotics (cephalosporins and fluoroquinolones) are more likely than narrow-spectrum antibiotics to cause *C. difficle*. The recommendations from the Health Protection Agency are such because of the waning of the immune system, and thereby increased risk, in elderly patients. Unfortunately, toxic megacolon and death can still happen despite treatment. Loperamide is not advised, as it is an antimotility medication, hence it could increase the risk of toxic megacolon. Although supportive treatment is important, there are other options, such as vancomycin, to help with this infection.

9 a The liver profile can be made worse if weight is lost too quick or if it is in the extreme. Statins aren't contraindicated, but it is important to measure function after starting treatment. There is an increased risk of hepatocellular carcinoma as compared with the general population. Metformin isn't specifically recommended, as trial results have been variable. NAFLD is no longer considered benign, but it does not fall within the criteria for the flu campaign.

10 a Reversible causes of faecal incontinence include rectal prolapse, third-degree haemorrhoids, irritable bowel disease, irritable bowel syndrome, gastrointestinal cancers and disc problems. Fluid intake should be 1.5 L per day; if up to 3 L there is a risk of hyponatraemia. Pelvic floor exercises could significantly improve the incontinence. Although patients with cognitive impairment may need psychogeriatric referral, they do often respond to the measures stated. Irrigation and stimulation are not usually first-line treatment but, rather, are more specialised treatments (www.nice.org.uk/nicemedia/live/11012/30546/30546.pdf).

Statement 15.3

Drug and alcohol problems

Alcohol misuse

www.ic.nhs.uk/webfiles/publications/003_Health_Lifestyles/Alcohol_2011/NHSIC_Statistics_on_Alcohol_England_2011.pdf

- There were 6584 deaths in 2009 directly related to alcohol.
- Around 18% of 11- to 15-year-olds drank in the week prior to the survey, and of these the average consumption was 11.6 units.
- The average weekly intake of alcohol for men is 16.4 units and for women, 8.0.

In men, alcohol consumption >300 g/week is associated with an increased blood pressure and stroke. Drinking of 1–4 units/day in men and 1–2 units/day in women on 5–6 days of the week appears to be protective against coronary heart disease and possibly stroke. Tackling those patients who misuse alcohol and getting them to recognise they are drinking too much is probably where we as GPs could make the biggest impact.

Brief intervention by a GP can be effective, depending upon where your patient is in the cycle of change. The *BMJ* editorial 'Tackling alcohol misuse in the UK' (*BMJ* 2008; 336(7642): 455) highlights the need for higher taxes and restricted availability.

Screening tools

The CAGE screening questionnaire and the Alcohol Use Disorders Identification Test (AUDIT) are the most widely validated methods of screening for alcohol use disorders.

CAGE screening questionnaire

- Have you ever felt you should **C**ut down?
- Have you ever been **A**nnoyed by someone criticising your drinking?
- Have you ever felt **G**uilty about your drinking?
- Have you ever had an **E**ye-opener (early-morning drink) to steady your nerves/get rid of your hangover?

A score of 2 or more has a high correlation with alcoholism but it has a low sensitivity and specificity.

AUDIT

This World Health Organization screening tool is thought to be a more suitable screening test for excessive drinking at the less severe end of the spectrum. It has been found to have a higher sensitivity and specificity than the CAGE screening questionnaire.

Fast Alcohol Screening Test

This is another quick screening test. Here the focus is on the frequency of risky levels of consumption of alcohol and asking the patient to rate the following:

- how often they drink
- to what extent they drink
- whether a friend or health professional has ever been concerned about the amount they drink.

FRAMES

This is an interventional model highlighted as important in the Royal College of General Practitioners curriculum.

Feedback: assessment and evaluation of the problem.
Responsibility: emphasising that drinking is by choice.
Advice: explicit advice on changing drinking behaviour.
Menu: offering alternative goals and strategies.
Empathy: the role of the counsellor is important.
Self-sufficiency: instilling optimism that the chosen goals can be achieved.

'Motivating young adults for treatment and lifestyle change', published in *Issues in Alcohol Use and Misuse in Young Adults* (University of Notre Dame Press, 1993) is also a useful document to read alongside this.

Drug misuse

Illicit drugs are used for their mind-altering effects, highs and in some cases (particularly relating to cannabis) symptom relief in some medical conditions, although this is not a legal use. The harmful effects from long-term use, both medically and socially, are well recognised, and are the driving force behind initiatives such as the National Drug Strategy and the National Service Framework for Children, Young People and Maternity Services (www.drugs.org.uk).

- In 2009/10, there were 5809 admissions to hospital with a primary diagnosis of a drug-related mental health and behavioural disorder.
- In 2009/10, 8.6% of adults had used one or more illicit drugs within the last year, compared with 10.1% in 2008/09.
- The total number of deaths related to drug misuse in England and Wales was 1738 in 2008; 78% of those who died were male. The most common underlying cause of death was from accidental poisoning for both males and females (597 and 166, respectively).

The Substance Misuse Management in General Practice website has the 2007 guidelines available for download (www.smmgp.org.uk/download/clinical/clinicalguidelines.pdf) for use as a framework to aid treatment. They are clear that it is not a case of 'one guideline for all' and that clinical judgement and experience are important.

The GP's role is primarily identification of patients who have and need specialist help, alongside the assessment of motivation. Although there has been an increase in the number of GPs providing specialist care (as part of enhanced services and as GPs with special interests) most still refer patients on. Of equal importance is the recognition of problems such as mental health complications, infections (e.g. human immunodeficiency virus and hepatitis) and thrombosis.

Although addicts want GPs to be involved in their treatment, doctors should not be pressured into accepting responsibilities beyond their level of skill. This has been brought to our attention again most recently where a GP was charged with manslaughter when a teenage patient of his died of a methadone overdose.

Drug and alcohol problems: questions

1 When interpreting an AUDIT score as part of a patient's assessment of alcohol use, what is the level above that which hazardous drinking levels are indicated?
   a. 8
   b. 4
   c. 20
   d. 16
   e. 2

2 Which of the following would not form part of the management of acute alcohol withdrawal?
   a. Spironolactone
   b. Thiamine
   c. Vitamin B
   d. Diazepam
   e. Information regarding the local alcohol support network

3 As part of ongoing assessment of benzodiazepine dependence, you could expect to find traces of the drug in the urine for up to how long?
   a. 4 days
   b. 3 days
   c. 12–14 hours
   d. 30 days
   e. 7 days

4 Which of the following is the most common cause of raised ferritin in primary care?
   a. Haemochromatosis.
   b. Excess alcohol intake.
   c. Obesity.
   d. Patients on long-term iron.
   e. Porphyria cutanea tarda.

5 Which of the following would not be considered an acceptable way of managing cannabis withdrawal in a patient?

a. Use of low-dose diazepam for agitation, for as long as the patient needs to enable them to withdraw from cannabis.
b. Advise gradual reduction in cannabis use prior to stopping.
c. Advise the use of nicotine replacement therapy if stopping smoking at the same time as stopping cannabis use.
d. Prescribe short-term sedation for management of insomnia.
e. Suggest delaying the first use of cannabis until later in the day.

For questions 6–10, the following points are known terminologies or side effects from cocaine drug use. Answer true or false for each statement.

6 Smoking 'free base' cocaine or crack is associated with gum disease.
7 Long-term use is known to cause dehydration.
8 Injection cocaine can increase the risk of endocarditis.
9 Anorexia.
10 'Speedballing' is when amphetamines and crack are used together.

Drug and alcohol problems: answers

1 a A total score of more than 8 indicates hazardous drinking; a score of 16–19 indicates harmful drinking or mild to moderate dependence; those with a score of 15 or higher should be considered for comprehensive assessment. Severe dependence is indicated where the score is above 20.

2 a This question is taken from the National Institute for Health and Clinical Excellence guidance on alcohol use disorders (www.nice.org.uk/nicemedia/live/12995/48991/48991.pdf).

3 d You could expect to find traces of benzodiazepines in the urine for up to 30 days. Heroin, for 1–3 days; amphetamines, for 2–4 days; methadone, for 2–4 days; and cannabis, for 5–7 days (although up to a month in heavy users).

4 b Although all are causes of a raised ferritin, alcohol is the most common cause.
Other causes include: thalassaemia and myelodysplastic syndrome (both of these would have a microcytic picture although not necessarily anaemia); underlying malignancy; infection or inflammation.

5 a The article 'Assessment and management of cannabis use disorders in primary care' (Clinical review *BMJ* 2010; 340: c1571) looks at physical and mental issues, management of withdrawal, minimising of harm and when to refer to a specialist. Diazepam for agitation would usually only be recommended for 3–4 days.

6 True Smoking cigarettes is also known to cause this problem.

7 False A risk with each use, there is an increased energy level and body temperature.

8 True The risk is higher with poor hygiene and groin access.

9 True Nausea and anorexia are recognised, with heroin use.

10 False Cocaine and heroin.

Statement 15.4

ENT and facial problems

ENT is one of the largest components of primary care. Although there is now a good evidence base for the more common ailments, it isn't quite as straightforward as it may seem and it is often the fourth-largest cohort of referrals into secondary care.

Sore throat

This is the most common, overtreated, controversial and mundane (or is it?!) symptom in general practice. Symptoms last for up to 10 days and may be associated with systemic features such as fever, malaise and vomiting.

A Cochrane review looked at antibiotics and complications with sore throats and concluded that antibiotics offered a small clinical benefit. They were found to reduce the risk of rheumatic fever by up to 30%, but this would be barely significant in the Western world. The incidence of acute otitis media was reduced by 25%. It is worth offering antibiotics to patients who have been unwell for 48 hours and who fit the Centor criteria (fever >38°C, purulent tonsils, tender anterior cervical nodes and no cough).

Public beliefs on antibiotics and respiratory tract infections: an Internet-based questionnaire study

Br J Gen Pract 2007; 57(545): 942–7

Patient expectations are one of the strongest predictors of antibiotic prescribing decisions. This study was based in the Netherlands and 20 questions were given to an Internet panel. Only 44.6% identified that antibiotics were effective against bacteria and not viruses. The study identified a misconception of the effectiveness of antibiotics for treatment of viral infections and highlighted that by prescribing, doctors positively reinforce the misconception.

Acute otitis media

- Around 66% of cases are due to *Haemophilus influenzae* and *Streptococcus pneumoniae*.
- Around 25% of cases are sterile (no organism can be isolated).
- Between 10% and 20% of cases are due to mycoplasma and anaerobes.
- About 4% are viral (although titres are raised in 25%, possibly preceding bacterial infection).

Use of antibiotics for otitis media

Several meta-analyses have shown that the effectiveness of antibiotics is limited in terms of clinical improvement. The advantages of antibiotics include the following:

- There is a bacterial aetiology.

- Antibiotics are cheap and relatively safe.
- There is a reduction in complications (e.g. mastoiditis).
- Use can reduce symptoms more quickly.

The disadvantages include the following:
- The cost escalates when you consider prescribing in mass numbers.
- It may discourage natural immunity.
- It may promote drug resistance.
- It may promote dependence on doctors by prescribing.

A randomized, double-blind, placebo-controlled noninferiority trial of amoxicillin for clinically diagnosed otitis media in children 6 months to 5 years of age

CMAJ 2005; 172(3): 335–41

This study randomly assigned 512 children aged 6 months to 5 years, with otitis media, to receive either amoxicillin (60 mg/kg daily) or placebo for 10 days. Follow-up was on days 1, 2 and 3 and for a final time between days 10 and 14.

At 14 days 84.2% of children receiving placebo and 92.8% of children receiving amoxicillin had clinical resolution of symptoms. More pain and fever was seen in the placebo group in the first 2 days. There was no difference in recurrence rates by 3 months. The cure rates were not substantially worse in the placebo groups than the treatment group.

One of the questions we need to ask is whether withholding antibiotics is justified when we know that they improve symptoms in children, especially in those who have systemic symptoms and those who are too young to express their symptoms, especially symptoms of pain.

Otitis media with effusion (glue ear)

This is the most common cause of conductive hearing loss in children aged 2–5 years. Up to 80% of children, by the age of 4 years, will have been affected with it at some time. Hearing loss has knock-on effects to speech development, school performance in writing and spelling and behaviour (which may be over-boisterous or clingy).

Around 50% of cases resolve spontaneously within 3 months and 95% resolve within 12 months.

Risk factors for developing otitis media with effusion include:
- passive smoking (environmental tobacco smoke)
- children attending day care (because of transmission rates of infection)
- bottle-feeding (breastfeeding may offer some preventive benefits)
- rhinitis, asthma and reflux.

Gastric reflux in children can mean that gastric juices reflux, via the Eustachian tube, into the middle ear. This can cause inflammation and ideal conditions for secondary infection.

Grommets (ventilation tubes) for hearing loss associated with otitis media with effusion in children

onlinelibrary.wiley.com/doi/10.1002/14651858.CD001801.pub3/abstract;jsessionid=4C994B4D7EAEFD9CEC28EF30F6255205.d03t03

This review assessed the effectiveness of grommet insertion compared with myringotomy or non-surgical treatment in children with otitis media with effusion. The outcomes studied were hearing level, duration of middle ear effusion, speech, language and cognitive development, behaviour and adverse effects.

The authors conclude that no evidence was available for long-term outcomes, benefits seemed to be small and diminished after six to nine months.

Screening for hearing defects

www.hearing.screening.nhs.uk/

- Around 840 children are born with permanent hearing impairment each year. This equates to approximately two babies in every 1000 born.
- Permanent hearing impairment impacts on communication skills, educational attainment and quality of life.
- If there is intervention by 6 months, the outcome for all of the communication skills, educational attainment and quality of life, as well as the cost to society, is improved.

The NHS Newborn Hearing Screening Programme screens all babies within 48 hours of birth. This is done by otoacoustic emissions testing (a test of cochlear function) and automated auditory brainstem response (assessment of sound transmission through the auditory nerve and brain stem). It has been known since the 1970s that for each sound heard by the ear, the ear produces a tiny corresponding sound (an 'echo') known as otoacoustic emission. This sound can now be measured by a computer and used clinically. Absence of an echo or a barely audible echo indicates the child has a hearing problem. Sensitivity is in the range of 80%–90%.

The National Deaf Children's Society (www.ndcs.org.uk/) is a charitable organisation and a good source of online information for professionals as well as for patients.

Early hearing screening: what is the best strategy?

Int J Pediatr Otorhinolaryngol 2007; 71(7): 1055–60

Although a number of factors increase the risk of hearing impairment (low birthweight, prematurity, perinatal hypoxia, jaundice and so forth), it can occur without any of these. This French study looked at screening after birth (before discharge) as compared with at 2 months in 5790 infants. Screening before discharge led to fewer false-positive results, which in turn had the knock-on effect of less maternal anxiety because of fewer false positives. It concluded that early neonatal screening was the better option (the article doesn't discuss the economics, but it would follow that fewer repeat tests must be more economic).

ENT and facial problems: questions

1 Collectively, what are the criteria for tonsillectomy more commonly known as?
   a. Centor criteria.
   b. Quinsy criteria.
   c. Paradise criteria.
   d. Utopia criteria.
   e. Herald criteria.

2 When counselling a patient with regard to tonsillectomy, which of the following is correct?
   a. Patients commonly experience chronic pain despite tonsillectomy.
   b. The risk of haemorrhage is 30%–35% immediately post-op.
   c. The risk of haemorrhage is 1%–2% immediately post-op.
   d. The risk of haemorrhage is 1%–2% and can occur up to 1 week post-op.
   e. The risk of haemorrhage is 1%–2% up to 4 weeks post-op.

3 Which of the following is not a legitimate differential for the discharging ear?
   a. Otitis externa.
   b. Otitis media.
   c. Acute perforation.
   d. Chronic perforation.
   e. Wax (especially when the patient has a temperature).

4 The patient shown in the image presents with a 2-week history of tonsillitis, lack of response to penicillins and extreme fatigue. Which of the following would be the most correct statement?

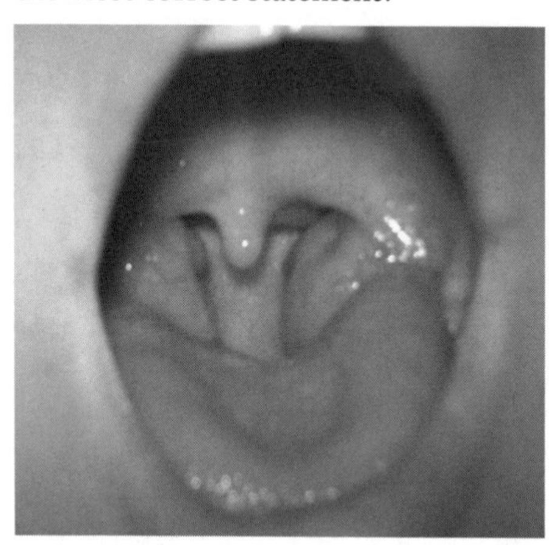

   a. This patient is developing chronic fatigue syndrome secondary to tonsillitis.
   b. This is a simple post-viral illness.
   c. They may go on to develop right upper quadrant pain and blood tests are needed.
   d. As penicillins haven't worked, you need to try an alternative antibiotic.
   e. Over-the-counter anti-inflammatories and paracetamol would be the best solution.

5 A 52-year-old male singer, who has never smoked, presents with a 4-week history of change in voice and dry cough after a cold. Which of the following is the best single answer?

a. He needs a course of co-amoxiclav 500/125 mg, one tablet three times a day, to clear any secondary bacterial infection.
b. He needs reassurance and analgesia, as everything will probably settle in the next couple of weeks.
c. He needs to stop work to allow his voice to rest.
d. He needs pulmonary function tests to look for airway disease and reversibility.
e. He needs an urgent chest X-ray.

ENT and facial problems: answers

1 c Paradise criteria, although may be considered arbitrary, help to stratify risk. A specialist referral should be considered:

- acutely if there is suspicion of a quinsy, airway obstruction or swelling causing dehydration
- routinely if there is a history of sleep apnoea, failure to thrive, five or more episodes of infection in the last 12 months for the previous 2 years (Paradise criteria) or they have guttate psoriasis caused by recurrent tonsillitis.

1 d The risk of haemorrhage (the most common complication is 1%–2% and can occur immediately or 5–7 days post-operatively).

3 b Otitis media, unless associated with a perforation, is enclosed and does not discharge into the external auditory canal.

4 c You need to be thinking glandular fever here, so, although all of the statements are vaguely true, you need to pick up on the need for a blood test. There is a very small risk of hepatic or splenic rupture in glandular fever.

5 e Although all of the answers may apply, he has had symptoms for more than 3 weeks (as per National Institute for Health and Clinical Excellence guidance) and by virtue of being a singer, previous laws around smoking in public places may mean that he has been exposed to a significant amount of cigarette smoke.

Statement 15.5

Eye problems

Age-related macular degeneration

Age-related macular degeneration (ARMD) is the most common cause of blindness in industrialised countries. It impairs central vision and it progresses slowly over a period of years; there is no cure. There are around 300 000 cases in the United Kingdom.

Legal blindness is vision <20/200 (6/60). This means a person can see at 20 yards (6 metres) when a normally sighted person can see at 200 yards (60 metres).

Dry ARMD is the most common form (85%–90% of cases). It is gradual in onset and is caused by drusen (thickening of Bruch's membrane between the retina and the choroids) and atrophy of the retinal pigment epithelium. Around 15% of cases of dry ARMD will progress to the exudative form, wet ARMD.

Possible protective factors

Although some factors cannot be modified – age, sex (men are seen to be at greater risk) or genetics (yet) – the following lifestyle changes have been found to be of importance in the possible prevention of ARMD:

- wearing sunglasses and brimmed hats in bright sunlight
- stopping smoking (smoking reduces antioxidants that can more than double the risk of ARMD)
- eating carotenoid-rich vegetables (green leafy vegetables) – lutein and zeaxanthin are the carotenoids found in the macula and are thought to be very important; a low-fat diet and a healthy approach to food underpin the general principles of beneficial nutrition.

Other possible protective factors:

- Statins have largely been discounted as possible protective factors, but it has been thought that they may help by reducing cholesterol (preventing deposition in Bruch's membrane), through antioxidant properties and by inhibiting endothelial cell apoptosis.
- Regular (every 2 years) eye tests would identify eye problems (tests are free for people over 60 years of age).

Wet ARMD accounts for 10% of cases, but it accounts for up to 90% of sight loss in ARMD. It occurs as growth of new blood vessels (stimulated by secretion of vascular endothelial growth factor) behind the retina leak blood and fluid, causing damage and more rapid loss of vision. This form of ARMD is amenable to treatment with photodynamic therapy or argon laser.

In photodynamic therapy with verteporfin dye, a non-thermal laser activates the dye once injected to close the new choroidal vessels (in exudative/wet ARMD). This treatment looks promising. There is no real evidence for radiotherapy or submacular surgery.

Eye problems: questions

1 Uveitis: which of the following is not a recognised complication of anterior uveitis?
   a. Glaucoma
   b. Cataract formation
   c. Posterior synechiae
   d. Papillitis
   e. Blindness

2 Sudden loss of vision: what is the most appropriate action in a 62-year-old man with sudden onset of flashing lights and partial loss of vision in the left eye?
   a. Review in 1 week.
   b. Review if sight doesn't return in 24 hours.
   c. A routine ophthalmology referral.
   d. An urgent ophthalmology referral.
   e. An emergency ophthalmology referral.

3 According to the National Institute of Health and Clinical Excellence guidance on glaucoma, above what intraocular pressure should ocular hypertension be formally diagnosed with a gonioscope?
   a. 12 mmHg
   b. 15 mmHg
   c. 19 mmHg
   d. 21 mmHg
   e. 35 mmHg

4 Which of the following statements with regard to glaucoma is correct?
   a. There are three genes known to be associated with glaucoma.
   b. Glaucoma is the cause of 60%–65% of all registrations for sight impairment in the United Kingdom.
   c. Diabetes is the most significant risk factor for developing glaucoma.
   d. By definition, the intraocular pressure in glaucoma would be >18 mmHg if untreated.
   e. Glaucoma is not known to affect visual fields.

For each of the conditions described in questions 5–7, select the single most appropriate answer from the following list. Each answer can be used once, more than once or not at all.

a. Glaucoma
b. Viral conjunctivitis
c. Wet macular degeneration
d. Cataract
e. Heterochromia

f. Diabetic retinopathy
g. Dry macular degeneration
h. Stye
i. Dacryocystitis

5 Is associated with progressive loss of cells and growth of blood vessels, it can be treated with ranibizumab.

6 After a phacoemulsification, Maxitrol eye drops are often used for several weeks.

7 Oral flucloxacillin is usually necessary to resolve this problem.

8 Which of the following is the single most appropriate statement regarding Marfan's syndrome?

a. All patients with a high-arched palate have Marfan's syndrome until proven otherwise.
b. A clinical diagnosis of Marfan's syndrome can only be made after careful assessment of ocular, skeletal and cardiovascular systems.
c. Marfan's syndrome is an autosomal recessively inherited condition.
d. Marfan's syndrome affects men more than women.
e. Dislocated lenses occur in up to 80% of patients by the age of 11 years.

9 What is the best course of action in this situation?

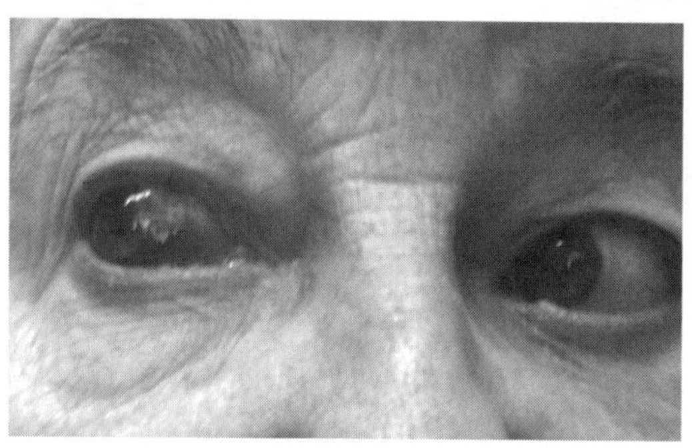

a. Emergency admission to the local eye clinic
b. Emergency admission to A&E
c. Maxitrol eye drops four times a day to the affected eye
d. Chloramphenicol eye drops five times a day to the affected eye
e. Reassurance

Eye problems: answers

1 d Papillitis is a variation of uveitis, not a complication, where the optic nerve is involved. (This question is taken from a *BMJ* Clinical Review article, 'Investigation and management of uveitis', *BMJ* 2010; 341: c4976). The uvea is the iris, ciliary body and choroids. Uveitis may also involve the retina (uveoretinitis), retinal blood vessels (retinal vasculitis), vitreous (vitritis) and the optic nerve (papillitis). Scarring around the iris causes glaucoma. Cataract formation is often because of the use of steroids in the treatment of uveitis. A posterior synechia is where the iris adheres to the lens causing distortion of the iris (it may not be apparent unless the pupil is dilated; the dilation will often break the synechia). Blindness can be caused not only by cataracts and glaucoma but also by cystoid macular oedema, vitreous opacities, chorioretinal scarring, inflammatory optic neuritis and retinal detachment.

2 e Retinal detachments, especially involving the macula, should be surgically repaired as soon as possible. Even if referred urgently, in some areas this surgical repair can take too long to be appropriate.

3 d (Note a quick reference guide is available online: www.nice.org.uk/nicemedia/live/12145/43791/43791.pdf)

4 a The three associated genes are MYOC (myocilin), OPTN (optineurin) and WDR36. There are also 20 known genetic loci. Glaucoma accounts for 10%–15% of registered blindness and it is the most significant risk factor in increasing age. Intraocular pressures are >22 mmHg.

5 c This form accounts for 10% of macular degeneration. Diabetic eye changes are usually treated with laser therapy.

6 d

7 i

8 b Marfan's syndrome is autosomal dominant and it affects lenses in 55% of children by the age of 11 years. The following issues may arise:

- Skeletal involvement: height over the 95th percentile for age, arm span > height and 70% of cases have a degree of scoliosis.
- Cardiovascular system: hypertension, aortic aneurysm and dissection, aortic valve and mitral valve regurgitation and arrhythmias can occur.
- Lungs: pneumothorax, bronchiectasis and bullae.
- Eyes: myopia, lens dislocation, retinal detachment and glaucoma.

9 e This is a subconjunctival haemorrhage. It is good practice to assess the blood pressure and other issues related to clotting problems; however, although it may look dramatic, it doesn't encroach on the vision and, as it will resolve, reassurance is all that is needed.

Statement 15.6

Metabolic problems

Diabetes

www.diabetes.org.uk

- The prevalence of diabetes in the United Kingdom is 4% (10% in those over 65 years of age).
- There are 33 000 deaths per year due to diabetes.
- Life expectancy is reduced by up to 20 years in type 1, and 10 years in type 2 diabetes.
- 70% of mortality in diabetes is related to cardiovascular disease.

Diabetes is a complex multisystem disease and for effective management you need, preferably, a coordinated patient-centred approach with set standards and a computerised register. It is a common disease, the incidence of which is estimated to rise by 25% over the next decade because of the ageing population, obesity, sedentary lifestyle and so forth.

Diagnosis

The criteria for diagnosis were agreed by the World Health Organization in June 2000 (there is currently some debate about the use of HbA1c diagnostically).

- **Diabetic symptoms** with random venous glucose concentration >11.1 mmol/L or fasting BM >7.0 mmol/L or 2 hour BM >11.1 mmom/L after 75 gm glucose tolerance test.
- **No symptoms** – do not diagnose on a single glucose measurement, but do a repeat plasma test (same values apply as above).

CURRENT CLASSIFICATION (ROYAL COLLEGE OF GENERAL PRACTITIONERS AND NHS DIABETES)

Diabetes:

- Type 1
- Type 2
- Genetic
- Other and unknown

Non-diabetic hyperglycaemia:

- Impaired glucose tolerance
- Gestational diabetes

The implications of these changes are that more people will be diagnosed as being diabetic (most will be diet controlled). Hopefully, long-term complications will be reduced but in the meantime the workload for primary care will remain substantial.

Research presented at the European Association of Diabetes in September 2001 emphasised that even the new World Health Organization guidelines on oral glucose tolerance test (for those with plasma glucose 6.1–6.9 mmol/L) would miss up to 20% of people with impaired glucose tolerance and recommended that oral glucose tolerance test be performed at 5.0–6.9 mmol/L. Even by using this range, 11% of diabetes could go undetected.

National Service Framework for Diabetes (2003 Delivery Strategy)
www.dh.gov.uk/en/Publicationsandstatistics/Publications/PublicationsPolicyAndGuidance/DH_4002951
This document states that 'all adults with diabetes will receive high quality care throughout their lifetime, including support to optimise the control of their blood sugar'. It includes 12 standards in nine areas of diabetic care.

1 Prevention of type 2 diabetes

- Multiagency approach to reduce the number of people who are inactive, overweight and obese.
- Physical education and a balanced diet need to be promoted from childhood.

2 Identification of people with diabetes

- Follow-up of those at increased risk – gestational diabetics, known family history, ischaemic heart disease, obesity and ethnicity.

3 Empowering people with diabetes

- Has been shown to reduce blood glucose and improve quality of life.
- Could involve structured education, personal care plans and patient-held records.

4 Clinical care of adults with diabetes

- Would include management of diabetes, hypertension, smoking cessation, all aimed at improving measurements and quality of life.

5, 6 Clinical care of children and young people with diabetes

- Similar high-quality care as with adults. It would also include physical, psychological, intellectual, educational and social development needs.

7 Management of diabetic emergencies

- Diabetic ketoacidosis, hyperosmolar non-ketotic syndrome and hypoglycaemia.

8 Care of people with diabetes during admission to hospital

- Outcome could be improved by better liaison between diabetes team and ward staff.

9 Diabetes and pregnancy

- Policies will be developed for women with pre-existing diabetes and those who develop diabetes to help achieve blood pressure control before and during pregnancy.

10, 11, 12 Detection and management of long-term complications

- Regular surveillance for long-term complications.
- Effective treatment and investigation for complications.
- Integrated health and social care.

Type 2 diabetes

The Management of Type 2 Diabetes

www.nice.org.uk/nicemedia/live/12165/44322/44322.pdf

Management of blood glucose

- HbA1c should be measured 2- to 6-monthly and should be individually defined, around 6.5% if possible but there may be no need to pursue this.
- Weight loss and physical activity should be encouraged if the patient is overweight.

Management of blood pressure and lipids

- An annual risk assessment should be made if there is no ischaemic heart disease. (Note that a significant number of doctors now treat cholesterol with statins, first line, despite this advice.)
- Blood pressure should be checked yearly; add treatment if >140/80 mmHg and lifestyle changes have not improved the blood pressure (130/80 if renal, eye or cerebrovascular disease).
- Measure lipids yearly. If cardiovascular risk is >20% for 10 years treat with simvastatin first line.

HbA1c levels: what is the evidence? (NICE suggests aiming for 6.5%, but not exclusively)

Although we aspire to good glucose control there are often practical problems with the medication and lifestyle, as well as the risk of hypoglycaemic episodes.

Effect of intensive glucose lowering treatment on all cause mortality, cardiovascular death and microvascular events in type 2 diabetes: meta-analysis of randomised controlled trials

BMJ 2011; 343: d4169

This article found limited benefits of intensive glucose monitoring on all cause mortality and cardiovascular deaths. Over a treatment period of 5 years 117–150 patients would need to be treated to avoid one myocardial infarction and 32–142 to avoid one episode of microalbuminuria. One severe episode of hypoglycaemia would occur in 15–52 patients.

It concluded that the risk benefit of intensive glucose monitoring remains uncertain.

Safety of tight glucose control in type 2 diabetes

BMJ 2008; 336(7642): 458-9

This editorial considers the glucose lowering arm of the ACCORD trial looking at people at risk of cardiovascular disease with type 2 diabetes; it has been stopped 18 months early because of safety concerns. Intensively lowering glucose <6% increased the risk of death as compared with the less intensive treatment (7%–7.9%). This was in contrast to the ADVANCE trial, which showed the opposite although in a smaller group of patients.

UK Prospective Diabetes Study 33

Lancet 1998; 352: 837-53, 854-65

The UK Prospective Diabetes Study (UKPDS) is a large, ongoing study of type 2 diabetes involving around 5000 patients set up in 1977. UKPDS 33 looked at newly diagnosed diabetics and treated them with diet for 3 months. If their HbA1c remained elevated they were entered into the trial.

Findings:

- Intensive treatment (average HbA1c 7% over the first 10 years) reduced the frequency of microvascular end points.
- Overweight patients with non-insulin-dependent diabetes then metformin and dietary improvement reduced the risk of diabetes-related end points by 32%, and diabetic deaths by 42%.
- Blood pressure control of <150/85 mmHg reduced microvascular complications and diabeties-related deaths (similar findings in the HOT study where blood pressure was reduced to <130/80 mmHg).
- Around 50% of diabetics had early signs of complications at time of diagnosis (this raises the importance of screening).

UK Prospective Diabetes Study 35

BMJ 2000; 321: 405-12

Each 1% reduction in HbA1c was associated with risk reduction of 21% for diabetic end points; 21% related to diabetic deaths; 14% for myocardial infarction and 37% for microvascular complications.

The case against aggressive treatment of type 2 diabetes: critique of UKPDS

BMJ 2001; 323: 854-8

The UKPDS grew out of the author's interest in the use of basal rather than post-prandial glucose. The first report was published in 1983. During the course of the study, length of follow-up has changed and end points have been redefined. The study is not blinded, the statistical analyses used have been questioned and the changes have not been in keeping with scientific principles.

Hypertension in diabetes

www.nice.org.uk/nicemedia/live/12165/44322/44322.pdf

Around 70% of adults with type 2 diabetes have hypertension and more than 70% have raised cholesterol levels.

- Target BP <140/80.
- If renal, eye or cerebrovascular disease present, treat to <130/80.

British Hypertension Society guidelines based on the HOT trial, 2000

- Start treatment if blood pressure is >140 mmHg systolic or >90 mmHg diastolic.
- Aim for a blood pressure 130/80 mmHg or 125/75 mmHg if there is proteinuria (this is more tight than the National Institute for Health and Clinical Excellence (NICE) guidance).
- Less than 30% of cases respond to monotherapy.
- ***Do not forget*** non-pharmacological treatment.

UK Prospective Diabetes Study 36 (and 49)

BMJ 2000; 321: 412-19

In type 2 diabetes the risk of diabetic complications is strongly associated with raised BP. Any reduction in BP is likely to reduce the risk of complications. The lowest risk seen is in those diabetics with a systolic BP <120 mmHg (**note that the BP-lowering arm of the ACCORD trial found outcomes <120 mmHg were not better than <140 mmHg**). Intensive BP control is at least as important (if not more so) than intensive blood glucose control.

Association of systolic blood pressure with macrovascular and microvascular complications of type 2 diabetes (UKPDS 36): prospective observational study

BMJ 2000; 321(7258): 412–19

For systolic blood pressure, each 10 mmHg decrease is associated with a risk reduction of 12% for any complications related to diabetes (15% for deaths related to diabetes, 11% for myocardial infarction and 13% for microvascular complications).

Effects of ramipril on cardiovascular and microvascular outcomes in people with diabetes mellitus: results of the HOPE study and MICRO-HOPE substudy

Lancet 2000; 355: 253-9

In the HOPE (Health Outcome Prevention Evaluation) and Micro-HOPE study, a total of 3577 diabetic patients aged 55 years and over were randomised to ramipril 10 mg/day or placebo and then vitamin E or placebo. Ramipril had a beneficial effect on cardiovascular events, which decreased by 25%–30%, and on overt nephropathy in people with diabetes. The benefit was greater than that attributable to the decrease in blood pressure. Ramipril showed vasculoprotective and renoprotective effects.

Obesity in diabetes

In 1973, following research by Sims, the term 'diabesity' was introduced, emphasising the link between diabetes and obesity. Up to 80% of type 2 diabetes is due to obesity (BMI > 27 kg/m^2), and the duration of obesity is significant. Weight loss improves morbidity (UKPDS 7).

Diet, lifestyle and the risk of type 2 diabetes mellitus in women

N Engl J Med 2001; 345(11): 790–7

A total of 84 941 female nurses aged 30–55 years were followed from 1980 to 1996. An important risk factor was a BMI > 35 kg/m^2. Poor diet, minimal exercise, smoking and abstinence from alcohol were all associated with significant risk of developing diabetes. It is no great surprise that lifestyle is a key risk.

Cholesterol and diabetes

The NICE guidance recommends:

- annual assessment of cardiovascular risk
- starting statins (simvastatin 40 mg) if over 40 years of age (unless risk using the JBS tables is <20% over 10 years)
- if triglycerides remain >2.3–4.5 mmol/L, treat with a fibrate (after excluding secondary causes and treatment of cholesterol).

Aspirin in diabetes

Given the cardiovascular risk seen in diabetes, aspirin has become considered a 'guardian drug'. NICE recommends offering aspirin to everyone over the age of 50 with diabetes (so long as BP is <145/90 mmHg); if there are cardiovascular risks, then can offer at any age. If aspirin is not tolerated, clopidogrel can be offered.

Aspirin for primary prevention of cardiovascular events in people with diabetes: meta-analysis of randomised controlled trials

BMJ 2009; 339: b4531

This meta-analysis could not find a clear benefit for use of aspirin in diabetes. The risk of major cardiac events was not significantly reduced as compared with placebo or no treatment.

Blood glucose

Self-monitoring of blood glucose in diabetes

Drug Ther Bull 2007; 45(9): 65–9

This topic was addressed because of the huge cost of glucose sticks to the NHS. Fluctuations in blood glucose can be significant and not always linked to symptoms; monitoring (especially when using insulin) can be a way of regulating and timing intake. Monitoring is not thought to be of benefit if patients are not acting on and interpreting the results correctly. Diabetes UK has advised (and DTB concurs) that in patients not using insulin, blood glucose monitoring may be useful as a supplement in certain situations (e.g. patients experiencing hypoglycaemia), where insulin monitoring is used 3–4 times a day to titrate insulin dose.

In pregnant women a seven-point testing approach may be needed, because of greater fluctuations and unpredictability. NICE does support the use of home monitoring as part of integrated self-care.

Efficacy of self-monitoring of blood glucose in patients with newly diagnosed type 2 diabetes (ESMON trial): randomised controlled trial

BMJ 2008; 336(7654): 1174–7

This study looked at 184 patients under 70 years of age. It found that there was no difference at 12 months in HbA1c, BMI, use of oral hypoglycaemics and reported hypoglycaemic episodes. There was an increase in the depression subscale of the well-being questionnaire. This trial finding has been found in previous randomised controlled trials.

Treatment for diabetes: metformin versus sulphonylureas

Risk of cardiovascular disease and all cause mortality among patients with type 2 diabetes prescribed oral antidiabetes drugs: retrospective cohort study using UK general practice research database

BMJ 2009; 339: b4731

This was a retrospective study from 1990 to 2005 looking at 91 521 patients with diabetes. Compared with metformin, monotherapy with first- or second-generation sulphonylureas was associated with a significant excess risk of all cause mortality. A total of 18 548 patients died during the course of the study; those receiving sulphonylureas were at a 61% greater risk than those receiving metformin. This guidance supports the NICE guidance that metformin should be the first-line treatment.

Glitazones/thiazolidinediones

These drugs enhance the effects of insulin in adipose tissue and skeletal muscle by acting as ligands that regulate gene expression (i.e. they reduce the body's resistance to insulin).

These drugs are topical because they are relatively new. There has been some concern regarding cardiovascular safety, rosiglitazone having been withdrawn relatively recently (because of increased risk of heart failure when used with insulin and increased fracture risk).

Pioglitazone has been shown to increase the risk of cardiac failure when used with insulin. It is contraindicated in patients with heart failure but still a prescribing option.

It is recommended that liver function tests are checked prior to starting treatment and then at 2-monthly intervals for the first year, stopping the drug if the liver enzymes rise three times the normal level or if the patient becomes jaundiced.

Secondary prevention of macrovascular events in patients with type 2 diabetes in the PROactive study (PROspective pioglitAzone Clinical Trial In macroVascular Events): a randomised controlled trial

Lancet 2005; 366(9493): 1241–2

In this study, 5238 patients with type 2 diabetes and evidence of macrovascular disease (i.e. high-risk patients) were randomised to either pioglitazone or placebo. Pioglitazone improved HbA1c by 0.8% (on average) and reduced all causes of mortality, non-fatal myocardial infarction and stroke.

Meglitinides/prandial glucose regulators

These are amino acid derivatives that are licensed for use with metformin in type 2 diabetes, where better control is needed, or where patients experience hypoglycaemia when treated with sulphonylureas.

The drugs are 'glucose responsive' so they induce insulin release when the patient eats by acting on the pancreatic beta-cells to stimulate a rapid, short-lasting release of insulin to a level dependent on the glucose concentration (i.e. where there is a post-prandial rise in glucose). This is thought to be beneficial where the patient has an erratic lifestyle (e.g. junior doctors).

As stimulation is not over 24 hours the endocrine function should be preserved.

Glucose tolerance and mortality: comparison of WHO and American Diabetes Association diagnostic criteria

Lancet 1999; 354(9179): 617–21

This study of 18 048 men and 7316 women over 30 years of age looked at risk of death according to different diagnostic glucose categories. There was a follow-up of 7.3 years.

It found that fasting glucose alone did not identify risk of death associated with hyperglycaemia. Mortality increased with increasing 2-hour glucose (i.e. post-prandial spike).

Dipeptidyl peptidase-4 inhibitors

This is a new class of oral hypoglycaemics that stop breakdown of incretin (an intestinal hormone that stimulates insulin release in response to food). Sitagliptin and vildagliptin are currently under investigation. Exanatide, a glucagon-like peptide is also now being used; this is a drug that simulates the effect of incretin when injected.

These drugs seem to reduce the risk of weight gain and hypoglycaemia.

Efficacy and safety of sitagliptin added to ongoing metformin therapy in patients with type 2 diabetes

Curr Med Res Opin 2008; 24(2): 537–50

This was a multinational, randomised, placebo-controlled, parallel-group, double-blind study of 190 patients non-insulin-dependent type 2 diabetics. Sitagliptin was found to reduce HbA1c (by 1%), fasting glucose and 2-hour post-prandial glucose at 18 and 30 weeks, all with statistical significance ($p < 0.001$). Sitagliptin was also found to be well tolerated.

Screening for diabetes

In 2030 it is estimated that half of the UK population will be diabetic and already up to half of the people with type 2 diabetes have vascular complications at the time of diagnosis.

Mass population screening would be costly and inefficient with low specificity, as less than 1% of undiagnosed cases were revealed by a British Diabetic Association study in 1994. Many organisations have published arguments for targeted approach of high-risk groups (e.g. obesity, family history of diabetes, ethnic groups, patients who have had gestational diabetes or impaired glucose tolerance, or hypertension).

Diabetes UK recommends opportunistic screening for those at high risk of diabetes, and slowly research into oral glucose tolerance testing is adding weight to the argument.

Screening for type 2 diabetes in primary care

BMJ 2009; 338: b880 p. 812

This paper looks at the use of a QDScore (Q = QResearch, D = diabetes) as a computer-based screening tool without the need for laboratory testing. The tool seems highly accurate in predicting risk with a 97% accuracy (having looked at 2 540 753 patients aged 25–79 years of age). The public can also use this tool (www.qdscore.org).

Should we screen for type 2 diabetes? Evaluation against National Screening Committee criteria

BMJ 2001; 322(9729): 986–8

This discussion paper looks at the role of the National Screening Committee in evaluating a screening programme for type 2 diabetes.

It summarises its findings as follows:

- Benefits of early detection and treatment of undiagnosed diabetes have not been proved.
- Disadvantages of screening are important and should be quantified.
- Universal screening is not merited, but targeted screening may be justified.
- Clinical management of diabetes should be optimised before a screening programme is considered.

No agreement was reached on how targeted screening could be achieved.

Acarbose

Acarbose for prevention of type 2 diabetes mellitus: the STOP-NIDDM randomised trial

Lancet 2002; 359(9323): 2072–7

People with impaired glucose tolerance treated with acarbose are 25% less likely to develop type 2 diabetes than those on placebo. It was concluded that acarbose could be used either as an alternative or in addition to lifestyle changes in patients with impaired glucose tolerance.

Vaccine

Beta-cell function in new-onset type 1 diabetes and immunomodulation with a heat-shock protein (DiaPep277): a randomised, double-blind, phase II trial

Lancet 2001; 358(9295): 1749–53

DiaPep277 is the first drug to successfully halt the immune system's destruction of pancreatic beta-cells. However, the intervals at which the vaccine should be given are not known. Phase III trials are in progress.

Insulin needs after CD3-antibody therapy in new-onset type 1 diabetes

N Engl J Med 2005; 352(25): 2598–608

This study of 80 people in Belgium showed that the monoclonal antibody preserved the remaining beta-cells in newly diagnosed diabetics. Patients diagnosed early would be ideal candidates for this type of treatment – opening again the debate on the need for a screening programme.

Islet cell transplant

In the United Kingdom, London and Oxford both have specialist laboratories to process islet cells from donors to develop a national transplant service. This is in the very early developmental stage.

Drugs for prevention of diabetes

This is an ongoing area of research and is not recommended that we prescribe. Metformin has long been recognised for its ability to help weight loss (although this is not a licensed use) and there was some work also looking at the combination of metformin and rosiglitazone at preventing the onset of diabetes, although given that rosiglitazone is effectively withdrawn, this is no longer an option.

Metabolic syndrome

Metabolic syndrome is known to be associated with cardiovascular disease and type 2 diabetes. There is a school of thought that all we are doing by labelling someone as having metabolic syndrome is medicalising obesity, when what we should be doing is tackling obesity to prevent impaired glucose tolerance and diabetes. Many feel that the term is imprecise and indeed there are a number of definitions.

THE INTERNATIONAL DIABETES FEDERATION (2005) DIAGNOSTIC CRITERIA

Essential requirements:

- Central obesity, waist measurement
  - Males >94 cm
  - Females >80 cm

Plus any two of the following:

- Raised fasting glucose >5.6 mmol/L (or previously diagnosed type 2 diabetes)
- Raised triglycerides >1.7 mmol/L (or on treatment) and/or
- Reduced HDL cholesterol
  - <1.03 mmol/L in men
  - <1.29 mmol/L in women
- Raised blood pressure
  - >130/85 mmHg (or on treatment for previously diagnosed hypertension)

Metabolic problems: questions

1. Diabetes: in a patient with type 2 diabetes, which of the following statements is considered correct?
   a. A patient with diabetes is always considered to be at high risk, even if they have never smoked.
   b. They should be offered aspirin 75 mg if over 50 years of age, even if there are no cardiovascular risk factors.
   c. If a statin is required, simvastatin 20 mg is to be recommended as the first-line treatment.
   d. If triglyceride levels remain at 2.3 mmol/L, despite dietary changes, omega-3 fish oils on prescription are recommended.
   e. If a diabetic patient is already being treated with statins and their triglyceride level continues to be 2.0 mmol/L, you should consider offering a fibrate.
2. It is considered unsafe to prescribe metformin in which of the following renal impairment categories?
   a. <30 mL/min/1.73 m^2
   b. <45 mL/min/1.73 m^2
   c. <60 with proteinuria mL/min/1.73 m^2
   d. <60 without proteinuria mL/min/1.73 m^2
   e. <90 mL/min/1.73 m^2
3. In a patient taking the maximum dose of metformin, whose HbA1c levels remain above 6.5%, which of the following statements is correct?
   a. There is no need to do anything, this is adequate.
   b. Start gliclazide 30 mg.
   c. Start pioglitazone 15 mg.
   d. Start gliclazide MR 30 mg.
   e. Consider secondary care referral for exenatide.
4. In management of diabetes, what level of albumin excretion is considered above normal (microalbuminuria) for an albumin-to-creatinine ratio in men?
   a. >1.0 mg/mmol
   b. >2.5 mg/mmol
   c. >3.5 mg/mmol
   d. >30 mg/mmol
   e. >50 mg/mmol
5. Which of the following has been identified as an independent risk factor for mortality in diabetic patients over 75 years of age?
   a. Estimated glomerular filtration rate (eGFR).
   b. Albumin-to-creatinine ratio.
   c. Creatinine level.
   d. Nitric oxide level.
   e. Insulin-like growth factor.
6. Hypothyroidism: consider the following thyroid results: thyroid stimulating hormone <0.01; Free T4, 25. In a 62-year-old man receiving 175 μg levothyroxine for hypothyroidism following a thyroidectomy for thyroid cancer, which of the

following options with regard to management of these results would be most appropriate?

a. Do nothing, maintain the patient at the same dose.
b. Increase the levothyroxine to 200 μg per day.
c. Decrease the levothyroxine to 150 μg per day.
d. Decrease the levothyroxine to 125 μg per day.
e. Stop the levothyroxine.

7 Hyperparathyroidism: select the single most appropriate answer from the following options.

a. Hyperparathyroidism can cause diarrhoea.
b. The most common cause of primary hyperparathyroidism is a solitary parathyroid adenoma.
c. Primary hyperparathyroidism is the most commonly seen where there is a familial case.
d. In primary hyperparathyroidism the parathyroid level could be expected to be between 1 and 3 pmol/L.
e. Because of the calcium levels, osteoporosis is uncommon.

8 Hyperthyroidism: in the presentation of each of the following symptoms, in which would you be advised to consider the diagnosis of hyperthyroidism?

a. Menorrhagia.
b. Sensitivity to the cold.
c. Constipation.
d. Eclampsia.
e. A macrosomic baby.

9 Hypopituitarism: with regard to the pharmacological management of hypopituitarism, which of the following statements is incorrect?

a. Steroid replacement with hydrocortisone 10 mg in the morning, 5 mg at lunch time and 5 mg in the evening would be considered sensible.
b. Steroid replacement may unmask a latent diabetes insipidus.
c. Steroid doses should be halved with co-morbid illness and major stress, taking into account endogenous production.
d. When treating with growth hormone, insulin like growth factor-1 levels can be used to guide therapy.
e. Oestrogen replacement in women up until the age of the menopause should not cause an increase in cancer risk.

10 Hyperkalaemia: which of the following ECG changes would be compatible with hyperkalaemia?

a. Tall peaked T waves, broad QRS complex and flattened p wave.
b. Flattened T wave, narrow QRS complex and tented p waves.
c. Narrow QRS complex, deep S wave and peaked T wave.
d. Narrow QRS complex, flattened T wave with a prolonged QTc.
e. Narrow QRS complex, flattened T wave with a shortened QTc.

Metabolic problems: answers

1 **b** So long as the blood pressure is controlled (<145/90), patients over the age of 50 with diabetes should be offered aspirin. This question has been written in light of the NICE guidance for type 2 diabetes (www.nice.org.uk/nicemedia/live/12165/44322/44322.pdf). A diabetic patient would only be considered low risk if all of the following apply: not overweight, normotensive (<140/80 on no treatment), non-smoker, no high-risk lipid profile and no family history of cardiovascular disease. First-line statin is simvastatin but the starting dose is 40 mg, not 20 mg. A fibrate is considered if the triglycerides remain 2.3–4.5 mmol/L despite statin treatment. Omega-3 fish oils and nicotinic acid are not routinely recommended.

2 **a** NICE and the British National Formulary advise avoiding where the eGFR is <30 mL/min/1.73 m^2 because of the increased risk of lactic acidosis (http://bnf.org/bnf/bnf/current/4186.htm). It is important to check the renal function before treatment and then at least annually (twice yearly if there is renal impairment).

3 **b** Technically above 6.5% is not adequate and a sulphonylurea is the next step. Exenatide is a third-line therapy, only considered if the BMI is greater than 35. If the BMI is under 35 it would only be considered where use of insulin would have significant occupational implications, or weight loss due to other co-morbidities would be beneficial.

4 **b** In women, the value would be >3.5 mg/mmol.

5 **b** Albumin-to-creatinine ratio has been found to be independently associated with increased risk of death at all levels of eGFR in diabetic patients over 75 years of age (in younger patients with lower eGFRs the association was less marked). Prognostic implications of the urinary albumin-to-creatinine ratio in veterans of different ages with diabetes are discussed in *Arch Intern Med* 2010; 170(11): 930–6.

6 **a** It is important to well and truly suppress the pituitary (without making the patient thyrotoxic) following thyroidectomy for thyroid cancer. In turn, this would mean any stray malignant cells would not be stimulated by thyroid-stimulating hormone.

7 **b** Constipation is common in those with hypercalcaemia. Eighty-five per cent of cases are solitary adenomas, 15% parathyroid hypertrophy with <1% being due to parathyroid carcinoma. It can be seen as a feature of multiple endocrine neoplasia but is generally not familial (if so there is usually a much more severe hypercalcaemia). The parathyroid level would be >3 pmol/L and osteoporosis is common despite the high serum calcium. Osteoporosis would be commonly seen because of the calcium release from the bone.

8 **d** In hyperthyroidism patients are more likely to get oligomenorrhoea, heat intolerance, tremor, sweating, tachycardia, atrial fibrillation, dyspnoea due to sympathetic nervous stimulation, as well as eye symptoms of Graves's disease. In pregnancy, patients can present with eclampsia, low birthweight and increased risk of miscarriage. There is also a risk of a thyrotoxic storm (hyperpyrexia,

tachycardia, abdominal symptoms and confusion); if this happens there is a 20%–30% risk of mortality.

9 c Steroid dose should be doubled in these instances. Steroid replacement should be started 24–48 hours prior to starting thyroxine replacement.

10 a Although 50% of patients with hyperkalaemia do not have ECG changes with a potassium >6.5 mmol/L. Sometimes the progression of ECG changes can be rapid and fatal.

Statement 15.7

Neurological problems

Stroke

This is defined as a sudden loss of neurological function (for which there is no other cause than a vascular one) lasting for more than 24 hours. A transient ischaemic attack (TIA) lasts for less than 24 hours.

- The incidence of stroke is 2 in 1000 (double this in 45- to 84-year-olds).
- It is the third most common cause of death in the United Kingdom and the greatest single cause of disability, affecting 130 000 people per year.
- Around 80% of all strokes are ischaemic.
- 50% of patients are physically dependent on others 6 months after the event.
- The incidence of TIA is 0.4 in 1000 (the future risk of stroke is 10% in the first year and 5% thereafter).
- There is a 1%–2% risk of a myocardial infarction following TIA.

A simple score (ABCD) to identify individuals at high early risk of stroke after transient ischaemic attack

Lancet 2005; 366(9479): 29–36

Deciding which patients need emergency assessment following a TIA is an important part of our initial management in general practice (although the gold standard is that all should be investigated within 7 days) and this outlines a simple scoring system to assist in decision-making.

ABCD	Meaning	Question	Score
A	Age	<60 years	0
		>60 years	1
B	Blood pressure	Systolic >140 mmHg and/or Diastolic > 90 mmHg	1
C	Clinical features	Unilateral weakness	2
		Speech disturbance, no weakness	1
		Other	0
D	Duration of symptoms	60 minutes	2
		10–59 minutes	1
		<10 minutes	0

A score >5/8 was predictive (in up to 24% of the 190 patients) of a subsequent stroke within 7 days of a TIA.

Interestingly, it doesn't use smoking history/pack-years; neither, as it is part of the initial assessment, does it include cholesterol.

Standard Five – Stroke, Older People's National Service Framework

Outcome for stroke patients is better, and their stay is usually shorter, if cared for by specialist teams in stroke units.

It specifically states the following:

- People who are thought to have had a stroke should have access to diagnostic and specialist stroke services.
- Subsequently they, and their carers, should participate in a multidisciplinary programme of secondary prevention and rehabilitation (e.g. speech therapy, occupational therapy, physiotherapy, social services, district nurse support and so forth).

National Stroke Strategy

The Department of Health has set a target to reduce the death rate from stroke and cardiovascular disease by 40% in people under 75 years of age. The development of the strategy included six key areas.

1. Public awareness and prevention – recognising emergency admission to hospital along with primary and secondary preventive measures.
2. TIA services – rapid access to diagnostics and treatment.
3. Emergency response – recognition that early treatment improves outcome.
4. Hospital stroke care – by specialist stroke units.
5. Post-hospital stroke care – rehabilitation in the community with long term services where needed.
6. Workforce – ensuring development of skills to allow implementation of the strategy.

Targeting risk factors in primary and secondary prevention

Hypertension

Hypertension accounts for up to 50% of ischaemic strokes. The British Hypertension Society guidelines state that hypertension persisting for over 1 month after a stroke should be treated (other sources state this should be from 2 weeks). Stroke risk can be reduced by up to 40% if the diastolic blood pressure is reduced by 6 mmHg or the systolic blood pressure is reduced by 10–12 mmHg (irrespective of whether the blood pressure is elevated or not).

Role of blood pressure and other variables in the differential cardiovascular event rates noted in the Anglo-Scandinavian Cardiac Outcomes Trial: Blood Pressure Lowering Arm (ASCOT-BPLA)

Lancet 2005; 366(9489): 869–71

Showed significantly lower rates of stroke in the amlodipine regime verses the atenolol regime. The significance was not fully understood and may be statistical rather than a real finding in this group of patients.

Heart Outcomes Prevention Study (HOPE)

N Engl J Med 2002; 347: 145–53

This was a ramipril study showing a 32% decrease in stroke incidence in patients with controlled blood pressure. Making the case for all patients having an angiotensin converting enzyme inhibitor irrespective of their blood pressure.

Antiplatelet drugs

Clopidogrel and Modified-Release Dipyridamole in the Prevention of Occlusive Vascular Events

www.nice.org.uk/nicemedia/pdf/word/TA090guidance.doc

The following are recommended after an ischaemic stroke or TIA.

- Dipyridamole and aspirin in combination for 2 years after the most recent event, thereafter (or if dipyridamole is not tolerated) aspirin should be used.
- Clopidogrel is recommended for patients who are intolerant of aspirin.

Give dipyridamole with aspirin instead of aspirin alone to prevent vascular events after ischaemic stroke or TIA

BMJ 2007; 334(7599): 901

This is an interesting article on changing our practice in medicine, specifically in relation to prescribing both aspirin and dipyridamole for patients following a stroke or TIA as this reduces the risk for vascular events by a fifth as compared with aspirin alone. The discussion is focused around the European Stroke Prevention Study and the European/Australasian Stroke Prevention in Reversible Ischaemia Trial, both of which show there is a reduction in vascular events by using aspirin with dipyridamole.

Medium intensity oral anticoagulants versus aspirin after cerebral ischaemia or arterial origin (ESPRIT): a randomised controlled trial

Lancet Neurol 2007; 6(2): 115–24

This was an international, multicentre trial where 2739 patients were randomly assigned after a TIA or minor stroke to either anticoagulants or aspirin. Anticoagulants were compared with the combination of aspirin and dipyridamole (200 mg twice daily) and there was a mean follow-up of 4.6 years. A primary outcome event (death from a vascular cause, non-fatal stroke or myocardial infarction or major bleeding) occurred in 99 (19%) patients on anticoagulants and in 98 (18%) patients on aspirin. Oral anticoagulants (target INR range 2.0–3.0) were not found to be more effective than aspirin for secondary prevention after TIA or minor stroke of arterial origin.

Anticoagulation in atrial fibrillation

Atrial fibrillation (AF) increases the risk of stroke sixfold. Warfarin was previously the drug of choice for prevention of stroke in AF. Several randomised controlled trials confirmed the benefit and low complication rate (0.4%). The number needed to treat to prevent one stroke was 11. For CHAD scoring and AF *see* Statement 15.1.

Systematic review of long term anticoagulation or antiplatelet treatment in patients with non-rheumatic atrial fibrillation

BMJ 2001; 322(7282): 321–6

This study found no added benefit in non-rheumatic AF. Previous meta-analyses had not included these trials. There were 3298 patients (thought to be too low a number, as around 5000 are needed). Individual trials were small and used slightly different international normalised ratios to monitor warfarin. Forty-five per cent of patients were more likely to bleed on warfarin (even within the controlled setting of trial). It was concluded that there was no obvious benefit to using warfarin.

Cholesterol

Statins are indicated as part of a secondary prevention treatment plan for patients following a stroke or TIA; however, guidance on statin use for primary prevention includes patients with a 10-year coronary heart disease risk of 20%.

The Heart Protection Study

Lancet 2002; 360: 7–20

This study of the treatment of high risk CHD looked at treatment of high-risk CHD patients with simvastatin and found that the latter reduced the incidence of stroke by up to 25%.

High-dose atorvastatin after stroke or transient ischemic attack

N Engl J Med 2006; 355(6): 549–59

This study compared atorvastatin 80 mg and placebo in 4731 patients over a follow-up period of 4.9 years. It found that there was a reduction in further TIA and other cardiovascular events (by 1.9%, $P = 0.05$) although this was slightly offset by an increased risk in haemorrhagic stroke.

Carotid endarterectomy

If there is a symptomatic stenosis the benefit of surgery relates to the degree of stenosis. This is classified as mild-moderate-severe (Cochrane Review 2003). Carotid endarterectomy for asymptomatic carotid stenosis reduces the risk of stroke by 30% over 3 years (Cochrane review 2005).

See also eGuidelines (www.eGuidelines.co.uk) for information based on the Royal College of Physician's guidelines for stroke management.

Parkinson's Disease, NICE (June 2006)

www.nice.org.uk/nicemedia/pdf/cg035niceguideline.pdf

Parkinson's disease (PD) affects over 100 000 people in the UK. National Institute for Health and Clinical Excellence (NICE) guidelines were published for the diagnosis and management of this condition.

The priorities are summarised as:

- referral to an expert for accurate diagnosis
- regular expert review and access to specialist nursing care

- access to physiotherapy, occupational therapy and speech therapy
- palliative care.

Pharmacologically the guidelines consider various drug treatments for both early and later PD. They don't advocate a specific treatment; rather they recommend discussion of the short- and long-term benefits and drawbacks, so making the decision in partnership. Avoid withdrawing medication suddenly (e.g. drug holidays or reduced absorption due to surgery) as this may cause acute akinesia or neuroleptic malignant syndrome.

Surgery

NICE has also published on deep brain stimulation for PD.

Bilateral subthalamic nucleus or globus pallidus interna stimulation may be used in patients that fit certain criteria, including that they are levodopa responsive.

Non-motor features of PD

Depression

This is common in PD (up to 50% of cases). It is thought to have neurobiological manifestations rather than being a purely emotional response to the disease (*J Neurol Neurosurg Psychiatry* 1999; 67(4): 492–6). NICE recommends that doctors have a low threshold for diagnosis.

Dementia

It is recognised that PD patients have an increased risk of developing dementia. Acetylcholinesterase inhibitors have been used successfully, but further research has been recommended.

Sleep disturbance

Poor sleep may improve with sleep hygiene; also, consider restless legs syndrome. Patients with sudden onset of sleep need to take care with driving.

Autonomic disturbance

Such as urinary dysfunction, weight loss, constipation, erectile dysfunction, excessive sweating, orthostatic hypotension and silarrhoea.

Prognosis of PD: risk of dementia and mortality: Rotterdam study

Arch Neurol 2005; 62(8): 1265–7

Found that the risk of dementia was more prevalent if patients carried the APOE episton allele. The dementia risk was also dependent on disease duration.

Parkinson's disease

BMJ 2007; 335: 441–5

Clarke writes a comprehensive and useful clinical review looking at differential diagnoses of tremor, practical applications of treatment options, management of psychosis in PD and the roles of professionals. Although there was a degree of criticism in other papers about GPs being excluded from the NICE guidelines, this review helps put us firmly in the picture – the main challenge being keeping abreast of developments.

Safety and tolerability of gene therapy with adeno-associated virus borne GAD gene for PD: an open label phase 1 trial

Lancet 2007; 369(9579): 2056–8

Phase 1 human trials are underway and this publication looked at 11 men and one woman, all with severe PD. Having transferred the gene to a virus it was then injected into the subthalamic nucleus region. One patient found his movements had improved by 65%. Although this is only looking at one genetic mutation in PD, results so far are encouraging.

Neurological problems: questions

1 Epilepsy: in a known epileptic patient who is having a tonic–clonic seizure, which of the following would be the most important action?
   a. Monitor the pulse because of the risk of tachyarrhythmias.
   b. Check the blood pressure.
   c. Record the ECG.
   d. Measure oxygen saturation.
   e. Protect the patient from injury.
2 Which of the following antiepileptic medications would be considered most suitable in an 18-year-old female patient?
   a. Sodium valproate
   b. Phenobarbitone
   c. Phenytoin
   d. Lamotrogine
   e. Levetiracetam
3 It is important to manage epilepsy proactively because fits are associated with which of the following?
   a. Tics
   b. Torsade de pointes
   c. Subarachnoid haemorrhage
   d. Sudden unexpected death
   e. Once treated patients will be able to drive 6 months after their last fit

For each of the scenarios in question 4–6, select the single most appropriate answer. Each answer can be used once, more than once or not at all.

   a. Myasthenia gravis
   b. Huntington's disease
   c. Giant cell arteritis
   d. Migraine
   e. Subarachnoid haemorrhage
   f. Cord compression
   g. Bell's palsy

h. Ischaemic stroke

4 A 64-year-old female presenting with bilateral lower leg paralysis.

5 Sudden onset of severe occipital headache.

6 A 72-year-old man presenting with a unilateral facial weakness and loss of ability to raise eyebrows.

7 Bell's palsy: which of the following is the current thinking for treatment of Bell's palsy?
   a. Prednisolone
   b. Prednisolone and aciclovir
   c. Prednisolone and famciclovir
   d. Vitamin E
   e. Carbamazepine

Neurological problems: answers

1 e This is really very simple, although rectal diazepam or buccal midazolam would be options depending on the situation you find yourself in out of hospital. An ECG is impossible and although observations are all very thorough there is little you are going to act on. You should try to place the patient in the recovery position but this might be technically impossible in the throws of a seizure. If the fit lasts for more than 5 minutes or there is a second fit within 24–48 hours, consider urgent referral to hospital. There will be some patients who this is the norm for regarding their clustering of fits, and hospital admission may be unnecessary.

2 e Valproate is probably the most teratogenic of the anti-epileptics although phenobarbital, carbamazipine, phenytoin, primidone and lamotrogine are all teratogenic. Other antiepileptics are not thought to be. It is often not safe to change medication once the patient is in pregnancy as the risk to mother and foetus of a fit may outweigh the risk of the medication. Folic acid supplementation is recommended at 5 mg. The chance of having a baby with no malformations is 90%, despite being on medication.

3 d Torsades de pointes can occur and is related to a short QT interval because of antiepileptics but it is specifically unexpected death prevention that needs prompt action. Subarachnoid is unusual but a subdural can occur following a fall. Patients with epilepsy can drive 12 months after their last fit, so long as there are no changes in medication after 6 months.

4 f This would be secondary to metastases.

5 e

6 g A stroke would spare the forehead because of bilateral cortical innervation of the upper facial muscles.

7 a Prednisolone increases the speed of recovery at 3 and 9 months, dose of 1 mg/kg/day for 5 days. Antivirals have not been shown to increase speed of recovery. They were used because of the viral aetiology theory.

Statement 15.8

Respiratory problems

Asthma

- Around 5.4% of the population are estimated to have asthma (www.lunguk.org).
- On average four people a day die from asthma.
- New diagnoses in children rose from 4% to 10% between 1964 and 1989.
- Approximately 1500 deaths per year are due to acute exacerbations of asthma.
- The annual cost of asthma to the NHS is £700 million (this does not include economic cost of working days lost).
- Children exposed to antibiotics in utero are thought to be more likely to develop asthma (by up to 43%), hay fever (by up to 38%) and eczema (by up to 11%). However, this has only been shown in one study.

Historically the second half of the twentieth century is when asthma diagnosis started to increase. Although British Thoracic Society (BTS) guidelines have been successful, asthma is still underdiagnosed and undertreated.

A recent government inquiry into asthma deaths concluded that many could have been prevented by more proactive GP care (not clear how much was patient and how much was GP). It cited the following problems:

- underuse of primary care services
- under-prescribing of oral steroids
- inadequate use of peak expiratory flow meters.

It also found only 12% of those that had died had attended a practice asthma clinic in the year before death.

Some recent work has looked at the use of nitric oxide, and pilot studies have found that patients with low nitric oxide levels have better asthma control and lung function. Another paper looked at the use of itraconazole versus placebo (58 patients who tested positive for fungal allergy were randomised and 60% taking the antifungal showed an improvement).

British Guideline on the Management of Asthma/Scottish Intercollegiate Guidelines Network/BTS Asthma Guidelines

www.brit-thoracic.org.uk/guidelines/asthma-guidelines.aspx

These guidelines, updated and published in 2011, aim to help us in achieving an accurate diagnosis and symptom control quickly by stepping up treatment and then stepping down treatment when control is good.

The guidelines are broken down into adults, children aged 5–12 years and children under 5 years. They suggest that there should be a method of identifying poorly controlled asthmatics so that they can be asked to come in for review or chased up if they fail to attend, as there is a higher mortality in this group of patients.

Organisation of care

All practices should have a list of people with asthma (now an easy task, given coding and computer databases).

Review

- This should be routine with a standard recording system.
- It should include inhaler technique, peak expiratory flow meters, current treatment, morbidity and a personal asthma action plan.
- It should be audited regularly.
- The best results are seen with nurses who have been trained in asthma management.

The following three questions should be asked:

1 Do you have difficulty sleeping because of your asthma?
2 Have you experienced your asthma symptoms during the day?
3 Has your asthma interfered with your usual activities?

Accessibility, clinical effectiveness, and practice costs of providing a telephone option for routine asthma reviews: phase IV controlled implementation study

Br J Gen Pract 2007; 57(542): 714–22

Initially we were able to offer telephone consultations (especially for patients who were well controlled and working, so unable to attend in normal hours) to fulfil the QOF requirements. This then became frowned upon despite good uptake and no suggestion that it compromised patient care.

This trial in Whitstable, Kent, randomised asthma patients receiving care to a telephone encounter (554), face-to-face consultation (659) or usual care (515) over a 12-month period. Morbidity was equivalent in the three groups; cost for telephone consultation was less than a face-to-face review. The study concluded that as well as being cost-effective, telephone consultations increased review rates, enhanced patient enablement and confidence with management.

Personal asthma action plans

- These should be customised and written.
- They should be offered to all patients with asthma.

Acute exacerbations

- Inpatients should be on specialist units.
- Discharge should be a planned and supervised event. It may take place as soon as clinical improvement is apparent.

Targeting care

Identify groups at risk, they include:

- children with frequent upper respiratory tract infections
- children over 5 years of age with persistent symptoms
- asthmatics with psychiatric disorders or learning disability
- patients who are using large quantities of beta-2 agonists.

If there is a suggestion or work-related asthma then patients should be referred.

Self-management plans for asthma

Since the revised 2003 BTS/Scottish Intercollegiate Guidelines Network guidelines, increasing importance is being placed with patients who have the education and the confidence to manage their own asthma, enabling them to live a symptom-free life, detecting and treating their exacerbations early. Personal action plans are intended for use in patients over 12 years of age. Self-management plans reduce exacerbations, hospital admission rates and time off work and although many asthma patients think their asthma is well managed, their symptoms (hence quality of life) could be improved. However, their use is still suboptimal.

Long-acting beta-2 agonists

Meta-analysis of increased dose of inhaled steroid or addition of salmeterol in symptomatic asthma (MIASMA)

BMJ 2000; 320(7246): 1368–73

Lung function was higher in patients who received salmeterol rather than steroids. Symptom-free days and nights were more frequent with salmeterol and rescue free days and nights higher with salmeterol. There were fewer exacerbations with salmeterol and the severity was less in those who did have an exacerbation.

Leukotriene-receptor antagonists

These are derived from arachidonic acid, the precursors of prostaglandins. By preventing prostaglandin release, they reduce bronchoconstriction, mucous secretion and oedema.

Improving asthma control in patients suboptimally controlled on inhaled corticosteroids and long acting beta-2 agonists: addition of montelukast in an open label pilot study

Curr Med Res Opin 2005; 21(6): 863–9

This is a real-life observational study of 313 Belgian patients already taking inhaled corticosteroids and long acting beta-2 agonists but who were inadequately controlled.

78.6% of the patients reported an improvement of their asthma with addition of montelukast.

Breathing exercises

The Butekyo method is a breathing technique developed by a Russian physician who believes that a significant amount of asthma is caused by hyperventilation. In the United Kingdom this can be provided by a trained physiotherapist and is recommended in the guidelines.

The body of evidence is increasing indicating that the breathing exercises work to reduce symptoms of asthma.

Tumour necrosis factor (TNF) blockers are being trialled, alongside usual treatment, for brittle asthmatics. Also being considered is an injection called omalizumab (a protein that blocks the immune response to allergens), which could prevent severe allergy-related asthma attacks. It would be administered by injection every 2–4 weeks.

Chronic obstructive pulmonary/airways disease

Chronic obstructive pulmonary disease (COPD) is recognised as a systemic disease. The systemic symptoms of muscle weakness and weight loss seem to relate poorly to lung function; hence, lung function should be only one of the tools we use to assess disease severity and progression.

British Thoracic Society definition

'A chronic slowly progressive disorder characterised by airflow obstruction that does not change markedly over several months. Most of the lung function is fixed although some reversibility can be produced by bronchodilator (or other) therapy.'

- COPD causes around 26 000 deaths per year (respiratory disease is now the biggest killer in the UK).
- It is responsible for 400–1000 per 10 000 consultations in general practice.
- Risk factors include smoking, pollution, occupation (cadmium and coal), lower social classes, genetic factors and chronic under-treatment of asthma.

In 2010 the National Institute for Health and Clinical Excellence (NICE) guidelines superseded the BTS guidelines.

Following recent publication in *Chest* (October 2005) it is thought that the UK BTS guidelines (now NICE) may miss 1.5% cases of COPD when compared with use of the European Respiratory Society guidelines (the difference being that BTS guidelines are fixed and ERS guidelines are weighted for gender).

Chronic Obstructive Pulmonary Disease (2010)

www.nice.org.uk/nicemedia/live/13029/49397/49397.pdf

This NICE document is available for reference and the summary is nice and concise. A new National Service Framework and stategy is also being developed (it is anticipated that GPs will be asked to screen high-risk groups).

Diagnosis of COPD

This is suggested by symptoms and established by objective measurements using spirometry, with a chest X-ray to exclude other pathologies. Spirometry is the most reliable means of confirming a diagnosis and assessing severity and reversibility. A trial of steroids (30 mg prednisolone for 2 weeks or 6 weeks beclomethasone 1000 μg per day), following baseline spirometry, is recommended in looking for reversibility. Reversibility is an increase of the forced expiratory volume in one second by 15% AND 200 mL above the baseline.

In October 2001, *GP News* looked at the potential savings that could be made identifying COPD patients on asthma registers and withdrawing inhaled steroids (following data presented at the eleventh European Respiratory Society Conference).

Steroid use in COPD

Inhaler and steroid use, amounts and best combinations, for symptom control and to reduce disease progression are always under debate. A validation study (*Respir Med* 2007; 101: 1313) of 749 randomly selected patients found that 90% of patients taking medication for their COPD do so based on trials for which they would not have been eligible for. Many studies have suggested that inhaled corticosteroids reduce exacerbation and improve health.

The prevention of chronic obstructive pulmonary disease exacerbations by salmeterol,fluticasone proprionate or tiotropium bromide

Am J Resp Crit Care Med 2008; 177(1): 19–26

The INSPIRE trial looked at 1323 patients with severe COPD and found that although the number of exacerbations were similar, those on salmeterol/fluticasone were more likely to need antibiotics while those on tiotropium tended to be treated with steroids. The fact that the drugs may have different and possibly synergistic effects is creating interesting debate that may lead to development of a triple inhaler.

Salmeterol and fluticasone proprionate and survival in chronic obstructive pulmonary disease

N Engl J Med 2007; 356(8): 775–89

This study was a 3-year, randomised, double-blind study in 6112 patients with COPD. It looked at the effects of combined salmeterol/fluticasone (50/500 μg) as compared with placebo, salmeterol or fluticasone. Salmeterol/fluticasone reduced moderate to severe exacerbations but not exacerbations requiring hospitalisation compared with salmeterol alone. The group on fluticasone alone were more likely to have pneumonia (number needed to harm, 17).

The study quotes the number needed to treat was four to prevent one exacerbation in 1 year. The number needed to treat was 32 to prevent one hospitalisation in seretide versus placebo (probably not the best comparison).

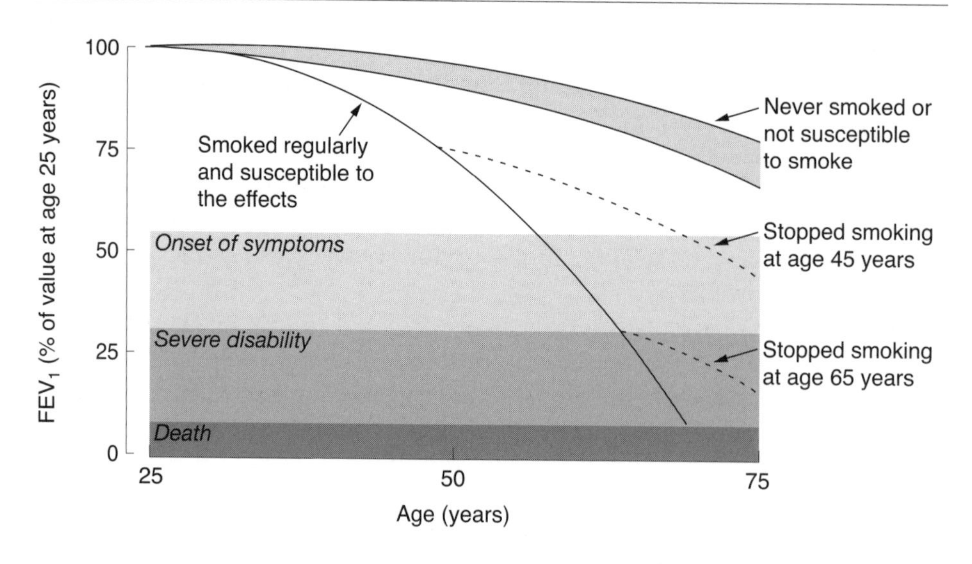

Smoking cessation

Reduces the rate of decline in lung function (Fletcher-Peto 1977 graph, www.spirometrie.info/img/fletcher.gif). Legislation in the United Kingdom means that people are no longer allowed to smoke in public places or work areas (including company cars).

Environmental tobacco smoke and risk of respiratory cancer and chronic obstructive pulmonary disease in former smokers and never smokers in the EPIC prospective study

BMJ 2005; 330(7486): 277–80

This was a prospective study of 303 020 people who had never smoked or who had stopped smoking at least 10 years ago, who provided information about environmental tobacco smoke. Controls were matched for sex, age, smoking status and country of recruitment. Over a 7-year follow-up the whole cohort had an increased risk of events (hazard ratio, 1.30; 95% confidence interval 0.87–1.95). It concluded that environmental tobacco smoke was a risk factor for respiratory diseases, especially in ex-smokers.

Long-term oxygen therapy

In hypoxaemic patients, long-term oxygen therapy (LTOT) prolongs life, but inappropriate use may cause respiratory depression. LTOT should be considered if PaO_2 <7.3 kPa. It is important to ensure that it does not cause carbon dioxide retention. Oxygen should be prescribed for 15–20 hours per day.

MRC trial

Lancet 1981; (i): 681–6

This trial showed that five patients would need to be treated for 5 years to avoid one death (number needed to treat, 5), where treatment involved administration of 15 hours oxygen per day. The difference was only evident after 500 hours. A

Cochrane review 2005 (2005; 4: CD001744) looked at six randomised trials and found improved survival in using oxygen where arterial $PaO^2 < 55$ mmHg.

Self-management plans for COPD

The principles follow the same lines as for asthma management plans.

Self-management reduces both short- and long-term hospitalisation in COPD

Eur Respir 2005; 26(5): 853–7

This Canadian study involving 191 patients who had been hospitalised with an exacerbation of their COPD involved a randomised issuing of the self-management programme 'Living with COPD' versus standard hospital care. At 2 years the intervention group showed a reduction from 26.9% to 21.1% cases of hospitalisation.

N-acetylcysteine

This is a mucolytic agent with antioxidant properties that has been found to reduce the exacerbations of COPD (number needed to treat, 6). It may also slow the rate of decline in lung function.

New developments in the treatment of COPD: comparing the effects of inhaled corticosteroids and N-acetylcysteine

J Physiol Pharmocol 2005; 56 Suppl 4: 135–42

The results of this complicated study showed that inhaled corticosteroids improved lung function in COPD. The N-acetylcysteine group showed a reduction in inflammatory markers.

Pulmonary rehabilitation

This is to become increasingly part of the holistic care approach we should have as GPs especially in patients who are disabled by their breathlessness (usually MRC 3 and above). It has been shown to reduce symptoms, increase mobility and improve quality of life. Exercise can reduce the risk of relapses requiring hospital admission by 50% (*Thorax* 2003; 58: 100–5).

Pulmonary rehabilitation and the BODE index in COPD

Eur Resp J 2005; 26(4): 630–6

The BODE index integrates body mass index, airflow limitation (forced expiratory volume in 1 second) dyspnoea and a 6-minute walking distance. It predicts mortality in COPD.

A total of 246 patients were divided into groups of patients who had received pulmonary rehabilitation and those who had not. BODE worsened by 4% over 12 months in those with no rehabilitation; mortality in this group was 39%. BODE improved by 19% following rehabilitation but returned to the original baseline after 2 years; mortality in this group was 7%.

It is thought that the BODE index change after pulmonary rehabilitation may provide valuable prognostic information.

Osteoporosis

There is a higher risk of osteoporosis in COPD than in asthma, even when patients have not had long-term steroid treatment (*Chest* 2003; 122: 1949–55). The cause of this is not completely understood although the multisystemic effects, poor nutrition and lower testosterone levels probably all contribute to the effect.

It is recommended that patients with COPD take a vitamin D supplement, the degree of vitamin D deficiency having been found to correlate with the severity of COPD in a Belgian study. This reduction could be due to skin ageing with smoking and reduced sun exposure from lack of exercise (outdoors) because of the severity of COPD.

National Strategy for COPD

July 2011

The strategy will aim to promote:

- respiratory health and good lung health
- early accurate diagnosis
- active partnership between healthcare professionals and people with COPD/asthma
- chronic disease management (and good control of symptoms)
- targeted evidence-based treatment for the individual.

The Outcomes Strategy identifies six objectives:

1. better prevention of COPD
2. reducing premature death
3. improving quality of life
4. improving safe and effective care
5. reducing the impact of asthma
6. reducing inequalities in access to and quality of services.

Tuberculosis

Tuberculosis (TB) is caused by mycobacterium tuberculosis and infects 9 million people, with 2 million deaths a year, worldwide. Depending where we work will determine whether we see TB or whether we just see an occasional letter telling us about a patient being in contact with a case diagnosed on the ward.

The annual report from the Health Protection Agency (www.hpa.org.uk/) outlines the following data, emphasising that the rate has dropped since 2009 but that this could be due in part to case reporting.

- There are currently 8587 cases a year in England (rate 13.9 per 100 000).
- Children aged 0–15 years represent 5% of cases.

Research into a TB vaccine as part of the ongoing drive to control and eliminate the disease is looking at:

- replacing the current BCG (Bacillus Calmette-Guérin) with an improved version, either by introducing genes (recombinant BCG30) or by delivering it orally
- boosting existing BCG
- developing an attenuated strain of TB.

Tuberculosis: clinical diagnosis and management of tuberculosis, and measures for its prevention and control
www.nice.org.uk/nicemedia/live/13422/53642/53642.pdf
This guidance was updated in March 2011 and supersedes the BTS guidance. It goes through screening, testing management of pulmonary and non-pulmonary TB, and the role of steroids.

Influenza

The influenza virus was first identified in 1933 and influenza A and B are estimated to cause 2000–4000 deaths per year in the United Kingdom, mainly from December to March. In the United States it is known that 10%–20% of their population will show a serological conversion, whether or not they are symptomatic, each year.

All through the influenza season the Health Protection Agency publishes a weekly report.

Immunisation against influenza

www.dh.gov.uk/prod_consum_dh/groups/dh_digitalassets/@dh/@en/documents/digitalasset/dh_129757.pdf
Immunisation of those at high risk of serious illness from influenza reduces hospital admissions and deaths. Immunisation can reduce mortality by up to 40% (up to 70% in repeated vaccination) and respiratory illness by up to 50%.

In October every year there is a fantastic influenza immunisation campaign run through primary care, the aim being to reduce morbidity and mortality. Currently work is looking into children and their role in transmission of the virus as well as how the illness affects them. They may be part of new inclusion groups in future campaigns that are sent out yearly by the Chief Medical Officer.

The Department of Health's Flu Campaign targets all people aged 65 years and all people over 6 months of age in the following risk groups:

- chronic respiratory disease, including children who have previously been admitted to hospital with lower respiratory tract infection
- chronic heart, kidney, liver and neurological disease
- diabetes
- pregnant women at any stage of pregnancy
- all those in long-stay residential and nursing homes, as well as other long-stay facilities
- people who are the main carer for an elderly or disabled person whose welfare may be at risk if their carer falls ill (added 2005)
- immunisation of healthcare workers (as part of what is called 'prudent winter planning'.

Patients who decline flu vaccine (this is from a collection of a number of different articles in the *Br J Gen Pract*):

- consider influenza a mild disease
- hope they won't get flu
- doubt the effectiveness of the vaccine

- fear the side effects of the vaccine and that it will give them flu
- lack campaign awareness
- are apathetic
- are unable to attend for immunisation (e.g. house bound or in residential care)
- find the timing of immunisation clinics inconvenient
- lack information about the vaccination.

Antiretroviral treatment for influenza

The neuraminidase inhibitors inhibit the replication of influenzas A and B. They should be started within 48 hours of symptoms and are designed to compliment the vaccination programme. Amantidine has been available since the 1970s but it is only effective against influenza A. If there were an influenza pandemic, of whatever strain, these drugs will be part of our management. It is not yet clear if they have a significant role to play in prophylaxis.

NICE *Influenza prophylaxis – amantadine oseltamivirand zanamivir*

http://guidance.nice.org.uk/TA158

Treatment advice for adults with symptoms of an influenza-like illness who can start treatment within 48 hours of the onset of symptoms is oseltamivir (zanamivir within 36 hours).

Advice for prevention is that these should be used if influenza A or B is circulating in the community for people over 13 years in the following groups:

- those in an at-risk group who have not had a flu jab this season, or had one too recently to have developed good protection
- who have been in close contact with someone with flu-like symptoms.

In this category of person they could start taking oseltamivir within 48 hours of contact.

The Department of Health has issued a pandemic framework (www.dh.gov.uk/pandemicflu) advising:

- Antiretrovirals are stockpiled to cover half of the UK population (currently 25%).
- Phoneline support for primary care with direct access to antiretrovirals (GPs only seeing cases with complications) to aid rapid diagnosis and treatment.
- Highlights secondary bacterial infections and advises consideration of antibiotics in adults with co-morbid diseases who are worsening or not improving over 48 hours.

The H5N1 strain of influenza

This has received much interest, causing the World Health Organization to declare an influenza pandemic in 2009/10. This is one type of avian flu that has been known about for over 10 years; H7N2 is another strain, which is less pathogenic. There were fewer than 500 deaths related to this in the United Kingdom, with a case mortality of 0.4 per 100 cases. Although the numbers are small, the proportion of deaths is extremely concerning and reflective of the virulence of the strain.

A lot of work has been done looking into whether a strain of H5N1 could be incorporated into the current influenza vaccine, replacing the strain of lower virulence.

Pneumococcal vaccine

This is a one-off vaccination (re-vaccinate after 5–10 years if antibody levels are likely to have declined). It can be given at the same time as the influenza vaccination but at different sites.

The Department of Health Pneumococcal Immunisation Programme was introduced in August 2003 as an all-year-round campaign. The age of eligibility for vaccination has gradually been reduced.

Current target groups include:

- all people over 65 years
- at-risk groups, from the age of 2 months (the main difference to the flu programme is that asthma is not included unless the patient needs frequent oral corticosteroids)
- individuals with cochlear implants
- individuals with the potential for cerebrospinal fluid leaks
- children under 5 years who have had a previously invasive pneumococcal disease.

Respiratory problems: questions

1 Asthma: which of the following would be considered the level below which is a life-threatening sign in an acute exacerbation of asthma according to the BTS guidelines?
   a. Oxygen saturation 98%
   b. Oxygen saturation 95%
   c. Oxygen saturation 92%
   d. Oxygen saturation 90%
   e. Oxygen saturation 88%

2 Influenza: which of the following vaccination regimes are recommended for an 8-year-old child with step 2 asthma, whose previous influenza vaccination history is unknown?
   a. Trivalent seasonal influenza, two 0.5 mL vaccinations 4–6 weeks apart.
   b. Trivalent seasonal influenza, one 0.5 mL vaccination.
   c. Pneumococcal conjugate vaccine (PCV), one 0.5 mL vaccination.
   d. Pneumococcal polysaccharide vaccine (PPV), one 0.5 mL vaccination.
   e. Both the trivalent seasonal influenza vaccination and the pneumococcal vaccination as per the green book guidance.

3 COPD: which of the following statements is considered correct with regard to inhaler use in COPD?
   a. Ipratropium should be used with tiotropium for maximal effect.
   b. Ipratropium should be used in preference to tiotropium in management of COPD, as per the NICE guidance.
   c. Ipratropium should only be prescribed after referral to secondary care.
   d. Ipratropium reduced the risk of cardiovascular disease in COPD.
   e. Ipratropium may increase cardiac risk in COPD.

4 Which of the following statements with regard to lung cancer is correct?
   a. Sixty per cent of male and 57% of female lung cancers are thought to be smoking related.
   b. An unexplained cough of 3 weeks' duration requires a chest X-ray to look for lung cancer pathology.
   c. Around 67% of patients with advanced lung cancer will present with malignant airway obstruction.
   d. Five per cent of all lung cancers will present with some form of haemorrhage.
   e. Patients with several episodes of haemoptysis should have a chest X-ray unless there are treatable signs of infection.

5 What is the acronym publicised in the COPD strategy?
   a. ACT
   b. CAN DO
   c. REACT
   d. BREATHE
   e. BREASTE EASI

TB: in the following table of features of extra-pulmonary TB, select the most appropriate answers for questions 6–9. Each answer can be used once, more than once or not at all.

Site	Percentage cases
6	29.4%
7	6.9%
8	4.1%
9	2%

   a. Central nervous system
   b. Spine
   c. Pleura
   d. Lymph nodes
   e. Skin

10 Considering LTOT, which of the following statements is correct?
   a. Reduces secondary polycythaemia.
   b. Arterial blood gas measurements should be made as soon as possible following the identification of hypoxaemia.
   c. It is important that patients only use the amount of oxygen they feel they need.
   d. Blood gas measurements should be made on at least two occasions, 1 week apart.
   e. If a patient has end-stage COPD and is using LTOT, it is acceptable for them to continue smoking as long as the oxygen is turned off while smoking.

Respiratory problems: answers

1 c Although options (d) and (e) would be considered significant, the question is testing your knowledge of the guideline value. This question is taken from the summarised version of the 2011 BTS/Scottish Intercollegiate Guidelines Network guidance. It is probably worth noting that the areas that the Royal College of General Practitioners have considered to be answered less well in the past are those in relation to acute management of emergency problems (www.brit-thoracic.org.uk/guidelines/asthma-guidelines.aspx). Signs would include a peak flow reduction of >33% normal, oxygen saturation <92%, partial pressure of oxygen <8 kPa, silent chest, cyanosis, arrhythmia, exhaustion and altered conscious level. If the $PaCO_2$ levels start to rise then that would be considered near fatal.

2 a Pneumococcal vaccination is not recommended at this stage of asthma. The influenza vaccine, at the first time of giving, needs two doses 4–6 weeks apart but thereafter just one dose. Given the vaccination history is unknown then you must consider the two vaccines.

3 e It is generally counterproductive to use ipratropium and tiotropium together, because of M3 receptor use of the drug. Tiotropium is recommended, not ipratropium, by NICE. There are a few studies coming out showing an increase in cardiovascular events in patients prescribed ipratropium in the previous 6 months. The latest paper has been published in *Chest* (40% increased in risk) although a *JAMA* study in 2009 showed up to an 80% increase in the risk of cardiovascular death. The MHRA Number 37 was published in 2008 saying the jury is still out although there is some evidence out there.

4 b In 90% of men and 83% of women, lung cancer is associated with smoke; it is rare under the age of 40 and it peaks at 80–84 years of age. NICE guidance (www.nice.org.uk/nicemedia/live/13465/54208/54208.pdf) recommends chest X-ray for cough of 3 weeks and all patients with haemoptysis. Between 20% and 30% of patients present with airway obstruction secondary to the tumour and 30% will haemorrhage.

5 c

- **R**espriatory health and lung health
- **E**arly accurate diagnosis
- **A**ctive partnership between healthcare professionals and people with COPD
- **C**hronic disease management (or good control of symptoms)
- **T**argeted evidence-based treatment for the individual.

6 d

7 c

8 b

9 a These questions are taken from UK data published in *GP* in a clinical review article on pulmonary TB (5 August 2011).

10 a This question is from the BTS and NICE guidelines for COPD. Blood gas measurements should be performed on at least two occasions at least 3 weeks apart. Blood gases are required once over an exacerbation or on maximal therapy. LTOT should be used for at least 15 hours a day to reduce mortality. Although realistically this will happen, the risk of burns to themselves and fire are significant. They are unlikely to get any benefit if they continue smoking.

Statement 15.9

Rheumatology and conditions of the musculoskeletal system (including trauma)

Osteoporosis

The NHS Consensus Development Conference defined this as a 'progressive skeletal disorder characterised by low bone mass and microarchitectural deterioration of bone tissue with a consequent increase in bone fragility and susceptibility to fracture'.

The World Health Organization definition is:

- Osteoporosis: bone density > 2.5 standard deviation below the mean (femoral neck).
- Osteopenia > 1 standard deviation below the mean.

Note that one definition is a pathological process and the other is an arbitrary point on a scale. The T-score criteria were proposed for epidemiological studies to compare populations and for defining thresholds in clinical trials. Unless stated otherwise the measurements will be from the femoral neck. They were not intended for diagnosis or management decisions in individual cases.

Recent research has identified the Maf gene that regulates creation of cells for bone formation in mice; regulation of expression of this gene may be able to be developed into a clinical application.

- It is estimated that up to 3 million women have osteoporosis in the United Kingdom.
- The prevalence increases from 2% at 50 years to 25% at 80 years (in women).
- Osteoporosis causes over 200 000 fractures per year (mainly wrist, vertebral and hip fractures) in England and Wales.
- It costs the government £1.73 billion per year (87% of this is because of hip fractures).
- One in five hip fracture patients die within 1 year, 50% have severely impaired mobility.
- A third of vertebral fractures cause chronic pain (i.e. there is a huge impact on morbidity and mortality).

Risk factors

Risk factors include the following:

- post-menopausal women

- early menopause (before 45 years of age, e.g. following a hysterectomy and oophrectomy)
- immobility
- long-term steroid use (it is suggested that this group receives preventive treatment)
- previous fragility fracture
- high systolic blood pressure (higher rate of bone loss).

Secondary causes (this will affect up to 50% of men and 10% of women):
- alcoholism
- thyroid problem (hypothyroidism and hyperthyroidism)
- liver disease
- malabsorption
- hypogonadism in men
- connective tissue disorders (e.g. rheumatoid and systemic lupus erythematosus).

Treatments

Monitoring the effect of treatment has usually been done with repeat DEXA scans, after at least 18 months of treatment. However bone turnover markers (such as P1NP) may be of more use in the short term and are currently being evaluated.

Prevention/lifestyle changes

- Stop smoking, avoid excess alcohol and take regular weight-bearing exercise.
- Fall prevention – assessment of safety in the home can be provided in primary care
- Protection of sites of high impact, hip protectors are of proven benefit with up to 50% reduction in some studies (residential care based).

Calcium supplements

- The recommended daily dose is 1 g for people over 50 years of age.
- There is no evidence that calcium reduces fractures unless it is taken with vitamin D.
- Calcium supplementation has been linked to an increased risk in cardiovascular disease, so some consideration needs to be given to its use outside of treatment for osteoporosis (*BMJ* 2010; 341: 260–1).

Vitamin D

- The recommended daily dose is 400 iU too low for fracture prevention, 800 iU would usually be used.
- Two trials have shown that vitamin D and calcium reduced risk of fracture by up to 50% over 5 years; the best results are seen in institutionalised frail elderly.

Bisphosphonates

These are now first choice in management of osteoporosis. A once-monthly preparation, ibandronate, has recently been released. Bisphosphonates have been identified as a cause of osteonecrosis of the jaw (1–3 years after starting treatment).

Strontium ranelate

This is a dual agent (like teriparatide) that improves bone mineral density by increasing bone formation and reducing bone resorption.

Hormone replacement therapy

A meta-analysis suggests that this yields a relative risk reduction of 40% (for fractures). However, the benefits are lost within 5 years of stopping hormone replacement therapy. This is a treatment option that is no longer recommended for treatment of prevention because of the risk factor profile.

Tibolone (bleed-free preparation of hormone replacement therapy)

This has been shown to increase bone mass density in the spine over 2 years.

Selective oestrogen receptor modulators (e.g. raloxifene)

These decrease the fracture rate by 30% over 3 years at best.

Osteoporosis: primary prevention of osteoporotic fragility fracture

www.nice.org.uk/nicemedia/live/11746/42486/42486.pdf

Alendronate is recommended for primary prevention in women with risk of fracture, and depending on their age an additional risk for low bone density, all with proven osteoporosis. It is important to recognise this is primary prevention of fracture related to osteoporosis, not primary prevention of osteoporosis.

Osteoporosis: secondary prevention

www.nice.org.uk/nicemedia/live/11748/42508/42508.pdf

The guidance for use of bisphosphonates, raloxifene and teriparatide standards for use are as follows:

- All women over 75 years of age who have fractured should be treated for presumed osteoporosis without the need for a DEXA scan.
- All women between 65 and 74 years of age should be treated if osteoporosis is confirmed by DEXA scan.
- Women younger than 65 years should be treated:
  - if they have a bone mineral density less than –3SD
  - if they have a bone mineral density of –2.5SD with one or more additional risk factors (BMI <19 kg/m^2, a family history of maternal hip fracture <75 year, untreated premature menopause, medical disorders associated with bone loss or conditions associated with prolonged immobility).

For treatment their preference are the bisphosphonates with raloxifene as an alternative. Teriparatide should be restricted for use in more severe cases.

Several articles have been published that raise concerns about the guidelines. Below are a number of issues that are often discussed:

- The guidelines are too restrictive and will exclude a lot of people who would benefit from treatment.

- The search omitted a number of European articles, casting doubt on the cost-effectiveness calculations.
- The T-score weighting means that under the guidelines patients need to be at a higher risk to qualify for treatment.
- It does not take into account the Royal College of Physician guidance (2002) that patients on long-term corticosteroids should receive treatment at a T-score of −1.5 standard deviation (−2.5 standard deviation in National Institute for Health and Clinical Excellence).
- The National Institute for Health and Clinical Excellence has now agreed that treatment can be given whilst awaiting a DEXA scan due to the long delays; how this would then affect their treatment if after scanning they were found to be just outside the treatment criteria, is not clear.

Screening

Fractures occur late and there are no symptoms prior to this. All women over 65 years of age in the United States are screened (it has been recognised that men are missing out on potential preventive advice). However, there is no universal policy in the United Kingdom. NICE guidance *Osteoporosis – primary prevention* (guidance.nice.org.uk/TA160) covers treatment for fragility fractures but as yet there is nothing which formerly addresses an active screening process within the UK.

Shifting the focus in fracture prevention from osteoporosis to falls

BMJ 2008; 336(7636): 124–6

This edition of the *BMJ* looks at several issues around falls and osteoporosis. No study to date has ever looked at whether preventing falls also prevents fractures with any sufficient power, and some randomised trials have reported a 50% reduction. The falls assessment looking at history, medical risk factors, movement, strength and gait are all part of how a GP should be assessing the risk of falling.

Royal College of Physicians guidelines 1999

These guidelines suggest DEXA scanning should be offered to individuals with risk factors, as well as those with a low bone mass density ($<19\,kg/m^2$) and those with a strong family history (despite the Finnish study concluding that genetics were not thought to be important).

Useful information can be obtained from the National Osteoporosis Society (www.nos.org.uk). There has been work around the QFractureScore (*BMJ* 2009; 339: 1291–5), as comparing it with FRAX, and it is seemingly valid and more accurate.

Back pain

- Around 60%–80% of the population will have back pain at some point in their life.
- Up to 85% of acute episodes resolve in 6 weeks; if they persist for 12 weeks or more it is a chronic problem.
- Around 7% of people consult their GP each year with back pain.
- A total of 120 million work days/year are lost as a result of back pain.

This information is based on 1998 data from the Office of National Statistics and ARC data from 2007.

Diagnosis and management

'Red flags' are symptoms and conditions that require urgent imaging, blood tests and referral. They include:

- a past medical history of carcinoma, tuberculosis, drug abuse and human immunodeficiency virus (cause of immunosuppression and infection)
- previous prescription drug use (e.g. steroids)
- symptoms of night sweats, fever and loss of weight
- a new structural deformity (e.g. kyphosis) suggestive of fracture
- widespread neurology.

Cauda equina symptoms need immediate referral as there is a risk of permanent damage and incontinence. These symptoms would include:

- loss of sphincter control
- bilateral neurological leg pain
- saddle loss of sensation.

Patients with simple back pain or isolated nerve root irritation can be managed conservatively. Multilevel or progressive neurological problems require urgent referral.

Clinical Evidence gives a comprehensive outline of current trial for each modality of treatment (www.clinicalevidence.com). Advice includes:

- simple analgesia regularly
- take regular exercise as soon as the pain allows
- muscle relaxants may help if there is a degree of spasm unresponsive to analgesia
- physiotherapy
- complementary therapy: chiropractor, osteopath and acupuncture may all be beneficial although there are no randomised trials confirming this.

Randomised controlled trial of exercise for low back pain: clinical outcomes, costs and preferences

***BMJ* 1999; 319(7205): 279–83**

This study showed that early access to a doctor (within 3 days) and physiotherapist (within 1 week) for exercise for new-onset back pain was associated with good outcomes. Early mobilisation increases the speed of recovery, reduces the length of time off work and reduces the number of recurrences.

Osteoarthritis

www.nice.org.uk/nicemedia/live/11926/39554/39554.pdf

Around 20%–25% of visits to GPs relate to the musculoskeletal system. Most of these cases are secondary to osteoarthritis. Osteoarthritis, by definition, cannot be cured but the previously held belief that it would inevitably progress is being challenged as the understanding of the metabolic process develops. Risk factors for development of osteoarthritis include being female, age, obesity, nutrition, bone density and muscle strength.

Management: diet

Other than weight loss, specific diets have no role to play in the management of osteoarthritis and rheumatic conditions. There are reports of vitamin C reducing rates of progression and improvements with certain seeds and cod liver oil.

Management: exercise and physiotherapy

Exercise improves muscular tone and joint function, so should not be avoided. Physiotherapy reduces pain, improves joint range and muscle strength as well as improving mobility and independence.

Investigation of clinical effects of high- and low-resistance training for patients with knee osteoarthritis: a randomised controlled trial

Phys Ther 2008; 88(4): 427–36

This paper from Asia compares the effects of high- and low-resistance strength training in elderly subjects with knee osteoarthritis. The study involved 102 patients who were assigned for 8 weeks of either treatment or none (the control group). Pain, function, walking time, and muscle torque were examined before and after intervention. Improvement for all measures was observed in both exercise groups, no significant difference between intensity.

Glucosamine

Glucosamine sulphate is a natural substance that forms proteoglycans (part of the articular cartilage). It is thought to be chondro-protective although the jury is still out on how clinically effective they are for pain relief. These are available as dietary supplements, which are expensive. There is an option to prescribe on an FP10 (a dose of 1500 mg/day) although availability will depend on the individual primary care trust.

Effect of glucosamine sulfate on hip osteoarthritis: a randomised trial

Ann Intern Med 2008; 148(4): 315–16

This study looked at whether glucosamine sulphate had an effect on the symptoms and progression of hip osteoarthritis during 2 years of treatment. The study involved 222 patients with hip osteoarthritis who were recruited by their general practitioner and randomised to 2 years of treatment with 1500 mg of oral glucosamine sulphate or placebo once daily. Glucosamine sulphate was no better than placebo in reducing symptoms and progression of hip osteoarthritis.

Local injections

Intra-articular hyaluronic acid gives symptomatic benefit. This has been confirmed in several randomised controlled trials. The lasting effect is uncertain as is the benefit compared to steroid injection (which is known to improve pain in both the short and the long term).

Intra-articular hyaluronic acid for treatment of osteoarthritis of the knee: systematic review and meta-analysis

CMAJ 2005; 172(8): 1039–43

This study included 22 trials published up to April 2004. It concluded that intra-articular hyaluronic acid injection has not been proven to be clinically effective and may be associated with greater risk of adverse events.

Rubefacients

Topical creams and gels are often used in patients, especially when they are unable to tolerate systemic treatments. This is often an area targeted in prescribing budgets because of relative lack of evidence and associated costs.

Systematic review of efficacy of topical rubefacients containing salicylates for the treatment of acute and chronic pain

BMJ 2004; 328(7446): 995–8

This study looked at randomised double-blind trials comparing rubifacients and placebo, all of which were fairly small in number. The conclusion was cautious but probably indicates that topically applied rubefacients containing salicylates are effective in treating acute pain. At best the number needed to treat is 5.3 (relative benefit, 1.5; 95% confidence interval 1.3–1.9).

Complementary therapies

These are all used regularly in subgroups of the population with good effect. Specific randomised trials are lacking.

Rheumatology and conditions of the musculoskeletal system (including trauma): questions

1 In a 54-year-old woman, previously fit and well, whose mother developed osteoporosis at the age of 70 years, which of the following statements are correct, assuming that she has never smoked and that she rarely drinks alcohol?
   a. She does not need a bone density scan.
   b. She needs a bone density scan every 3 years.
   c. She needs a bone density scan every 5 years.
   d. She should be treated prophylactically with a bisphosphonate.
   e. She should be treated prophylactically with hormone replacement therapy.

2 A 68-year-old man presents with a painful, swollen, hot knee. He is systemically well and apyrexial. Which of the following is the most likely diagnosis?
   a. Psoriatic arthropathy.
   b. Rheumatoid arthritis.
   c. Pseudogout.
   d. Gout.
   e. Septic arthritis.

3 Which of the following would be considered one of the criteria for inflammatory arthritis?
   a. Cystic changes seen on X-ray of the hands.
   b. Early-evening stiffness.

c. Early-morning stiffness lasting 5–10 minutes.
d. ESR of 24 mm/first hour in women.
e. ESR of 24 mm/first hour in men.

4 In tennis elbow which anatomical site is affected?
a. The insertion of extensor digitorum and extensor carpi radialis brevis.
b. The medial epicondyle.
c. The lateral malleolus.
d. The medial malleolus.
e. The olecranon bursa.

For each of questions 5–8, select the single most appropriate answer. Each answer can be used once, more than once or not at all.
a. Patella/quadriceps tendinitis
b. Plica
c. Prepatellar bursitis
d. Osgood Schlatter's
e. Patellofemoral malalignment
f. Osteochondritis dissecans
g. Chondromalacia patellae
h. Patellofemoral joint osteoarthritis

5 This may be seen in adolescents with effusion of the knee and pain on patellofemoral movement.

6 Pain would be specifically over the tibial tuberosity.

7 This happens because of overuse or trauma and it is a palpable band from the medial femoral condyle to the patella that may snap on movement.

8 This is usually seen in adolescent girls with a history of overuse, there is pain and grinding with movement of the knee.

9 Which of the following would be the most appropriate treatment to reduce the destructive effects of psoriatic arthritis overall?
a. Ibuprofen
b. Diclofenac
c. Prednisolone
d. Methotrexate
e. Anti-TNFs

10 What is the most likely diagnosis in this picture? The patient is essentially pain free unless there is overuse, the only problem being lack of strength in the hands and cosmetic issues.

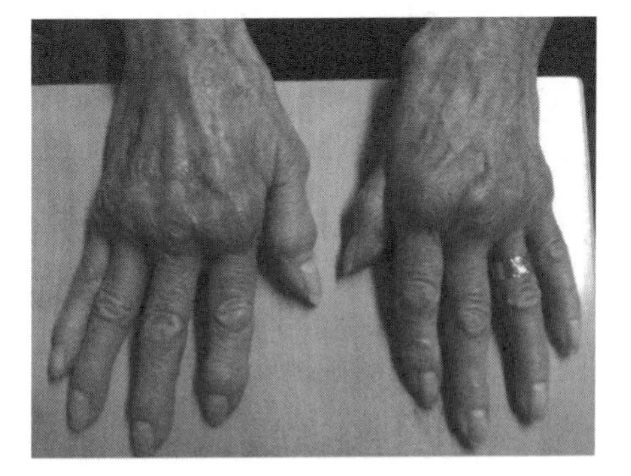

a. Systemic lupus erythematosis
b. Osteoarthritis
c. Rheumatoid arthritis
d. Psoriatic arthritis
e. Rheumatoid negative inflammatory arthritis

Rheumatology and conditions of the musculoskeletal system (including trauma): answers

1 a Using the 10-year risk assessment models (for example, www.sheffield.ac.uk/FRAX) her risk is <5%. There is no evidence with the above information that a bone density scan is needed. No medication is warranted (hormone replacement therapy would no longer be recommended as first-line therapy if it was) although sensible calcium intake (up to 1 gm/day) and vitamin D, regular weight-bearing exercise and not drinking to excess (more than 3 units per day in the FRAX model) should be recommended.

2 d Gout is more common than pseudogout. Inflammatory parkers and uric acid may be raised. Joint aspiration would show birefringent monosodium urate crystals (whereas pseudogout would show calcium pyrophosphate dehydrate crystals). Treatment for a one-off attack would be anti-inflammatories or colchicines, if recurrent >3 times a year then allopurinol would be considered.

3 e This question was taken from a 'Hand On' article produced by the ARC. The screening tool for inflammatory arthritis (*Ann Rheum Dis* 2003; 62(2): 187) identifies the following as indicative of inflammatory arthritis:

- early morning stiffness lasting >1 hour
- characteristic distribution for inflammatory joint disease
- first-degree relative with inflammatory joint disease
- clinical evidence of synovitis
- ESR >20 mm/first hour in men, >30 mm/first hour in women
- erosions on hand or feet X-rays
- benefit from non-steroidal anti-inflammatory drugs or steroids.

4 a These muscles insert onto the lateral epicondyle, the medical epicondyle would be golfer's elbow.

5 f

6 d

7 b

8 g

Questions 5–8 were adapted from Update February 2006 'Ten-minute consultation Anterior Knee Pain' by James and Tindall. Their table is summarised here.

Condition	History	Examination	Treatment
Patellar/quadriceps tendonitis	Overuse activities	Pain on palpation of the tendon	Rest, NSAIDs, ice
Pica	Direct trauma or overuse	Palpable band from the medial femoral condyle to patella	Rest, NSAIDs, ice
Prepatellar and pes anserinus bursitis	Repetitive kneeling activities or trauma	Erythematous swollen area over the bursa. Movement intact	Ice, rest. If infected may need antibiotics or surgical drainage

(*continued*)

Condition	History	Examination	Treatment
Osgood Schlatter disease	Athletic adolescent male	Tender, prominent tibial tubercle	Rest, brace
Patellofemoral malalignment	Over use, trauma, may be insidious onset with no clear history	Assess the patellar tracking	Physiotherapy, taping and brace. May need arthroscopic lateral release
Osteochondritis dissecans	Adolescents, history of trauma	Effusion, locking. May come and go	MRI – young patients conservative approach, older patients need arthroscopy
Chondromalacia patellae	Adolescent girls, there may be a history of over use	Grinding pain on flexion and pain on patellofemoral movement	Rest, physio, NSAIDs, bracing Arthroscopy if these measures fail
Patellofemoral joint osteoarthritis	Chronic pain, usually in the elderly	Pain and crepitus	Physio, arthroscopy, possible patellofemoral joint replacement

9 e Although methotrexate is a disease-modifying drug, the effects are not as wide-ranging as the anti-TNFs which improve not only the arthritis but also skin and nail changes, axial disease, dactylitis and enthesitis. (Reports on Rhuematic Disease 2009 series 6 number 3, Psoriatic Arthritis.)

10 c This was rheumatoid, the arthritis having burnt out so caused no inflammatory pain although sometimes a functional pain with over use.

You can see the metocarpophalangeal joint changes, which are characteristic. The Heberden's nodes are the lesser problem of osteoarthritis so would not be the correct answer here.

Statement 15.10

Skin problems

Understanding dermatology is about taking an interest in the history, reading around and looking at many pictures. There are some excellent update courses and diplomas available, but I think that it always comes down to personal interest and practical experience on the ground. Dip in and out of the picture books, learn from your referrals and consider some of the online sites such as DermIS.net (www.dermis.net/dermisroot/en/home/index.htm). You'll know you've got it cracked when you don't break out in a sweat every time a rash walks into the consulting room.

I've tried many ways to write this part of the curriculum, but I come back to pictures every time. The pictures here are of my patients who have agreed for me to use their photographs.

Skin problems: questions

1 On biopsy this rash proved to be a discoid lupus reaction. Which of the following medications that this patient is taking is the most likely cause?

a. Terbinafine
b. Aspirin
c. Ramipril
d. Tamsulosin
e. Bisoprolol

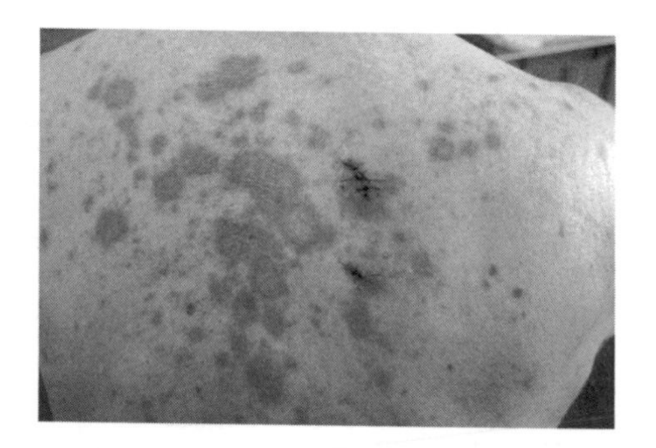

2 What is the most likely diagnosis in the picture shown?

a. Erythrasma
b. Hyperhidrosis
c. Bromhidrosis
d. Severe scarring acne
e. Hidradenitis suppurativa

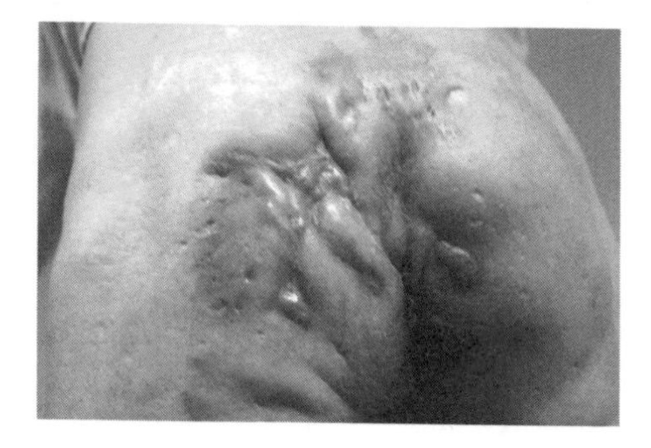

3 In hyperhidrosis, if aluminium chloride products have failed to help symptoms there are many other options. Which of the following options below would not be considered worthwhile?

a. Iontophoresis
b. Driclor

c. Botox
d. Endoscopic thoracic sympathectomy
e. Retrodermal curettage of the axilla

4 What is the most appropriate treatment for this enlarging lesion on a 4-month-old child's torso?
a. Laser treatment
b. Surgical excision
c. Hydrocortisone (0.5%)
d. Vaniqa cream for 3 months
e. No treatment is needed

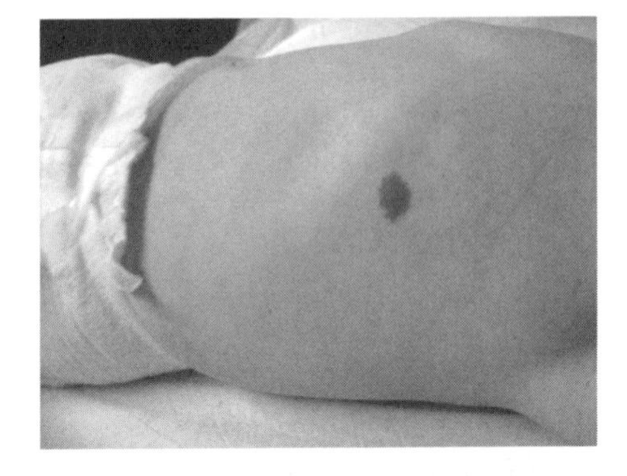

5 What is the diagnosis in this picture?
a. Benign intradermal naevi
b. Multiple sebaceous cysts
c. Neurofibromatosis
d. Basal cell carcinomas
e. Pustular psoriasis

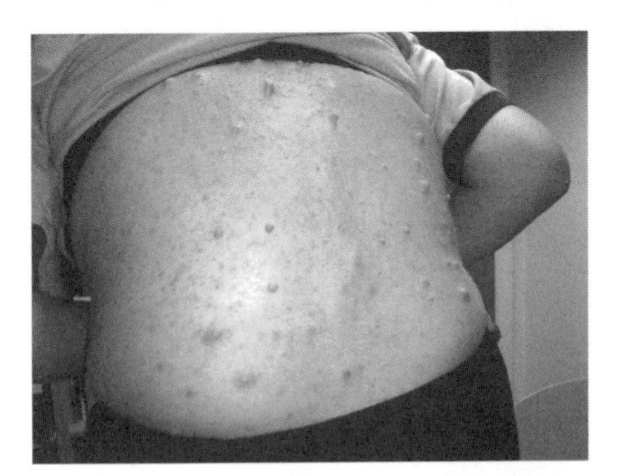

6 What is the diagnosis of these lesions in a young woman on the combined oral contraceptive pill?
a. Erythema nodosum
b. Henoch–Schönlein purpura
c. Wegener's vasculitis
d. Discoid lupus
e. Systemic lupus erythematosis

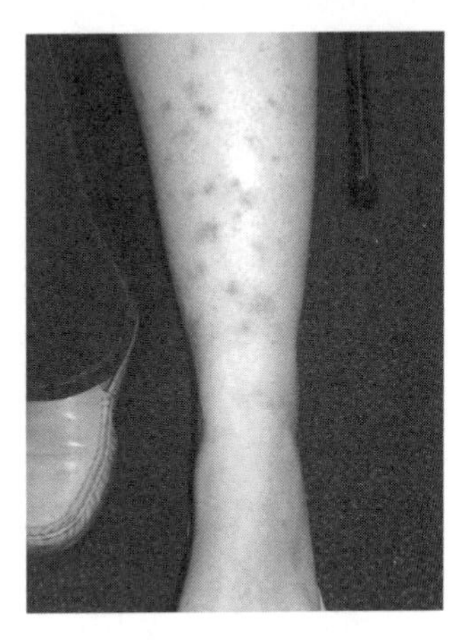

7 Which of the following is not a recognised treatment for alopecia areata?
a. Intralesional steroids
b. Topical tretinoin
c. Topical minoxidil

d. Topical hydrocortisone
e. Topical Rogaine

8 Which of the following is the best solution to the problem seen?
a. Tea tree oil
b. Betnovate scalp application
c. Cocois scalp application
d. Permethrin scalp application
e. T/Gel shampoo

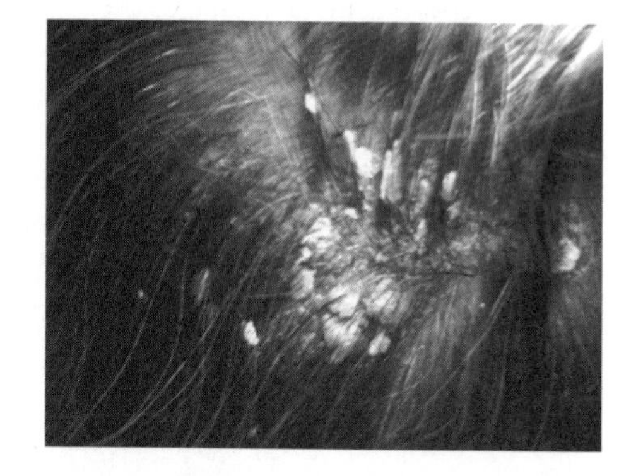

9 This patient attended for a second opinion regarding this long-standing lesion. What is the most likely diagnosis?
a. Lipoma
b. Subdural haematoma
c. Cranial haematoma
d. Epidermoid cyst
e. Sebaceous cyst

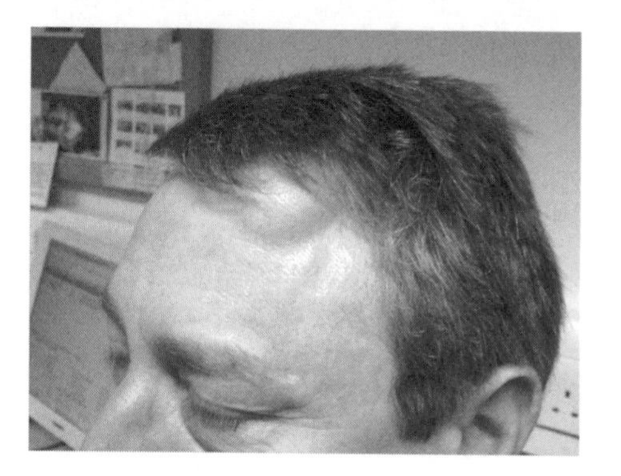

10 An epidermoid cyst presenting before puberty can be associated with which of the following?
a. Eczema
b. Polyposis coli
c. Hereditory hemangiomata
d. Steatocystoma multiplex
e. Hyperhidrosis

Skin problems: answers

1 a Terbinafine was the cause in this patient. Beta blockers are known to cause lupus-like reactions, but not usually discoid lupus – more malar flush.

2 e Erythrasma is caused by corynebacteria infection and fluoresces coral pink in Wood's light. Hyperhidrosis is excessive sweating. Bromhidrosis is body odour caused by sweat being broken down by bacteria on the skin. Hidradenitis is a chronic inflammatory condition of the apocrine sweat glands. It heals leaving scarring and is most likely to be due to *Streptococcus milleri.* Treatment with antibiotics is often adequate, although acitretin is sometimes needed, as is surgical excision of the affected glands. This man's hidradenitis was slowly progressive despite intensive treatment. He had several surgical procedures to debride and treat abscesses. He went on to develop osteomyelitis and a psoas abscess needing a hind-quarter amputation, which then went on to change cell type and became squamous cell carcinoma at the edges – probably as severe as it gets.

3 b Driclor is aluminium chloride and you are given in the question that it has not been successful. Iontophoresis is where hands are placed on metal plates covered with gauze in either water or water and glycopyrronium bromide solution (you can get this in wipes online). An electric current is passed in one direction through the plates and then reversed. Tap water alone works in 85% of cases. Botox can be repeated every 3 months. Sympathectomy and curettage are a last resort but can be helpful in some cases.

4 e This is a strawberry naevus. It will enlarge and will then regress over the next 3–4 years or so. No treatment is needed unless it encroaches on the orbit, in which case it may affect orbital development. If there are multiple haemangiomas it is sometimes prudent to scan the liver and skull with ultrasound for arteriovenous malformations that may rupture and where prophylactic treatment may be needed.

5 c Neurofibromatosis is more common than you may think. It can crop up in genetics (autosomal dominant), paediatrics with screening issues and the counting of café au lait spots, medicine and surgery depending upon complications from the neuromas.

6 a Erythema nodosum – tender purple patches. Unfortunately they didn't resolve on stopping the pill with this woman. A subsequent X-ray and bloods showed sarcoidosis.

7 d Hydrocortisone is too weak. You would need dermovate or betnovate to really have any effect (used daily for 3 months). Intralesional steroids, usually triamcinolone, can be used as a first-line treatment where there is persistent hair loss affecting <5% of the scalp.

8 c This is scalp psoriasis and the cocoas will soften up the plaques. Although T/Gel shampoo and betnovate scalp application may give some effect, the Xamiol (betamethasone and calcipotriol) would give the best effect and may also be used as an alternative option to the Cocois. Premethrin is used as lyclear for head lice. This was not pityriasis amiantacea, where the plaque and scale grow out along the hair follicle.

9 a There is little to expand upon here; subdural would be exactly that (i.e. inside the skull), the size and lack of punctum or bruising means lipoma is the differential of choice.

10 b (Gardner's syndrome). However, it can also be associated with basal cell naevus syndrome. Steatocystoma multiplex are small skin-coloured papules that are inherited autosomal dominantly.

Statement 15.11

The rest of general practice

The title doesn't involve general for nothing – this is 'proper doctor'. If you don't know something it is your responsibility to find out, learn, ask a colleague or refer, depending on the problem. Similarly, it is your professional responsibility to keep learning and updating long after the exam has been and passed. Everything that is noted here in the curriculum can be found in a textbook but you will probably already know that anything can crop up.

Chronic kidney disease

www.renal.org.uk

Having estimated glomerular filtration rates (eGFRs) reported on all our renal results has meant we are screening these cohorts for renal disease more actively than ever in the past. As chronic kidney disease is an independent risk factor for vascular disease and increases mortality and morbidity, this is going to be an area of our routine work that can only expand.

Stage	Description	eGFR (mL/min/1.73 m^2)
1	Kidney damage (dip positive for protein, microalbumin or blood) with normal or increased eGFR	**>90**
2	Kidney damage with mild decreased eGFR	**60–89**
3	Moderate decreased eGFR	**30–59**
4	Severe decreased eGFR	**15–29**
5	Kidney failure	**<15 or dialysis**

The estimated glomerular filtration rate

As up to 50% of renal function is usually compromised before any increase in creatinine is seen, the eGFR allows us to identify issues and to enable us to take action sooner. The gold standard for renal function is inulin clearance. This is costly and time-consuming – certainly not practical for primary care numbers.

This thankfully comes calculated for us (there is an automatic calculator we can use online (www.renal.org.uk). The calculation of eGFR is based on:

- age
- sex
- ethnicity (not sure how the lab really knows this)
- creatinine.

$$eGFR = 186 \times [(creatinine / 88.4) - 1.154] \times [age - 0.203] \times [0.742 \text{ (if female)}] \times [1.21 \text{ (if black)}]$$

Problems that may give misleading eGFRs:

- There are lab variations.
- Anything >90 will not be exact as not accurate in extremes.
- May be falsely low if following high protein meal (i.e. fasting sample best).
- If elderly or extreme body mass may be inaccurate.
- Must be stable (over 3 months).

It is important not to interpret eGFRs out of context.

Effects of statins in patients with chronic kidney disease: meta-analysis and meta-aggression of randomised controlled trials

BMJ 2008; 336(7645): 645–51

This meta-analysis of 30 144 patients (pre-dialysis and transplant patients) looked at the benefits versus the harm with statin treatment. It found that although lipid concentration was reduced and cardiac outcomes improved, all causes of mortality showed no improvement. It concluded that the role of statins in primary prevention was uncertain and the renoprotective effects of statins as uncertain.

Chronic fatigue syndrome/myalgic encephalomyelitis

www.nice.org.uk/nicemedia/pdf/word/CG53NICEGuideline.doc

Chronic fatigue syndrome (CFS), also known as myalgic encephalitis, is defined as disabling fatigue associated with other symptoms, e.g. musculoskeletal pain, sleep disturbance, impaired concentration and headaches. The cause is not understood; a polypeptide involved in the antiviral response was more common in CFS but this has no clinical application.

- The overall population prevalence is 0.2%–0.4%.
- In a practice of 10 000 patients, around 40 will have CFS.
- The World Health Organization classifies it as a neurological condition.
- Communication is the key to good management, providing:
  - acceptance and understanding
  - information about the illness
  - assistance with occupational and social care issues.

Treatment of CFS/myalgic encephalitis

- Function and quality-of-life management:
  - sleep management to avoid napping
  - rest periods
  - exercise, encourage pacing and not overdoing things on a good day
  - healthy diet
  - consider cognitive behavioural therapy.
- Pharmacological intervention:
  - low-dose tricyclic for pain (e.g. amitryptiline)
  - melatonin may be considered in young people who have sleep difficulties.

- Setbacks and relapse:
  - management is about understanding the experience and going back to the basics set out above.
- Ongoing review – as with any chronic disease.

Chronic fatigue syndrome or myalgic encephalomyelitis

BMJ 2007; 335(7617): 411–12

The guidelines have been criticised for not being sufficiently evidence based, but this editorial is somewhat more optimistic (they have taken 11 years to come together). It highlights the message that this is a recognised condition (interestingly a significant number of doctors still do not believe it exists) with positive treatment options. Rehabilitation trials for CFS are underway by the UK Medical Research Council.

What to do about medically unexplained symptoms

Drug Ther Bull 2001; 39(1): 5–8

Around one in five new consultations are by patients with physical symptoms for which there is no organic cause (and one in 10 children). In a third of cases the symptoms persist and can cause distress and disability.

General practice is about dealing with symptoms that don't fit the disease model. Don't make the mistake of labelling symptoms 'MUS' until a thorough clinical assessment and appropriate investigations have been carried out; if no physical explanation can be found the psychological and emotional issues need to be considered. Malingering is rare; the definition mainly used being 'deliberate simulation or exaggeration of physical or psychiatric symptoms for obvious and understandable gain.'

It is thought that, although by definition the cause is unknown, they probably are due to a complex interaction of biological, psychological, social and cultural factors. Although seen in all specialities this is addressed mainly in psychiatry probably due to the links with anxious personality types and the tendency to develop psychological symptoms (www.rcpsych.ac.uk).

Understanding the narratives of people who live with medically unexplained illness

Patient Educ Couns 2005; 56(2): 205–10

This paper identified three features of the patient's narrative: a chaotic history of the illness narrative; concerns that their symptoms were all in their mind; and their status as medical orphans. There was genuine concern to secure some form of ongoing medical and social support.

Management

It is important to acknowledge the symptoms and distress, as well as to provide continuity of care.

Management of medically unexplained symptoms

BMJ 2005; 330(7481): 4–5

This is a discussion of some of the issues and options available. It highlights that some of the essential elements in medical models are: to make the patient feel understood, then to broaden the agenda and finally to negotiate a new understanding of the symptoms including psychosocial factors.

Antidepressants

These can be useful especially if the patient is experiencing pain or difficulty in sleeping, whether or not they are depressed. Benefit is usually seen within 1–7 days (i.e. quickly!). The number needed to treat is three.

Reattribution

This involves demonstrating understanding of the patient's complaints by taking a history of related physical, mood and social factors. It is making the patient feel understood and making the link between symptoms and psychological problems (i.e. make the patient feel understood).

Cognitive behavioural therapy

This has been shown in systematic review to be beneficial particularly in reducing physical symptoms.

Recent developments in the understanding and management of functional somatic symptoms in primary care

Curr Opin Psychiatry 2008; 21(2): 182–8

Fink and Rosendal consider the training in primary care and recent stepped care approaches (that they explain need further evaluation). They feel names that 'presuppose a mind-body dualism (such as somatisation, medically unexplained)' should not be used and that treatment offered must be professional as in any other condition.

Frequent attenders

This is usually a different group of people to those with unexplained symptoms. The average general practice attendance per patient is three to four times per year. Part of the problem can include lack of reassurance, loss of confidence with the doctor, fear and concern.

Characteristics of high attenders include:

- multiple health problems
- lower social class
- medically unexplained symptoms
- belief that re-attendance is necessary to get the right treatment.

Is frequent attendance in primary care disease-specific?

Fam Pract 2006; 23(4): 444–52

This study looked at a random sample of 1000 adults in North Staffordshire, in nine general practices, who had attended at least once in the last 12 months. It then categorised them as either frequent (high or very high), moderate or low frequency consulters. It found that frequent attenders were not statistically limited to specific diseases although certain pathologies did consult more frequently.

Air travel

www.dh.gov.uk/en/Publicationsandstatistics/Publications/PublicationsPolicyAndGuidance/DH_4005997

When booking our holidays and long-haul flights few of us will give much thought to our health, but increasingly as GPs we will be asked questions on risk and recommendations for prevention of, for example, deep vein thrombosis. Deep-vein thrombosis (DVT) in association with air travel has been reported since the 1950s and in response to the House of Lords report on health and air travel (November 2000), the Department of Health has published advice for passengers.

The absolute risk of thrombosis is small (one case in every 6000 journeys that last for 4 hours or more). The longer the duration of travel the higher the apparent risk, although there is no lower limit below which it is safe. As the risks for thrombosis are additive, short sequential flights probably increase the risk.

Factors that put people at risk on long haul flights include cramped conditions, varying air pressure and oxygen concentration, dehydration with or without excess alcohol consumption. Certain other factors put some people at higher risk than others; these include obesity, heart disease, pregnancy, the pill, hormone replacement therapy, a family history of DVT, recent major leg surgery and increasing age.

Sensible advice is lacking in evidence, but the general consensus is:

- move around in the seat and in the cabin as much as possible
- rotate ankles and flex calf muscles regularly
- avoid alcohol and caffeine
- avoid dehydration (i.e. drink plenty of water).

Air travel and venous thromboembolism: a systematic review

J Gen Intern Med 2007; 22(1): 107–14

This systematic review was to determine the efficacy of preventive treatments from 25 trials over a 40-year period. It compared duration of travel (less than 6 hours to 6–8 hours; 27 pulmonary emboli were diagnosed per million flights and 0.05% risk of venous thromboembolism, diagnosed through ultrasound.

Graduated pressure stockings helped prevent venous thromboembolism in four out of the six studies ($p < 0.05$), but aspirin did not. The study concluded that all travellers should avoid dehydration and should exercise leg muscles. If a flight is less than 6 hours and there are no known risk factors, no DVT prophylaxis is needed. Travellers with one or more risk factors should consider stockings for travel longer than 6 hours.

Thromboembolic deterrent stockings

Mediven travel stockings (which exert a pressure of 20 mmHg at the ankle) have been shown to reduce the incidence of DVT in travellers. There is no evidence for the use of lower compression stockings.

Aspirin

The benefits of aspirin are arterial rather than venous. To my knowledge, no published study has shown any reduction in risk of thrombosis in travellers. It is important to be aware of the gastrointestinal haemorrhage risk, and that some clinics are advising taking 150 mg of aspirin the day before travel.

Subcutaneous heparin

This is indicated in high-risk patients and does reduce the risk of DVT. Usually one injection 2–4 hours before travelling is adequate. If the patient is on warfarin there is no additional benefit.

Airogym

This is an inflatable cushion placed under the feet that simulates walking when pressed. The results so far are encouraging, but as yet there are no published outcome trials.

Chronic disease management

Chronic diseases are the main cause of morbidity and mortality in developed countries (having overtaken infectious diseases) and account for almost a quarter of GPs' workload, according to recent statistics. Managing these conditions effectively helps to reduce complications and deterioration, overt a potential crisis, and reduce acute admission and referral rates to secondary care.

Meeting the needs of chronically ill people

***BMJ* 2001; 323(7319): 945–6**

This editorial reiterates that the best outcomes depend upon competent self-management and decision-making by patients, as well as clinical treatments. It also brings to the forefront the frequent co-occurrence of mental disorders.

Management programme

Elements of a chronic disease management programme would usually include the following:

- clinical guidelines
- patient-friendly information that is accessible
- continuous quality improvement and clinical audit
- access to specialist care
- resource management techniques and systems
- case management
- patient education and counselling

- tracking systems
- national disease registers.

Having chronic disease morbidity registers allows audit of standards such as compliance and prescribing. This enables better planning of services and necessary changes. The data extracted is dependent on accuracy of diagnosis and coding. A number of chronic diseases form part of specific indicators in the new General Medical Services contract.

Further issues

- Care must be organised. If a system is methodical it reduces the risk of error. This is helped further with the use of computers in terms of speed (once the data has been input) as well as for audit when trying to improve quality. Protocols need to be in place, but flexible enough to allow for patient-dependent factors.
- The patient should be the most important member of the team; it is their life and in essence we are there in an advisory capacity.
- Ethical issues when giving the diagnosis of a chronic disease and then motivating them with regard to best management and compliance, when they still consider themselves to be a 'normal healthy adult'.
- Economic and political issues in funding screening programmes and chronic disease clinics in an evidence-based way (medical care, equipment, administration, audit and so forth).
- No doctor, or member of the primary healthcare team, should make the mistake of underestimating the psychological impact a chronic disease could have on a person's life. It should not be trivialised but wherever possible we should help that person keep things in perspective as best we can.

Support for self care for patients with chronic disease

***BMJ* 2007; 335(7627): 968–70**

Self-care is defined as actions taken 'to lead a healthy lifestyle; to meet their social, emotional and psychological needs; to care for their long term condition'. The Department of Health has a three-tier approach – case management, disease management and self-care support – a critical part of the support being the expert patient programme.

The Expert Patient: a new approach to chronic disease management in the 21st century

Published in 2001, this proposed that every primary caregiver should have a lay-led training course in self-management for chronic diseases for patients. Approximately £2 million is being invested for the pilot schemes and to mainstream the programmes through the NHS by 2007.

The gold standard for this was a six-session group intervention led by laypeople who have the disease, or experience of it, to help improve skills and confidence of other patients.

Although people have needs specific to their individual disease they have a core of common requirements:

- knowing how to recognise and act upon symptoms
- dealing with acute attacks or exacerbations of the disease
- making the most effective use of medicines and treatment
- understanding the implications of professional advice
- establishing a stable pattern of sleep and rest and dealing with fatigue
- accessing social and other services
- managing work and resources of employment services
- accessing chosen leisure activities
- developing strategies to deal with the psychological consequence of illness
- learning to cope with other people's response to their chronic illness.

How effective are expert patient (lay led) education programmes for chronic disease?

BMJ 2007; 334(7606): 1254–6

This analysis reflects on four randomised controlled trials and that although they increase patients' confidence they are unlikely to reduce significant targets such as admission. They are not recommended over other programmes at this stage.

Integrated/alternative medicine

Complementary medicine (which focuses on health and healing) and conventional medicine (which focuses on disease and treatment) have traditionally been distinct from each other, but recently they have become increasingly integrated. This means complementary medicine will have to be subject to similar clinical, scientific and regulatory standards as is applied to conventional healthcare.

The *ABC of Complementary Medicine* estimates that 30% of the UK population use alternative medicines and 40% of GPs offer access to complementary treatment. Furthermore, you are unlikely to see review articles that don't feature herbal remedies to some degree, as they are becoming an increasingly used (despite lack of evidence on effectiveness) method of self-treatment.

Public awareness of complementary medicines has meant that the use has increased dramatically over the last 10 years, but many complimentary practitioners remain unregulated.

Regulating herbal medicines in the UK

BMJ 2005; 331(7508): 62–3

This editorial discusses the use of a specific committee to help consumers distinguish between unproven herbal therapies as compared to pharmaceutical treatments proven to have an effect. Currently in the United Kingdom the Medicines and Healthcare Products Regulatory Agency is consulting on a proposal for a herbal medicines committee.

Perceptions about complementary therapies relative to conventional therapies among adults who use both: results from a national survey

Ann Intern Med 2001; 135(5): 344–51

A total of 831 people in the United States who use alternative/complementary medicine were surveyed.

- Around 80% thought the combination of both complementary and conventional medicine was superior to either alone.
- Most saw a conventional doctor first.
- Around 70% did not subsequently disclose they were seeing a complementary therapist as it was not thought to be any of the doctor's business rather than it being for fear of criticism.

Acupuncture

www.medical-acupuncture.co.uk

On the basis of current evidence, acupuncture is effective in treating nausea and vomiting, back pain, dental pain and migraine. The incidence of adverse reactions to acupuncture is relatively low. It is the most popular form of complementary therapy amongst GPs (used by 47%). This popularity has only emerged in the United Kingdom over the last 20 years, although it has been used for many thousands of years in Chinese medicine.

Non-medical acupuncturists should be members of the British Acupuncture Council, which has strict educational criteria and a code of practice. Physiotherapists may belong to the Acupuncture Association of Chartered Physiotherapists, and doctors usually belong to the British Medical Acupuncture Society.

Adverse events following acupuncture: prospective survey of 32 000 consultations with doctors and physiotherapists

BMJ 2001; 323(7311): 485–6

This study (there is an accompanying editorial) found no adverse events were reported after 34 407 acupuncture treatments from data collected over a 4-week period. It did not look at patients' experiences of adverse events, but it is encouraging and reassuring research.

Herbal remedies

The European Union's Traditional Herbal Medicinal Products Directive came into force in October 2005. It means that all unlicensed herbal remedies sold in the UK will become regulated; companies will have to prove that new products have a traditional use and have accompanying safety data.

Again popularity in the UK means sales are increasing by 20% a year. The users often have the belief that 'herbal' means that something is natural and is both safe and cheaper than conventional medicine and with no side effects. Many herbal products do have side effects and can interact with other drugs.

As there is little legislation for control, doses of preparations can vary widely, even in the same product. Some products may also contain conventional medicines (e.g. recently one eczema cream was found to contain high doses of dexamethasone, having been advertised as a natural product).

- **Ginseng**: is teratogenic, it increases INR and may also increase blood pressure. It also interacts with digoxin. There are several varieties, the active ingredients (ginsenosides) are antioxidants and enhance nitrate production.
- **St John's wort**: this is a weak selective serotonin reuptake inhibitor and antiviral. It is a liver enzyme inducer so may reduce the concentrations of digoxin, carbamazipine, warfarin and the oral contraceptive pill. It also interacts with several drugs.
- **Ginkgo biloba**: this is used to delay clinical progression of dementia. It is a potent inhibitor of platelet-activating factor so can increase the risk of bleeds (including intracerebral bleeding) in patients on aspirin or warfarin.

The herbal advice line is staffed by members of the National Institute of Medical Herbalists (www.nimh.org.uk). They can give advice on remedies, interactions and use in children and during pregnancy.

Homeopathy

This needs to be distinguished from herbal remedies. Homeopathic remedies contain minute or non-existent amounts of the original substance and are prepared by successive dilutions. Although to our knowledge there are insufficient randomised controlled trials to advocate the use of homeopathic treatments in specific conditions, many people report having benefited.

Are the clinical effects of homeopathy placebo effect? Comparative study of placebo-controlled trials of homeopathy and allopathy

Lancet 2005; 366(9487): 726–32

This meta-analysis of 110 trials concluded that their results were not compatible with the hypothesis that the clinical effects of homeopathy were completely due to placebo effect. There was weak evidence for a specific effect of homeopathic remedies but the findings were compatible with the notion that the effect was that of placebo.

Homeopathy: a guide for GPs

From the British Homeopathic Society, this describes a range of NHS services that are now available and details on how GPs can refer patients. The Glasgow and London homeopathic hospitals are the two leading bodies in research of this field, but funding is severely lacking. The British Homeopathic Society website (www.britishhomeopathic.org/) is a good source of information.

Antioxidants

These include ginseng, B-carotene, vitamins C and E, minerals such as zinc and copper, flavonoids and so forth. Most of the evidence available is in the form of cohort studies. As yet there seems to be insufficient evidence that taking antioxidants offers much in the way of benefits to healthy people.

Mortality in randomised trials of antioxidant supplements for primary and secondary prevention: a systematic review and meta-analysis
JAMA 2007; 297(8): 842–57
This analysis considered 68 trials of 232 606 patients and found that there was a significant increase in the risk of mortality, especially with beta-carotene and vitamins A and E. Vitamin C and selenium had no effect on mortality.

The rest of general practice: questions

1 Which of the following albumin-to-creatinine ratio results would equate to a significant microalbuminuria?
   a. 1.0 mg/mmol in a male.
   b. 2.2 mg/mmol in a female.
   c. 2.2 mg/mmol in a male.
   d. 2.7 mg/mmol in a female.
   e. 2.7 mg/mmol in a male.

2 On a case-by-case basis, which of the following is least likely to cause an eosinophilic blood picture?
   a. Giardia
   b. Schistosomiasis
   c. Asthma
   d. *Streptococcus* pneumonia
   e. Penicillin

3 Chronic kidney disease: which of the following is the correct classification for a patient with an estimated glomerular filtration rate of 40 mL/min/1.73 m^2?
   a. Stage 2
   b. Stage 3a
   c. Stage 3b
   d. Stage 4
   e. Stage 5

4 What would be accepted management in the acute presentation of the problem shown in this picture?

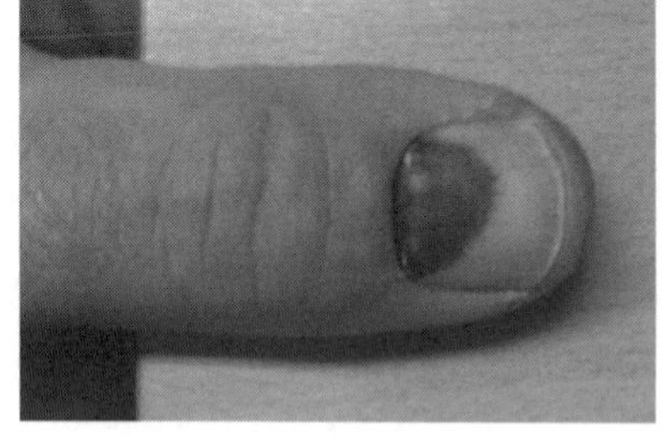

   a. Refer to the 14-day cancer initiative because of the suspicion of melanoma.
   b. Refer to chiropody for nail avulsion.
   c. Refer to dermatology for advice on permanent damage to the nail bed.
   d. Refer to orthopaedics to release the pressure to help prevent permanent damage.
   e. Heat a paperclip in a flame and pierce the nail to allow the blood to drain.

5 Which of the following would be considered a risk factor for venous thromboembolism?
   a. A past history of bowel cancer.
   b. A platelet count of 64×10^9/L.
   c. Use of triadene medication.

d. Hyponatraemia.
e. Age over 50 years.

6 With regard to venous ulceration with oedema, which of the following statements is correct?

a. Four-layer compression, in a patient with an ankle-brachial pressure index of 0.57 in the affected leg, would be the best treatment and increase speed of resolution.
b. Four-layer compression, in a patient with an ankle-brachial pressure index of 1.46 in the affected leg, would be the best treatment and increase the speed of resolution.
c. If secondarily infected, the use of maggots is superior and known to have fewer side effects than antibiotics when it comes to speeding the healing process.
d. If secondarily infected the use of vinegar works better than antibiotics and prevents pseudomonas infection.
e. You must consider a biopsy, especially when the ulcer is not responding to treatment.

Haemochromatosis can be either secondary or genetic. Consider the points in questions 7–10 and answer true or false.

7 Venesection as a form of treatment is only used when the patient is symptomatic.

8 It is a known cause of diabetes.

9 In haemoglobinopathies such as B-thalassaemia, intestinal absorption of iron may lead to a secondary haemochromatosis.

10 Hook osteophytes are a known association.

The rest of general practice: answers

1 e Albumin-to-creatinine ratio >2.5 mg/mmol in men and >3.5 mg/mmol in women would be significant. Protein-to-creatinine ratio isn't used for microalbuminuria. Proteinuria would be >30 mg/mmol for albumin-to-creatinine ratio and >50 mg/mmol for protein-to-creatinine ratio (www.renal.org.uk).

2 d Investigation of an incidental finding of eosinophilia (*BMJ* 2011; 342: d2670 1147–8). The most common causes of eosinophilia are parasitic infection, drugs (sulfonamides, penicillins, carbamazipine), allergy and hypersensitivity disorders. These account for 95% of cases. Less common causes are Churg–Strauss syndrome, connective tissue and autoimmune disease and other infections (bacterial, fungal).

3 c

- Stage 1: >90 mL/min/1.73 m^2
- Stage 2: 60–89 mL/min/1.73 m^2
- Stage 3a: 45–59 mL/min/1.73 m^2
- Stage 3b: 30–44 mL/min/1.73 m^2
- Stage 4: 15–29 mL/min/1.73 m^2
- Stage 5: <15 mL/min/1.73 m^2 (5D on dialysis).

4 e If this presents acutely (often because of being hit with a hammer or trapping a finger in a door), if the patient will allow you the heat from the paper clip will burn a hole through the nail (painless) and the blood will drain (warm running water helps). Like many things, probably not evidence based but helps pain significantly and probably, by releasing the pressure, reduces permanent nail bed trauma that would otherwise affect the appearance of the nail.

5 c Triadene is a triphasic oral contraceptive pill. Past cancer is not a risk but active cancer and cancer treatment is. A low platelet count (<75) is associated with a risk of bleeding. Hyponatraemia isn't a risk, but dehydration is. And aged over 60 years is a risk.

6 e Ankle-brachial pressure index when low can indicate arterial disease, which would be a contraindication; similarly, when high it can indicate atherosclerosis. Both options should be considered for vascular referral for angiography. Maggots and vinegar both have a use in treatment of ulceration but they are not used regularly and can cause inter-team issues and be difficult for patients to accept. In a non-healing ulcer you must consider squamous cell change and the need for biopsy.

7 False Venesection prevents the patient becoming not only symptomatic but developing the secondary effects of iron overload. These answers use the *Oxford Textbook of Medicine* coupled with experience from the first patient I diagnosed and became involved in helping manage. I have included this question as it is the type of diagnosis that requires clinical suspicion and awareness as, like amyloidosis, it can present in many varied ways.

8 True As iron accumulates in the B-cells of the pancreatic islets.

9 True Due to iron overload.

10 True Seen on X-ray, arthritis can affect any joint but it is usually the metacarpophalangeal joints.

Applied Knowledge Test: introduction

The Applied Knowledge Test (AKT) (www.rcgp-curriculum.org.uk/nmrgcp/akt.aspx) is a 3-hour, computer-based, multiple-choice exam. Approximately 80% of the exam will be on clinical medicine, 10% on critical appraisal and evidence-based medicine and 10% on health informatics and administrative issues (with 200 questions in total). It is important to read the Royal College of General Practitioners information prior to revising for and sitting the exam, as this information may change. The sample paper provided on the college website gives you a stem from which you then have to select the single best answer, extended matching questions, flow charts and picture spots to identify. You can view the exam format online (www.pearsonvue.com/rcgp/).

For AKT multiple-choice question exams, it is important to know how to interpret certain phrases. The following definitions are from the college guidelines, but you will find almost identical definitions in most multiple-choice question books.

- **Diagnostic, characteristic, pathognomonic, in the vast majority**: implies that the feature would occur in 90% of cases.
- **Typically, frequently, significantly, commonly, in a substantial majority**: implies that the feature would occur in 60% of cases or more.
- **In the majority**: implies that the feature would occur in 50% of cases or more.
- **In the minority**: implies that the feature would occur in less than 50% of cases.
- **Low chance, in a substantial minority**: implies that a feature may occur in up to 30% of cases.
- **Has been shown, recognised, reported**: all refer to evidence found in authoritative medical text.

It is good practice, both here and with other AKT books, to set aside a period of time to simulate the exam, as your concentration may be quite different when working on a paper this way than when dipping in and out of questions.

Applied Knowledge Test: questions

1 Heart failure: serum natriuretic peptides are used diagnostically in heart failure. Which of the following would not affect interpretation of the results?
   a. Obesity can increase the B-type natriuretic peptide (BNP) level.
   b. An estimated glomerular filtration rate of <30 can lower the BNP level.
   c. Tachycardia can lower the BNP level because of the increased glomerular filtration rate.
   d. Sepsis can increase the BNP level.
   e. Diuretics can reduce the BNP level.
2 Cardiovascular disease assessment: which of the following is not used to assess cardiovascular risk in the QRISK assessment tool?
   a. Total cholesterol : high-density lipoprotein ratio
   b. Postcode
   c. Being on blood pressure treatment
   d. Body mass index
   e. Waist circumference
3 Other risk factors for cardiovascular disease: which of the following is thought to have a future role as an indicator for cardiovascular disease?
   a. Fibrinogen
   b. Calcium level
   c. Homocysteine
   d. C-reactive protein
   e. Nitric oxide
4 In assessing cardiovascular disease risk in a 42-year-old female, which of the following factors would prompt you to offer professional lifestyle intervention in a patient with a cardiovascular disease risk of >20%?
   a. A waist circumference of >94 cm in a Caucasian woman
   b. A blood pressure of 136/80 mmHg
   c. A fasting glucose of 5.2 mmol/L
   d. An ex-smoker with a 20-pack-year history
5 In atrial fibrillation, which of the following factors is not included in the HAS-BLED scoring system?
   a. Elderly, over 60 years
   b. History of hypertension
   c. Renal function
   d. Previous stroke
6 Which of the following medications is/are not considered appropriate for patients with atrial fibrillation?
   a. Warfarin

b. Statins
c. Aspirin
d. Sotolol
e. Amiodarone

For questions 7–10 regarding the UK screening programme for cervical screening, choose the most appropriate answer from the following list. Each option can be used once, more than once or not at all.

a. Over 65 years
b. Over 60 years
c. 50–64 years
d. 30–40 years
e. 20–35 years
f. 20–49 years
g. 25–49 years
h. 25 years
i. 21 years
j. 18 years
k. 3-yearly invitation
l. 5-yearly invitation

7 What is the age at which cervical screening is first offered?
8 What is the frequency of invitation of cervical screening at 47 years?
9 What is the age at which cervical screening invitation ceases?
10 What is the frequency of invitation when cervical screening first starts?
11 Which of the following has not been identified as a priority group for smoking cessation?

a. Pregnant women who smoke
b. Adults with mental health problems
c. Prisoners
d. Patients suffering from anxiety and depression
e. Patients who have a high rate of smoking, such as those from ethnic minority groups

12 Which of the following is not regarded as a true statement with regard to prostate cancer screening?

a. It may detect cancer at an early stage when treatments may be available.
b. Forty-eight men will undergo treatment in order to save one life.
c. The speed of increase of prostate-specific antigen (PSA) reflects how aggressive a prostate cancer will be.
d. PSA testing may do more harm than good by identifying slow growing tumours that would never have created a negative effect.
e. PSA testing can miss cancer and provide false reassurance.

13 Which of the following is not known to have an association with obesity?

a. Postmenopausal breast cancer
b. Endometrial cancer
c. Renal cancer

d. Type 2 diabetes
e. Childhood type 1 diabetes

14 Which of the following statements is not true of Wernicke's encephalopathy?
a. Wernicke–Korsakoff's syndrome develops in patients who drink in hazardous ways and are thiamine deficient.
b. It comprises global confusion, eye signs and ataxia.
c. It may progress to Korsakoff's psychosis.
d. Patients who drink to harmful levels but eat a normal diet cannot develop a Wernicke's encephalopathy.

15 Which of the following would be appropriate first-line management for a patient with delirium tremens?
a. Carbamazepine
b. Diazepam
c. Phenytoin
d. Clomethiazole
e. Lorazepam

16 When considering blood alcohol concentration, which of the following statements is true?
a. Blood alcohol concentration varies according to the phase of the menstrual cycle, being highest premenstrually and at ovulation.
b. After drinking on an empty stomach, blood alcohol levels peak at around 15–20 minutes.
c. Effects of alcohol persist longer if a person has a higher body fat concentration because of storage within and slow release from the adipose tissue.
d. All organs and tissues are exposed to the same concentration of alcohol as that found in the blood, given that alcohol is water-soluble.
e. Although the rate of absorption differs, the blood concentration achieved drinking 1 unit of alcohol is the same whether drunk on an empty stomach or with a carbohydrate-rich meal.

For questions 17–20 choose the most appropriate answer from the following list of blood alcohol levels.

a. 4.4
b. 3.3
c. 17.4
d. 21.7
e. 15.2
f. 86.8
g. 90.2
h. 104

17 What is the level of alcohol in mmol/L known to be potentially fatal?

18 What is the rate in mmol/hour at which alcohol is removed from the body?

19 What is the level of alcohol in mmol/L at which the UK drink-driving limit is set?

20 What is the level of alcohol in mmol/L at which a person becomes garrulous, elated and aggressive?

For each of the statements in questions 21–24, select the most likely causative agent from the following list. (Drugs that we understand to be illicit are known to have negative clinical effects on the heart.)

a. Heroin (diamorphine)
b. Cocaine
c. Amphetamine and methamphetamine
d. Ecstasy (methylenedioxymethamphetamine)
e. GHD (gamma-hydroxybutyric acid)
f. Ketamine
g. LSK (lysergic acid diethylamide)
h. Poppers (nitrites)
i. Volatile substances (glue, solvents)

21 An anaesthetic agent that may increase the heart rate and blood pressure, there is no evidence that it leads to problems concerning the heart or blood vessels.

22 This agent causes vasodilatation that in turn causes flushes and low blood pressure and, although the effects are short-lived, it can contribute to falls.

23 This agent is known to lower heart rate and respiration. If this drug has been injected, especially if contaminated, it can lead to endocarditis and deep-vein thrombosis.

24 This agent is a powerful vasoconstrictor increasing blood pressure and may contribute to a heart attack if used.

For questions 25–29 regarding the childhood immunisation schedule in the UK, select the single most appropriate vaccination for each scenario that would be recommended from the following list.

a. *Haemophilus influenzae* type B and pneumococcal vaccination
b. *H. influenzae* type B, pneumococcal vaccination, diphtheria, tetanus, polio and whooping cough
c. Meningitis C and *H. influenzae* type B vaccination
d. Diphtheria, tetanus, polio, whooping cough and meningitis C vaccination
e. Diphtheria, tetanus, polio, whooping cough, meningitis C and pneumococcal vaccination
f. Diphtheria, tetanus, polio, whooping cough, *H. influenzae* B, meningitis C and pneumococcal vaccination
g. Measles, mumps and rubella vaccination
h. Measles, mumps and rubella and pneumococcal vaccination
i. Measles, mumps and rubella, meningitis C and pneumococcal vaccination
j. Diphtheria, tetanus, whooping cough, polio and measles, mumps and rubella vaccination
k. Pneumococcal vaccination
l. Nothing

25 What is the ideal combination of vaccines given to a 2-month-old child?

26 Which vaccinations should be offered at 12 months of age?

27 Which vaccinations should be offered to a 13-month-old child who has previously had a red patch on his leg following a pneumococcal vaccination?

28 What is the routine schedule offered to a 4-month-old child?

29 What vaccinations should be offered to a well 6-month-old child who has no known vaccination history and is new to the UK?

30 In a 26-week pregnancy of an otherwise well mother, which of the following would be the most appropriate investigation if reduced foetal movement was reported?
   a. Ultrasound scan
   b. CTT (cardiotocography)
   c. Umbilical artery Doppler assessment
   d. Umbilical artery Doppler velocimetry
   e. Foetal vibroacoustic stimulation test
   f. Handheld Doppler assessment

31 Which of the following treatments is the most effective at clearing plantar warts (verrucae)?
   a. Five per cent self-applied salicylic acid
   b. Cyrotherapy treatment
   c. Bazzucca
   d. Scholl Seal and Heal
   e. Not one of the above is more affective that the others

32 Which of the following would you expect to see in patients being treated with antipsychotic drugs?
   a. Hyperprolactinaemia
   b. Breast lumps
   c. Hypertension
   d. Shortening of the QT interval
   e. Reduction in weight
   f. Hypoglycaemia

33 Dermatology: a scaly itchy scalp can be commonly seen in several scalp conditions. Which of the following would be most helpful in making the diagnosis of scalp psoriasis?
   a. Onycholysis
   b. Scarring alopecia
   c. Beefy red erythematous plaques
   d. Weeping areas
   e. Flakes of dandruff visible through the hair

34 Dermatology: there are many options for management of psoriasis. Which of the following options would be considered a third-line treatment known to increase the risk of skin cancer?
   a. Psoralen and ultraviolet A radiation (PUVA)
   b. T/Gel shampoo, if used daily
   c. Dithranol
   d. Calcipotriol
   e. Calcipotriol with betamethasone

35 Impetigo: with regard to a classical case of bullous impetigo, which of the following is the best course of treatment in an adult patient?
   a. Flucloxacillin 250 mg four times a day for 7 days
   b. Co-amoxiclav 375 mg three times a day for 14 days
   c. Fucidin H topically twice a day
   d. Fucibet topically twice a day
   a. Erythromycin 250 mg four times a day for 7 days

36 Schizophrenia: when considering starting an antipsychotic treatment for a patient with a new presentation of schizophrenia, which of the following would be a contraindication?
   a. A QTc interval of 0.42
   b. A QT interval of 0.46
   c. A cardiovascular risk Q score of 28%
   d. A total cholesterol of 6.8 mmol/L
   e. A strong family history of ischaemic heart disease

37 Drug interactions with antidepressants: which of the following statements is correct?
   a. Selective serotonin reuptake inhibitors are contraindicated when patients are using aspirin.
   b. SSRIs would be the treatment of choice for depression if patients also needed to take triptans for migraines.
   c. When patients are using flecainide, fluoxetine would be the preferred antidepressant.
   d. If taking theophylline, either sertraline or citalapram would be acceptable antidepressants.
   e. When patients are taking warfarin the INR can be expected to decrease.

38 Pre-eclampsia: which of the following is a risk factor for pre-eclampsia?
   a. Second pregnancy
   b. Age <40 years
   c. Pregnancy interval of >5 years
   d. Body mass index >25 kg/m^2 at booking
   e. Twin pregnancy

39 Pre-eclampsia: which of the following is the correct advice regarding the use of aspirin (although unlicensed) if there are two moderate risk factors or at least one high-risk factor for pre-eclampsia?
   a. Advise 75 mg aspirin a day from week 12 until birth.
   b. Advise 300 mg aspirin a day from week 12 until birth.
   c. Advise 75 mg aspirin a day from conception until week 12.
   d. Advise 75 mg aspirin a day from conception until birth.
   e. Advise 75 mg aspirin a day prenatally (with folic acid) until week 12.

40 Breast cancer: which of the following statements regarding human epidermal growth factor receptor 2 (HER2) is correct?
   a. Trastuzumab (Herceptin) is considered a first-line treatment in women who are HER2 positive.
   b. HER2-positive patients are known to have a better long-term prognosis.

c. A rare side effect of treatment with Herceptin for HER2-positive patients is cardiotoxicity.
d. All patients with a cardiac function (left ventricular ejection fraction) of <80% should be excluded from Herceptin treatment.
e. Herceptin is given orally every 3 weeks for 1 year or until disease recurrence.

For questions 41–45 regarding contraception, select the single most appropriate treatment choice for each scenario from the following list.

a. PC4
b. Levonelle One Step 1.5 gm
c. EllaOne
d. Microgynon
e. Dianette
f. Nexplanon
g. Implanon
h. Multiload copper coil
i. Mirena coil
j. Cerazette

41 A woman wanting postnatal contraception who is breastfeeding and is not certain about her future family plans or long-term contraceptive choice.

42 A 17-year-old who would like no periods, would like contraception and has a variable routine with a hectic social life.

43 A 22-year-old, currently on Cilest with pustular acne, needing contraception.

44 A 37-year-old woman who has completed her family, needs contraception and has heavy periods with flooding on days 2 and 3 of her menses.

45 An 18-year-old woman on Cerazette who is nulliparous, not in a stable relationship and who has missed one of her pills this pack.

For questions 46–48, select the single most appropriate cause for each of the scenarios presented.

a. Uveitis
b. Conjunctivitis
c. Acute closed-angle glaucoma
d. Cataract
e. Retinal detachment

46 A 34-year-old female presenting with sudden onset of a photophobic red eye and blurred vision.

47 A 52-year-old male presenting with transient flashing in the right eye and with a linear loss of vision laterally.

48 A 22-year-old male with bilateral red eyes with mucous discharge.

49 Tonsillitis: which of the following is not one of the Centor criteria when considering the diagnosis of a quinsy?

a. A fever above 38°C
b. Tonsils touching in the midline
c. Purulent tonsils

d. Tender anterior cervical lymph nodes
e. No cough

50 Diabetes: which of the following treatments should you consider prescribing in a 55-year-old male diabetic who is of Afro-Caribbean descent and has a blood pressure of 162/94 mmHg?
a. Bendroflumethazide
b. Olmesartan
c. Olmesartan and bendroflumethazide
d. Ramipril and doxazosin
e. Ramipril and amlodipine

51 Diabetes: which of the following could be correctly diagnosed as diabetes?
a. A random HbA1c of 7.0%
b. An asymptomatic patient with a first fasting glucose of 6.7 mmol/L and a second of 6.9
c. An asymptomatic patient with a first fasting glucose of 7.2 mmol/L and a second of 6.7
d. A symptomatic patient with a first fasting glucose of 7.1 mmol/L
e. A fasting glucose of 6.1 mmol/L 2 hours after a glucose load in an oral glucose tolerance test

52 Diabetes: in the management of diabetes, above what level of albumin excretion is considered above normal (microalbuminuria) for an albumin-to-creatinine ratio in women?
a. >1.0 mg/mmol
b. >2.5 mg/mmol
c. >3.5 mg/mmol
d. >30 mg/mmol
e. >50 mg/mmol

53 Constipation: which of the following is most useful in helping to diagnose idiopathic constipation?
a. Abdominal ultrasound scan
b. Gastrointestinal endoscopy
c. Plain abdominal radiograph
d. Transit studies
e. None of the above

54 Developmental dysplasia of the hip: with regard to a child who has been found to have signs suggestive of developmental dysplasia of the hip, which of the following would be the most appropriate action to take?
a. Irrespective of age, repeat the Ortolani and Barlow test/leg crease assessment (checking for clinical instability) the following week.
b. If <4.5 months old, arrange an anteroposterior pelvic X-ray (well positioned).
c. If <4.5 months old, arrange an ultrasound scan.
d. If >4.5 months old, arrange an ultrasound scan.
e. If >4.5 months old, arrange both an ultrasound scan and an anteroposterior pelvic X-ray.

For questions 55 and 56 regarding neonatal jaundice, consider the table showing bilirubin levels for a baby 12 hours old.

Bilirubin level (μmol/L)				
a	b	c	d	e
<50	>100	>150	>200	>300

55 At what level of bilirubin should phototherapy be considered alongside a repeat bilirubin in 6 hours?

56 At what level of bilirubin should an exchange transfusion be performed?

57 Motor development: at what age would you expect a child to be able to balance on one foot?
- a. 18 months
- b. 2 years
- c. 4 years
- d. 6 years
- e. 9 years

58 In-toeing: which of the following is not a cause of or associated with in-toeing?
- a. Bow legs
- b. Femoral anteversion
- c. Internal tibial torsion
- d. Metatarsus adductus
- e. Knock knees

59 Child protection: which of the following would not reassure that a child who has noticeable bruises has not been subject to physical abuse?
- a. A history of a haematoma after a routine vitamin K injection
- b. A history of an unexplained nosebleed at 18 months of age
- c. A history of a heavy bleed from the umbilical stump at birth
- d. A family history of haemophilia
- e. A 7-year-old boy with unexplained bruises down the front of his shins

60 Attention deficit disorder: which of the following would be an appropriate choice of medication to consider for a child with attention deficit disorder where the maximum dose of methylphenidate has been ineffective?
- a. Gradual titration of the methylphenidate dose up to a maximum of three times the recommended dose
- b. Atomoxetine
- c. Diazepam
- d. Clonazepam
- e. Melatonin

For questions 61 and 62, consider the desmopressin diagram shown.

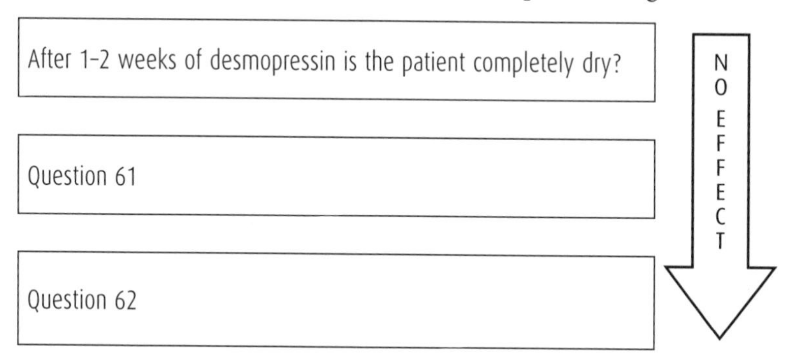

61 Which of the following would be suggested at this stage?
- a. Increase the dose of desmomelts to 240 μg.
- b. Increase the dose of desmotabs to 400 μg.
- c. Encourage bladder retraining, including delayed micturition through the day.
- d. Encourage routine lifting in the night.
- e. Consider stopping desmopressin treatment.

62 Which of the following would be suggested at this stage?
- a. Stop desmopressin.
- b. Encourage routine lifting in the night.
- c. Refer to a paediatrician.
- d. Consider taking the desmopressin at bedtime.
- e. Consider taking the desmopressin 1–2 hours before bed.

63 Pandemic influenza: a pregnant woman (10 weeks) should be offered which of the following vaccination regimes when influenza A(H1N1) is pandemic?
- a. Celvapan 0.5 mL, two doses at least 6 weeks apart
- b. Pandemrix 0.5 mL, one stat dose
- c. Celvapan 0.25 mL, two doses at least 3 weeks apart
- d. Pandemrix 0.25 mL, two doses at least 3 weeks apart
- e. None of the above – it is not considered safe at this stage of pregnancy

For questions 64–67, regarding school exclusion for infection, select the most appropriate duration of school exclusion when advising parents. Each answer can be used once, more than once or not at all.
- a. None
- b. 24 hours from last episode
- c. 48 hours from last episode
- d. 5 days from last episode
- e. 24 hours from start of episode
- f. 48 hours from start of episode
- g. 5 days from start of episode
- h. Should only be having homeschooling for the remainder of the school term

64 Conjunctivitis

65 Gastroenteritis

66 Meningitis

67 Chickenpox

68 Obsessive-compulsive disorder: the Yale–Brown Obsessive Compulsive Scale can be used to assess the severity of obsessive-compulsive disorder. Which of the following would be considered a significant response?
a. I only have to check the doors are locked twice before going to bed.
b. If I don't double check the toilet has been flushed and is clean I am unable to get off to sleep.
c. I have no problems with my friends, as they all understand me.
d. If I avoid the house cleaning I'm not worried and don't need to repeatedly wash my hands.
e. My bedroom is cluttered and untidy.

69 Disseminated intravascular coagulation: with regard to severe disseminated intravascular coagulation in a 28-year-old primigravida woman at 32 weeks, what is the most appropriate emergency action?
a. Intravenous steroids (e.g. hydrocortisone)
b. Oral steroids (e.g. prednisolone)
c. Vitamin K intramuscularly
d. Magnesium intravenously
e. Caesarean section

70 *Escherichia coli*: which of the following is true of *E. coli* 0151 (VTEC)?
a. There is usually an increase in numbers of infection in the summer.
b. It can cause renal failure in 25%–37% of cases.
c. Symptoms can last for up to 2 months.
d. Non-steroidal anti-inflammatories would be the drug of choice for fever.
e. Antibiotics should not be used.

71 Urinary tract infection: which of the following antibiotics would be best used for a 62-year-old woman with a symptomatic, dip positive UTI who reports an allergy to septrin? She is known to have an estimated glomerular filtration rate of 32 mL/min/1.73 m^2.
a. Ciprofloxacin
b. Nitrofurantoin
c. Trimethoprim
d. Ofloxacin
e. Amoxicillin

72 Turner's syndrome: in women with Turner's syndrome, which of the following is correct regarding involvement of the gastrointestinal tract?
a. Ulcerative colitis is seen less frequently.
b. Crohn's disease is seen less frequently.
c. Coeliac disease is seen less frequently.
d. Patients may present with iron deficiency anaemia due to bowel telangiectasia more frequently than would be expected.
e. Patients with Turner's should be screened for liver disease every 5 years.

73 Menopause: which of the following treatments for hot flushes is known to be better than placebo when going through the menopause, and has no additional risk of breast cancer?

a. Evening primrose oil
b. Clonidine
c. Kliovance
d. Tibolone
e. Premique Cycle

74 Infertility: when considering causes of infertility in a couple, what percentage of cases are found to be unexplained?

a. 75%
b. 50%
c. 25%
d. 6%
e. <1%

75 Obstetrics: which of the following is the correct advice to give a pregnant woman having been exposed to varicella?

a. Chickenpox only poses a risk to the foetus.
b. Exposure to shingles does not pose any risk.
c. Even if a patient has had chickenpox, varicella zoster immunoglobulin is recommended if exposure to chickenpox occurs.
d. Live attenuated varicella vaccination should be offered to all seronegative women in pregnancy.
e. If they are known to have had chickenpox in the past and are exposed to chickenpox in pregnancy, then no further action would be needed.

76 Diabetes: which of the following treatment options should you consider prescribing in a 55-year-old male diabetic who is of Afro-Caribbean descent with a blood pressure of 162/94 mmHg?

a. Bendroflumethiazide
b. Olmesartan
c. Olmesartan + Bendroflumethiazide
d. Ramipril + doxazosin
e. Ramipril + amlodipine

Considering atrial fibrillation, chose the single most appropriate answer for each of questions 77–83. Each answer can be used once, more than once or not at all.

a. Beta blockers
b. Aspirin
c. Clopidogrel
d. Warfarin
e. Aspirin and clopidogrel
f. Aspirin and warfarin
g. Amiodarone
h. Dronedarone
i. Direct current cardioversion
j. Digoxin

77 What is the most effective choice to slow heart rate in atrial fibrillation?

78 What has been shown to reduce the risk of stroke by 32%–47%?

79 In completely new presentations of atrial fibrillation it would be appropriate if this treatment were instigated immediately.

80 Is contraindicated in patients with heart failure.

81 Has been shown to reduce the risk of stroke by 22% in patients with atrial fibrillation.

82 Should be offered to all patients with a CHAD score of 1.

83 Should be offered to all patients with a CHAD score of 3.

84 Epilepsy: with regard to epilepsy, which of the following is correct?

a. Patients with epilepsy must never drive again.
b. A patient can drive 6 months after an initial fit if there has only been one fit.
c. A patient with nocturnal epilepsy can drive 6 months after diagnosis so long as there are no daytime fits.
d. A person with epilepsy cannot drive heavy goods or passenger vehicles.
e. If there is a change in antiepileptic medication, the patient can drive 3 months after any changes, so long as they have been fit free.

85 Adenomas: according to current National Institute for Health and Clinical Excellence guidance, in patients with adenomas, which of the following would be considered a high-risk case needing follow-up colonoscopy at 1 year?

a. One adenoma 30 mm in size
b. Two adenomas less than or equal to 10 mm in size
c. One adenoma greater than 10 mm
d. Two adenomas, if one is greater than 10 mm
e. Five adenomas smaller than 10 mm

Select the single most appropriate answers for each of questions 86–88. Each answer can be used once, more than once or not at all.

a. Urticaria
b. Contact dermatitis
c. Angioneurotic oedema
d. Eczema
e. Nodular prurigo
f. Dermatofibroma
g. Cheiropompholyx

86 This problem could be described as having a red, puffy area, the severity of which can rapidly deteriorate causing death.

87 This is a vesicular itchy rash seen on the palms and the soles, more often in adults than children.

88 This could be described as having a firm base, often excoriated.

89 Hay fever: with regard to hay fever, which of the following falls outside current guidance/advice/licence?

a. Loratidine 10 mg a day
b. Local honey, 1 teaspoon a day
c. Betterbar

d. Desensitisation immunotherapy
e. Montelukast 10 mg a day

90 Atrial fibrillation: which of the following would be the medication of choice to maintain sinus rhythm in paroxysmal atrial fibrillation?
a. Amiodarone
b. Sotolol
c. Diltiazem
d. Warfarin
e. Verapamil

91 Hirsuitism: which of the following is not considered an appropriate treatment option for hirsuitism?
a. Vaniqa
b. Eflornithine
c. Finasteride
d. Yasmin
e. Femodene

For each of questions 92–94, regarding prosthetic heart valves, select the single most appropriate answer. Each option can be used once, more than once or not at all.
a. Bileaflet mechanical valve
b. Ball-and-cage mechanical valve
c. Bioprosthetic porcine valve
d. Homograft from a human cadaver
e. Both mechanical and bioprosthetic valves
f. None of the above

92 In isolation, with no other co-morbidities, which valve type requires bacterial endocarditis prophylaxis?

93 Which are the most frequently used valves?

94 Which valve type needs long-term anticoagulation in the range 2.0–3.0 lifelong?

For each of questions 95–100, regarding diabetes, choose the correct figure from the following options. Each answer can be used once, more than once or not at all.
a. 20–40
b. 28
c. 10
d. 22–66
e. 5
f. 0.5
g. 0.1–0.4

95 What is the percentage of diabetics with peripheral neuropathy?

96 What is the percentage of diabetics with Charcot's neuropathy each year?

97 What is the weight, in grams, of the monofilament used in a diabetic foot check?

98 What is the percentage of diabetics who develop a foot ulcer each year?

99 What is the percentage of diabetics with foot ulcers that develop osteomyelitis?

100 What is the percentage of diabetics who have an amputation each year?

101 Hyponatraemia: which of the following is correct in a case of hyponatraemia?
a. When associated with diuretic use, stopping the diuretic is always possible to resolve the problem.
b. When there is suspected association with adrenal insufficiency, admission for intravenous saline should correct the problem.
c. The prognosis for hyponatraemia is poor in acute cases and good in chronic cases.
d. There is a known association of hyponatraemia with hyperglycaemia.
e. Urinary sodium levels are not helpful in diagnosing the underlying cause.

102 Menorrhagia: which of the following would be considered a risk factor for endometrial carcinoma in women with menorrhagia?
a. Age >45 years.
b. A patient who has had no response/improvement with the use of a copper coil.
c. A woman with a history of a subserosal fibroid.
d. A woman with a history of a chocolate cyst.
e. A woman with a history of hypothyroidism.

For questions 103–105, advise which would be considered worthwhile and correct treatments for menorrhagia – answer true or false.

103 Although a Mirena coil could be used, it would only be licensed for 4 years for treatment of menorrhagia.

104 Tranexamic acid 2 gm three times a day.

105 Norethisterone 5 mg three times a day from day 5 until day 26.

106 Hyperemesis gravidarum: which of the following statements, with respect to hyperemesis, is correct?
a. It can affect up to 50% of pregnancies.
b. The definition is vomiting in pregnancy with weight loss of 0.5 kg.
c. Onset is usually week 12–14.
d. Hypokalaemia due to excess fluid intake may occur.
e. Vitamin B_1 deficiency can occur, leading to Wernicke's encephalopathy (without any link to alcohol).

107 In a case of jaundice with an isolated unconjugated bilirubin of 40 μmol/L, which of the following is the most likely diagnosis?
a. Non-alcoholic fatty liver
b. Gilbert's syndrome
c. Pancreatic carcinoma
d. Crigler–Najjar's syndrome
e. Autoimmune hepatitis

For each of questions 108–111, select the single best answer from the following options. Each option can be used once, more than once or not at all.
a. Gilbert's syndrome
b. Alcoholic hepatitis
c. Non-alcoholic fatty liver
d. Gallstones
e. Haemolytic uraemic syndrome

f. Haemochromatosis
g. Pancreatic cancer
h. Thalassaemia
i. Hepatitis B
j. Hepatitis A
k. Crigler–Najjar's syndrome

108 What is a rare autosomal recessive disorder affecting bilirubin metabolism?

109 In a patient presenting with abnormal liver function tests, having returned from Cuba 3 weeks before.

110 This can cause recurrent episodes of self-limiting jaundice related to periods of stress, especially when associated with a reduction in calorific intake.

111 If untreated this will lead to cirrhosis, liver failure and the need for liver transplant.

112 Anaemia: which of the following blood pictures would be indicative of anaemia of chronic disease?

a. A reduced haemoglobin with an increased mean cell volume and reduced ferritin.
b. A reduced haemoglobin with a reduced mean cell volume and mean cell haemoglobin.
c. A reduced haemoglobin, normal mean cell volume, normal ferritin but reduced serum iron.
d. Normal haemoglobin with a reduced mean cell volume.
e. Normal haemoglobin with a reduced mean cell volume and an increase ferritin.

113 Sunburn: which of the following would not be sound advice in sunburn avoidance and treatment?

a. Avoid midday sun.
b. Apply sunscreen every 6–8 hours.
c. Wear loose clothes, sunglasses that reflect ultraviolet radiation and a wide-brimmed hat.
d. Silver sulphadiazine is contraindicated in pregnancy.
e. Vomiting and confusion are signs associated with sunburn.

114 Cardiomyopathy: which of the following inherited cardiovascular conditions has a prevalence of 1 in 500, can develop in adolescence (although is known to develop in adults as well) and would have a systolic outflow murmur?

a. Dilated cardiomyopathy
b. Brugada's syndrome
c. Marfan's syndrome
d. Hypertropic cardiomyopathy
e. Arrythmogenic right ventricular cardiomyopathy

115 Alopecia: which of the following would be an indication of poor prognosis is alopecia?

a. Nail pitting
b. Late age of onset
c. A 1 cm patch of loss

d. Slow progressive loss
e. Alopecia in pregnancy

116 Group B Streptococcus: which of the following statements regarding Group B Streptococcus is correct?
a. Group B Streptococcus is routinely screened for in pregnancy in the United Kingdom.
b. Group B Streptococcus cannot be acquired through vertical transmission.
c. Seventy-two per cent of babies who develop Group B Streptococcus die.
d. Once infected with Group B Streptococcus, colonisation is lifelong.
e. Group B Streptococcus infection is the most common cause of life-threatening infection in newborns.

117 Methicillin-resistant *Staphylococcus aureus* superbug (MRSA): which of the statements below, regarding MRSA, is correct?
a. MRSA in hospitals is continuing to increase.
b. MRSA screening has been introduced for all patients, in any capacity, attending hospital.
c. Chlorhexidine wash for 7 days does not help reduce colonisation.
d. Taking antibiotics increases your risk of MRSA carriage by a factor of 10.
e. Quinolones triple the risk of MRSA colonisation.

118 Chronic kidney disease: how often should a patient with stable CKD 3 have their renal function retested?
a. Monthly
b. 3 monthly
c. 6 monthly
d. 12 monthly
e. Testing is not needed if stable

119 Fitness to fly: following an episode of acute heart failure, which of the following would be correct advice regarding air travel?
a. They may fly 6 weeks after symptoms have stabilised.
b. They may fly 10 days after symptoms have settled.
c. They may fly 2 days after symptoms have settled.
d. They may fly 3 days after symptoms have settled.
e. There are no restrictions to air travel.

120 Which of the following is currently advocated in the United Kingdom for human immunodeficiency virus post-exposure prophylaxis?
a. Zidovudine and ritonavir
b. One Truvada (tenofovir and emtricitabine) tablet and two Kaletra (lopinavir and ritonavir) tablets
c. Rifampicin and didanosine
d. Zidovudine, ritonovir and didanosine
e. Maraviroc, ritonovir and enfuvirtide

For questions 121–128, choose the most appropriate answer from the following list of options.
a. No precautions needed

b. 7
c. 14
d. 5
e. 19
f. 21
g. 3

121 A patient needing post-coital contraception has presented too late for Levonelle-2. If she has a regular 28-day cycle, up to what day of her cycle is it acceptable to use an intrauterine device?

122 Cerazette (a progestogen-only contraception) is started on day 1 of your patient's period. How many days should you advise that she uses additional contraception?

123 A patient is 4 hours late taking her Loestrin-20 contraceptive pill. How many days extra precautions are required?

124 Your patient is changing from a combined contraceptive pill to Noriday, without a break between pill packs. How many days' extra precautions are required?

125 Your patient is breastfeeding and needs contraception. How many days post partum can the progestogen-only pill Femulen be started.

126 If your post partum woman wanted to start Micronor (her usual progestogen-only pill), when can this be started from?

127 Within how many days (after unprotected sexual intercourse) should Levonelle-2 be taken, to be in licence, to be effective as post-coital contraception?

128 A patient calls having missed two of her Microgynon pills (day 10 and 11 in her pill pack). How many days does she need to use extra precautions for?

For questions 129 and 130, consider which would be the most appropriate measure for each from the following list of options.

a. Case fatality
b. Prevalence
c. Incidence
d. Mortality
e. Median survival

129 A measure of the number of new cases of tuberculosis within 1 year in the United Kingdom.

130 Number of patients in your practice with coronary heart disease who died within 6 months of stopping clopidogrel.

131 Select the single best diagnosis for the picture shown.

a. Pigmented basal cell carcinoma
b. Junctional naevus
c. Malignant melanoma
d. Spitz naevus
e. Seborrhoeic keratosis

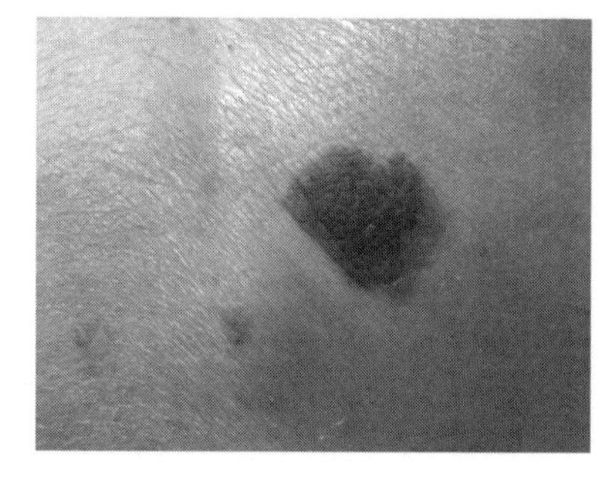

132 What is the best cause of action for the lesion in the picture shown for question 131?

a. Plastic surgery referral for excision under the 14-day-wait cancer initiative
b. If it is itching and catching wide local excision
c. If it is catching and itching curettage and hyphercation
d. If it is catching and itching diclofenac gel twice daily
e. If it is catching and itching 5-fluorouracil at night

133 Given that the condition shown in the picture not only affects the hairline but extends onto the scalp as well and is associated with a rash in both the axilla and around the anus, which of the following is the most likely diagnosis?

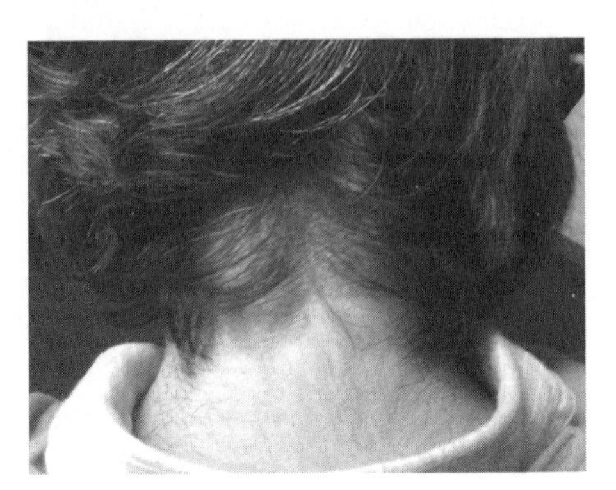

a. Seborrhoeic dermatitis
b. Psoriasis
c. Allergic dermatitis
d. Pityriasis rosea
e. Eczema

134 Which of the following would cause a Hyperuricaemia by reducing excretion of uric acid, so predisposing to gout?

a. Chemotherapy treatment
b. Bendroflumethiazide
c. Leukaemia
d. Multiple myeloma
e. Alcoholism

135 Which of the following is not a test that can be used to analyse data?

a. Student's t-test
b. Mann–Whitney
c. Confidence intervals
d. Chi-squared
e. u-test

For questions 136–138, select the single best option from the following list. Each answer can be used once, more than once or not at all.

a. Benzylperoxide
b. Zineryt
c. Lymecycline
d. Roaccutate
e. Dianette
f. Metrogel
g. Psoralen and ultraviolet A radiation (PUVA)
h. Laser

136 A 16-year-old boy with comedones and oily skin. There are no pustules or pigmentation.

137 A 19-year-old girl who has had no improvement of her acne with antibiotics, topical agents or cyproterone. She has one or two pitted scars on her forehead.

138 A 46-year-old man with a new presentation of redness and blind spots around his nose.

139 Which of the statements with regard to restless legs syndrome is correct?

a. Restless legs syndrome is usually trivial and not of concern to patients.
b. Diagnosis is based on one simple criterion: the urge to move your legs.
c. There is nothing to gain from doing blood tests.
d. Treatment with paracetamol is usually adequate.
e. Treatment with dopamine agonists is an option.

140 In an 8-year-old patient with atopic eczema on the face, there has been no response to emollients, hydrocortisone, montelukast or piriton. Assuming that there is no secondary infection, which of the following options would be the most worthwhile step in reducing the severity?

a. Protopic topically
b. Atarax
c. Synalar
d. Dermovate
e. Eurax hydrocortisone

141 A patient has presented with a discomfort in their ears and on looking at the tympanic membrane you see a cholesteotoma. What is the single best course of action?

a. Sofradex drops
b. Gentamicin hydrocortisone drops
c. Oral erythromycin
d. Oral co-amoxiclav
e. Referral to ENT

142 In the assessment of a patient, in line with the Driver and Vehicle Licensing Agency guidance on fitness to drive, which of the following patients should be advised not to drive and the Driver and Vehicle Licensing Agency informed?

a. An 89-year-old woman
b. Two weeks post-laporascopic cholecystectomy
c. A patient who has had an episode of angina at rest
d. A patient with dementia Mini Mental State Examination score 21/30
e. A patient who, 10 months previously, had an unprovoked seizure where no cause has been found.

143 Which of the following is correct with regard to carbocisteine use?

a. It is known to increase sputum viscosity, in turn improving the ease of expectoration.
b. It is known to reduce winter exacerbations by 21%.
c. It has no known impact on quality of life.
d. It is best prescribed in a once-daily dose to aid compliance.
e. It is known to increase activation of neutrophils, so reducing exacerbations.

144 Your practice is broken into and several sets of Lloyd George notes are missing, having been used for insurance reports. What is your obligation under the Data Protection Act 1998?

a. You must inform the relevant patients.
b. You must inform the primary care trust (or equivalent).
c. You must inform the Information Commissioner's Office (ICO).
d. You must inform the patient, the ICO and the primary care trust.
e. You must inform the patient, the ICO and your Defence Union.

For each of questions 145–148, select the treatment option that would be most appropriate in the management of the migraine problem described. Each answer can be used once, more than once or not at all.

a. Dissolvable paracetamol and aspirin
b. Migraleve
c. Propanolol
d. Amitriptyline
e. Pizotifen
f. Topiromate
g. Methysergide
h. Zolmitriptan orodispersible
i. Clonidine
j. Cocodamol 30/500

145 A patient has had a flare-up of their focal migraines; they are currently once every 2–3 weeks and last <24 hours.

146 A patient, who is regularly sick with migraines, is suffering once every 2 weeks or so when they are at their worst.

147 A patient who is getting headaches and anxiety symptoms every few days because of stresses at work.

148 A patient who responds well to triptans but is getting migraines every few days.

149 In a pregnant patient with Crohn's disease, controlled on mesalazine, what is the correct advice?

a. It should be stopped and prednisolone tablets used to control symptoms.
b. It should be stopped and rectal steroid enemas used to prevent flare-ups.
c. It should be stopped and flare-ups managed if they occur.
d. It is relatively safe to continue in pregnancy.
e. It should be stopped and balsalazide used instead.

150 For a homosexual male, what is the guidance on being a blood donor?

a. If there has been a 12-month period since oral or penetrative sex with another man, they are able to donate blood.
b. There is no restriction on donation.
c. If they are in a stable, monogamous relationship they are able to donate blood.
d. They will never be able to donate blood, even if there has been only one episode.
e. If they have had a human immunodeficiency virus test within the last 12 months they are able to donate blood.

151 Which of the following conditions is most likely, in a 32-year-old woman, to cause a situation where you would be physically unable to pass a speculum for a cervical smear.

a. Vaginismus
b. *Chlamydia* infection
c. Bacterial vaginitis
d. Lichen sclerosis
e. Lichen planus

152 In a patient with osteoarthritis, post myocardial infarction, which is the most appropriate analgesic to consider?

a. BuTrans patch
b. Cocodamol 8/500 two tablets four times a day
c. Celebrex 100 mg twice a day
d. Ibuprofen 400 mg three times a day
e. Diclofenac 50 mg three times a day

153 An ultrasound report following the scan of a patient's shoulder reads: 'the appearances are consistent with calcific tendinitis.' Given that previous physiotherapy and a subacromial Depo-Medrone injection have failed to improve the pain, which of the following would be the best course of action?

a. Referral for an MRI scan to confirm the extent of the problem.
b. Referral to orthopaedics for a further injection.
c. Referral to rheumatology for further injection.
d. Referral to radiology for ultrasound guided barbotage.
e. A further injection, into the glenohumeral space, in primary care.

154 In a child who is allergic to egg and who has had a reaction to the first MMR vaccination, which of the following statements is correct?

a. Future MMR vaccine booster is contraindicated.
b. It is acceptable to give the MMR booster in primary care under steroid cover.
c. It would be acceptable to give the MMR booster in primary care, as all necessary resuscitation equipment is available.
d. It is acceptable to give the MMR booster in primary care with steroid and adrenaline cover.
e. It is acceptable to give the MMR booster under hospital supervision.

155 In a patient on methotrexate and with an uncomplicated urinary tract infection, which of the following is relatively contraindicated?

a. Sodium citrate
b. Amoxicillin
c. Trimethoprim
d. Cephalexin
e. Nitrofurantoin

156 Which of the following blood pictures would be the lowest expected for a polycythaemia vera?

a. A haematocrit of 0.32 (32%)
b. A haematocrit of 0.40 (40%)
c. A haematocrit of 0.42 (42%)

d. A haematocrit of 0.50 (50%)
e. A haematocrit of 0.76 (76%)

157 What is the most likely cause of a mean cell volume of 130 fL?
a. Alcohol abuse
b. Hypothyroidism
c. Iron deficiency anaemia
d. Vitamin B_{12} deficiency
e. Post-partum routine bloods following haemorrhage needing transfusion

158 When considering calcium supplementation in a patient, which of the following would be sensible advice based on the following data?

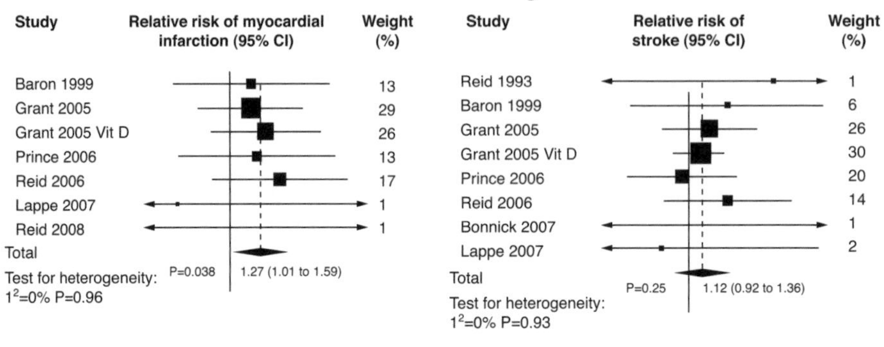

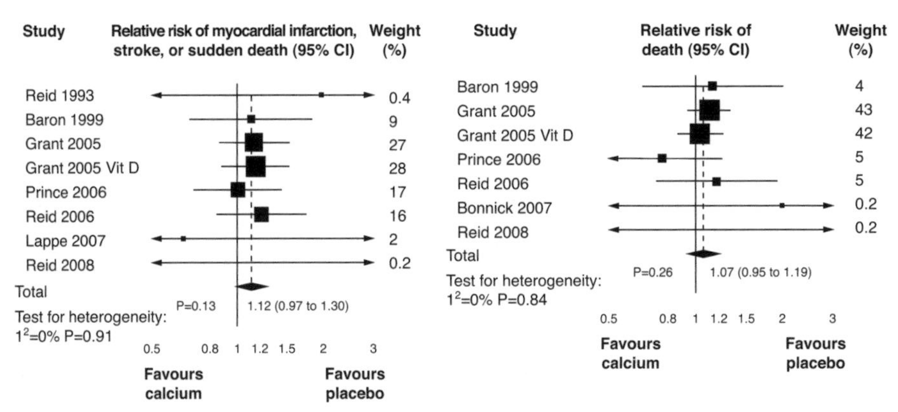

a. When using calcium and vitamin D supplementation there is an increased risk of myocardial infarction.
b. When using calcium supplements there is no increased risk of myocardial infarction.
c. When using calcium supplements there is no increased risk of renal stones.
d. When using calcium supplements, they may increase the risk of myocardial infarction.
e. When using calcium and vitamin D supplements they may increase the risk of myocardial infarction by up to 30%.

159 In the understanding of cluster headaches, which is the single best response?
a. In using oxygen, 100% (10–12 L/min) with a non-rebreathable mask should be ordered.

b. In using oxygen, 24% (2–4 L/min) with a non-rebreathable mask should be ordered.
c. Aura is not uncommon.
d. Pain tends to be occipital.
e. Beta blockers are recommended first line to reduce severity and frequency.

160 In an osteopenic patient who has stopped taking Didronel PMO because of dyspepsia, what would be the best course of action at their medication review?
a. Change to irandronic acid 150 mg
b. Change to alendronic acid 70 mg
c. Change to alendronic acid 10 mg
d. Add in a proton pump inhibitor
e. Start Calceos, one tablet three times a day

For each of questions 161–163, select the single best option from the following list. Each answer may be used only once or not at all.
a. Gaviscon infant
b. Colief
c. Colefac
d. Infracol
e. Continue with normal feeds
f. Domperidone
g. Ranitidine
h. Omeprazole
i. Emergency admission
j. Paediatric referral

161 A 7-week-old baby has been bottle-fed and is regularly vomiting despite mum's change of formula. The vomit is non-projectile and after feeds. The baby is not gaining weight as would be expected.

162 A baby 10 days old is occasionally vomiting and uncomfortable after feeds. This settles with winding and growth is as would be expected.

163 A 5-week-old baby, born to consanguineous parents, has started vomiting after feeds the last few days and is rapidly losing weight.

164 What is the best management plan in a patient with a sodium of 124, in a patient with low mood, slowly losing weight but otherwise well?
a. Fluid restriction to 1 L and repeat the blood tests in 10–14 days.
b. Arrange for an urgent chest X-ray to look for small cell carcinoma of the lung.
c. Arrange for an emergency admission.
d. Restrict fluid to 2 L and arrange urine osmolality testing.
e. Restrict fluid to 800 mL and arrange for both plasma and urine osmolality.

165 Which of the following statements are correct?
a. A corneal arcus is a predictor of ischaemic heart disease.
b. A corneal arcus is a predictor of death.
c. Xanthelasmata are predictive of myocardial infarction.
d. Both corneal arcus and xanthelasmata are predictive of myocardial infarction and death.

e. Corneal arcus, xanthelasmata and tendon xanthomas are predictive of myocardial infarction and death.

166 In a terminal palliation of distressing oral secretions in a patient with oesophageal carcinoma, where the patient is still active and mobile, which of the following would be the most acceptable method of control?

a. Hyoscine 400 mg subcutaneously, every 4 hours
b. Glycopyronium subcutaneously every 4 hours
c. Speech therapy to improve tone and swallowing ability
d. Scopoderm patches
e. District nurse referral for provision of appropriate bibs and wipes.

167 Which of the following immunology tests are diagnostic of myasthenia gravis?

a. Anti-glomerular basement membrane antibody
b. Anti-acetylcholine receptor antibody
c. Antigliadin antibody
d. Anti-endomysial antibody
e. Anti-Ro antibody

168 Which of the following is not known to be effective in the treatment of myaethenia gravis?

a. Prednisolone
b. Mycophenylate
c. Azathioprine
d. Methotrexate
e. Pyridostigmine

169 Which of the following would be the most expected finding in hyperprolactinaemia secondary to a macroprolactinoma?

a. A homonymous hemianopia
b. A bilateral scotoma
c. An optic neuritis
d. A bitemporal hemianopia
e. A lower motor neurone facial nerve weakness

170 In a patient who is hypothyroid having had a thyroidectomy for thyroid cancer, which level of thyroid-stimulating hormone (TSH) would be the most appropriate to run at?

a. TSH 5.0–10.0
b. TSH 2.0–3.0
c. TSH 1.0–2.0
d. TSH <1.0
e. TSH <0.01

171 Which of the following is specifically associated with hypocalcaemia?

a. A positive Chvostek's sign, where tapping over the medial nerve elicits a tingling in the middle finger.
b. A positive Trousseau's sign, where carpel tunnel spasm is created when a blood pressure cuff is inflated above the patient's own systolic pressure in the same arm.
c. A positive Tinel's sign, where carpel tunnel spasm is created when a blood

pressure cuff is inflated above the patient's own systolic pressure in the same arm.
d. A positive Phalen's manoeuvre, where the wrist is held in forced flexion.
e. A positive Trendelenburg's sign

172 Which of the following tests would give an indication of ovulation in a lady with a 28-day cycle?
a. Day 14 FSH/LH ratio
b. Day 21 FSH/LH ratio
c. Day 14 progesterone
d. Day 21 progesterone
e. Sex hormone-binding globulin

173 A woman has been given an expected delivery date (EDD) of 14 March for the birth of her baby. She is usually a 36-day cycle and has conceived naturally. Which of the following statements is correct?
a. Her real EDD is 22 March.
b. Her real EDD is 6 March.
c. Her real EDD is 14 March and would only be adjusted if her dating scan showed more than a 7-day difference in growth.
d. If not in labour by 14 March you would expect her to be booked for induction within 10 days of that date.
e. If not in labour by 24 March she should be listed for a caesarean section.

174 If a ROSIER score = 1, what is the most likely cause?
a. A transient ischaemic attack
b. Bell's palsy
c. Brain stem death
d. A stroke
e. Hypoglycaemia

For each of questions 175–178, select the single best option. Each answer can be used once, more than once or not at all.
a. Cardiac arrest
b. Transient ischaemic attack
c. Stroke affecting the anterior circulation
d. Stroke affecting the posterior circulation
e. Micturition syncope
f. Carotid sinus syncope
g. Vasovagal syncope
h. Subarachnoid haemorrhage
i. Thunderclap headache

175 A patient who loses consciousness while undergoing a tilt test.

176 A patient who loses consciousness after the sudden onset of an occipital headache.

177 A patient who initially loses consciousness but after coming around is ataxic and has a homonymous hemianopia.

178 An elderly man with benign prostatic hyperplasia and hypertension who passes out in the night when going to the toilet.

179 Which of the following could be considered the most appropriate antipyretic interventions in a feverish child?

a. Having a cold bath
b. Antipyretic drugs such as paracetamol
c. Antipyretics such as ibuprofen
d. Keeping a child well wrapped up to sweat out the fever.
e. Keeping the child completely stripped off

For questions 180–184, consider the following ophthalmological problems and choose the most appropriate answer for the stems below. Each answer can be used once, more than once or not at all.

a. Pinguecula
b. Scleritis
c. Dendritic ulcer
d. Blepharitis
e. Pterygium
f. Conjunctivitis

180 What would be seen as wing-shaped fibrovascular tissue arising from the conjunctiva and extending to the cornea?

181 The lid margin is seen to have scaling and some crusting; there may be some thickening of the eyelid.

182 Prominent features include severe pain and exquisite tenderness on palpation of the globe of the eye.

183 What is seen with acne rosacea and seborrhoeic dermatitis?

184 Would present as a painful, red, photophobic eye, often associated with herpes simplex (type 1).

Obesity is an ever-increasing public health concern. Consider the following stems, as applied to adults, when answering the questions 185–189. Each stem may be used once, more than once or not at all.

a. Healthy weight
b. Overweight
c. Obesity I
d. Obesity II
e. Obesity III
f. Waist circumference 94–102 cm
g. Waist circumference more than 102 cm
h. Waist circumference 80–88 cm
i. Waist circumference more than 88 cm

185 Which would be representative of a BMI 30–34.9?

186 For a male classified as Obesity I, what waist circumference would equate to a high risk?

187 Using the classification for obesity, what would be the advised earliest point at which you could start drug treatment in a patient with hypertension?

188 For a female classified as overweight, what waist circumference would equate to increased risk?

189 In a patient with no co-morbidities, at what level (assuming other measures have been unsuccessful) would you consider a surgical opinion?

190 Consider the following questions and the requirement/current advice for BCG vaccination for tuberculosis. Who of the following should be vaccinated?
   a. Contacts of tuberculosis who have no evidence of vaccination and are Mantoux negative
   b. New entrants to the United Kingdom, with no evidence of previous vaccination, who are younger than 65 years of age
   c. A booster vaccination for healthcare workers working with people with active tuberculosis, where their original vaccination was more than 20 years previously
   d. All school children (unless contraindicated) at the age of 14 years
   e. Rural police officers clearing roadkill such as badgers

191 Concerning febrile convulsions, which of the following statements are correct?
   a. Febrile convulsions are seen in 1%–3% of children aged 0–8 years.
   b. The fever is usually at least 40°C.
   c. Sixty per cent of children will have recurrent febrile convulsions.
   d. There is a 1% increased chance of developing epilepsy after a febrile convulsion.
   e. It is important to rapidly reduce the temperature to gain control of the seizure.

192 Regarding shingles (herpes zoster) infection, select the single most correct statement.
   a. Herpes zoster typically affects a single dermatome, crossing the midline.
   b. Antivirals are only effective if started within 24 hours of the appearance of the blisters.
   c. Classically there is a prodrome of pain and paraesthesia before the appearance of the rash.
   d. Use of steroids early in treatment is known to reduce post-herpetic neuralgia.
   e. Tricyclic antidepressants are only useful for the chronic pain of post-herpetic neuralgia.

193 A 42-year-old school teacher with known haemachromatosis and associated arthritis develops an intermittent dilated left pupil with a weakness and intermittent patchy paraesthesia affecting her limbs. Which of the following is the most likely diagnosis (select only one)?
   a. Diabetes
   b. Myaesthenia gravis
   c. Horner's syndrome
   d. Multiple sclerosis
   e. Holmes–Adie pupil

194 A 78-year-old woman being treated on the following medications develops swollen ankles and since the swelling started, itching over her lower limbs. Which of the medications is the most likely culprit?
   a. Aspirin E/C

b. Simvastatin
c. Ramipril
d. Felodipine
e. Bendrofluazide

For questions 195–197, select the most likely diagnoses. Each answer can apply once, more than once or not at all.
a. Testicular tumour
b. Testicular torsion
c. Varicocoele
d. Epididymitis
e. Epididymal cyst

195 A painful scrotum with swelling and positive Prehn's sign.

196 A 10-year-old boy with a painful, swollen scrotum.

197 A 24-year-old man with a painless lump that transluminates with a pen torch.

198 Paget's disease is a condition of increased bone turnover causing pain. Which of the following statements is correct?
a. The risk in the United Kingdom is rare under the age of 40 years, with an overall prevalence estimated at 25%.
b. Bone biopsies are essential in correctly diagnosing Paget's disease.
c. Classical problems include tibial bowing and spontaneous fractures.
d. Raised calcium and alkaline phosphatase are usually seen.
e. There is no increased risk of developing osteosarcomas in Paget's.

199 Consider the following statements regarding tuberculosis in the United Kingdom and select the single most correct answer.
a. The recent increase in tuberculosis is due to improved air travel and foreign holidays in third world countries.
b. The Mantoux test is diagnostic of tuberculosis.
c. Children aged 14 years are routinely offered the BCG vaccination (earlier if at risk).
d. Only pulmonary tuberculosis is highly contagious.
e. With supervising medication drug resistance in tuberculosis is much less of a problem.

200 Which of the following problems is seen with human immunodeficiency virus infection?
a. Pneumocystis carinii
b. Persistant lymphadenopathy
c. Pityriasis versicolor
d. Eczema
e. Constipation

Applied Knowledge Test: answers

1 **d** See *Chronic Heart Failure: management of chronic heart failure in adults in primary and secondary care* (August 2010) (www.nice.org.uk/nicemedia/live/13099/50526/50526.pdf). Obesity, diuretics, angiotensin-converting enzyme (ACE) inhibitors, beta blockers, angiotensin receptor blockers (ARBs) and aldosterone antagonists can reduce levels. High levels can be caused by left ventricular hypertrophy, tachycardia, pulmonary embolus, estimated glomerular filtration rate <60, sepsis, chronic obstructive pulmonary disease, diabetes, age >70 years and cirrhosis. B-type natriuretic peptide (BNP) and N-terminal-pro BNP is found at high levels in patients with impaired left ventricular systolic function (because of increased pressure or volume overload of the myocardium). There are conflicting studies related to practical use, as there is a low positive predictive value (other factors that increase BNP are age, renal failure and drugs such as beta blockers or ACE inhibitors). A role may develop for their use in helping to determine who to send for echocardiography as well as for monitoring treatment.

2 **e** *See* section 15.1 for explanations.

3 **c** The British Heart Foundation (February 2007) looked at novel risk factors (homocysteine, C-reactive protein and fibrinogen). To be clinically valuable they must be reliably quantifiable and they must help predict more accurately the risk of developing coronary heart disease. At present there is insufficient evidence to use any of these methods, but homocysteine seems to be the most promising. In 2002, the British Cardiovascular Society presented research showing that elevated homocysteine levels (>12 mmol/L) doubled the risk of a second coronary event but high levels in the UK population are probably because of lack of folate and vitamin B. C-reactive protein, fibrinogen, nitric oxide and vitamin D all have some following in this area but to a lesser degree than homocysteine. Calcium supplementation risks discussed recently do not correlate with calcium levels and are not applicable to this question. Homocysteine is an amino acid that stimulates platelet aggregation and thrombus formation (hence atherosclerosis). It is produced as a breakdown product from the animal protein we digest (methionine). The use of folic acid is being considered; the government is currently looking into adding folate to flour as a general public health measure. The current main points are as follows:

- In 2002, the British Cardiovasacular Society presented research showing that elevated homocysteine levels (>12 mmol/L) doubled the risk of a second coronary event.
- High homocysteine levels in the general population are mainly due to insuf-

ficient folate and vitamin B concentrations (hence the role of folic acid in the polypill).

- There is not enough evidence to recommend levels as part of the routine coronary heart disease risk assessment.
- Guidelines from the International Atherosclerosis Society recommend screening in high-risk patients (not agreed by the National Screening Committee). If the levels are checked and are found to be raised, treatment with diet or 400 μg folic acid should be initiated and the test repeated after 3 months. If still raised, higher doses of folate, vitamin B_6 and vitamin B_{12} are advocated.

4 a Professional lifestyle and risk management should be offered to achieve defined targets (*Joint British Societies' Guidelines on the Prevention of Cardiovascular Disease in Clinical Practice: risk assessment*, summarised in the British Heart Foundation FactFile 2006) and should be focused on achieving the following: smoking cessation, body weight distribution (waist circumference <102 cm in men and <88 cm in women, <92 cm in Asian men and <78 cm in Asian women), body mass index (BMI) <25, blood pressure (BP) <130/80, total cholesterol <4 mmol/L (or 25% reduction, whichever achieves the lower cholesterol), low-density lipoprotein cholesterol <2 mmol/L (or 30%), fasting glucose <6 mmol/L and HbA1c <6.5% (in diabetics only).

5 a HAS-BLED (*Chest*, 2010) is a suggested scoring system to assess an atrial fibrillation patient's risk of having a major bleed within 12 months. Hypertension; abnormal renal or liver function; stroke; bleeding history; labile INR; elderly, over 65 years; history of drug use (aspirin and non-steroidal inflammatory drugs); and alcohol are all used by the system.

6 b Statins used in patients with atrial fibrillation show no additional benefit (you must differentiate here between lone atrial fibrillation and other primary or secondary preventive reasons for using statins). See 'Effects of statins on atrial fibrillation: collaborative meta-analysis of published and unpublished evidence from randomised controlled trials' (*BMJ* 2011; 342: d1250).

Cervical screening: protocol for cervical screening

Age group	Frequency
25	First invitation
2–49	3-yearly invitation
50–64	5-yearly invitation
Over 65	Only if the last three tests include an abnormal result or if patient has not been screened since the age of 50

7 h This used to be 21 years but changed because of unnecessary treatment that was being undertaken because of human papillomavirus changes that would have otherwise resolved. Despite this, ongoing surveillance means that age at start and end of screening is always being reviewed.

8 k

9 a

10 k

11 d Although smoking cessation is important for everyone, depression and anxiety have not been identified specifically, although they could come under the umbrella of mental health issues.

12 c While this was thought to be a good indication, a recent trial, 2742 men (*Eur Urol* 2009; 56: 753–60) has disproved this. This has since been followed by a US study of 616 men with the finding that yearly increasing prostate-specific antigen was more likely to be associated with prostate cancer. This is still an undecided fact and therefore not a true statement. There is a helpful information sheet for men considering a prostate-specific antigen test available online (www.cancerscreening.nhs.uk/prostate/prostate-patient-info-sheet.pdf). Also *see* Statement 5.

13 e See 'Obesity and cancer' (*BMJ* 2007; 335(7630): 1107–8). This editorial discusses the work commissioned by the International Agency for Research on Cancer to look at epidemiological, clinical and experimental data to evaluate the risk between weight and cancer. As previously discussed, there was an association with postmenopausal breast cancer, endometrial cancer, kidney cancer and adenocarcinoma of the oesophagus. Higher BMI was also significantly related to leukaemia, multiple myeloma, non-Hodgkin's lymphoma and pancreatic and ovarian cancers.

14 d This question is taken from the National Institute for Health and Clinical Excellence (NICE) *Alcohol-Use Disorders* (June 2010) (www.nice.org.uk/nicemedia/live/12995/48991/48991.pdf). These patients can still develop an encephalopathy but they are at lower risk.

15 e See *Alcohol-Use Disorders* (www.nice.org.uk/nicemedia/live/12995/48991/48991.pdf).

16 a This question is taken from the *ABC of Alcohol* (fourth edition). It is true that menstrual cycle affects absorption. Alcohol peaks after 1 hour when drunk on an empty stomach. Alcohol is water-soluble; very little enters fat, as it is poorly fat-soluble. The liver is exposed to the greatest concentration, as blood is received directly from the stomach. When drinking with a carbohydrate-rich meal, absorption can be up to three-quarters less. The liver eliminates 90% of alcohol, and 2%–5% is excreted in urine, sweat and breath.

17 f (This is equivalent to 400 mg/100 mL.)

18 b (This is equivalent to 15 mg/100 mL/hr.)

19 c (This is equivalent to 80 mg/100 mL.)

20 d (This is equivalent to 100 mg/100 mL.)

21 f Ketamine. Questions 21–24 were taken from a FactFile produced by the British Heart Foundation on the effects of illicit drugs on the heart (www.bhf.org.uk/healthcare-professionals/resources/factfiles.aspx).

22 h Poppers, such as nitrites, amyl nitrite and butyl nitrite.

23 a Heroin.

24 b Cocaine – amphetamines have a similar effect but are less potent than cocaine.

25 b *Haemophilus influenzae* type B, pneumococcal vaccination, diphtheria, tetanus, polio and whooping cough.

26 c Meningitis C and *H. influenzae* type B. The measles, mumps and rubella (MMR) vaccine is not offered until 13 months of age; if given early then inadequate immunity would develop and an additional dose thought necessary.

27 h A red patch is not a contraindication for the pneumococcal vaccination; this is just the body mounting an immune response.

28 f Diphtheria, tetanus, polio, whooping cough, *H. influenzae* type B, meningitis C and pneumococcal vaccinations should all be offered.

29 b Although the child is 6 months old, because no vaccination history is known and the child is well, you start at the beginning.

30 f See *Antenatal Care* (www.nice.org.uk/nicemedia/live/11947/40145/40145.pdf). Ultrasound scan may be appropriate as an additional investigation within 24 hours of a Doppler if there are additional risk factors, auscultation is unsatisfactory or persistence of reduced movement on two or more occasions. CTT (cardiotocography) would be appropriate if over 28 weeks and then for only 20 minutes to assess foetal well-being. However, handheld Dopplers are the best first choice. If there are other risk factors (such as hypertension, diabetes, previous poor obstetric history, small for gestational age) then the patient should be referred. Kick charts and formal counting should no longer be used.

31 e All the treatments have a similar outcome to a 'watch and wait' policy. Obviously this may not be appropriate if hard callus is developing and the callus may need to be rubbed down. See 'Cryotherapy versus salicylic acid for the treatment of plantar warts: a randomised controlled trial' (*BMJ* 2011; 342: d3271).

32 a This question is taken from a therapeutics article in the *BMJ*, 'Atypical antipsychotic drugs' (*BMJ* 2011; 342: d1126). Raised prolactin levels are common. Hypotension may occur, and QT intervals may increase (may cause arrhythmias such as torsade de pointes). Weight often increases and blood profiles often show raised glucose and lipids.

33 c This question was developed following a *MIMS Dermatology* article, 'Psoriasis: management of scalp psoriasis in primary care' (2011; 1017(2): 26–30). The differential diagnosis of scaly scalp conditions include: psoriasis, eczema, contact/allergic dermatitis, discoid lupus, sarcoid and seborrhoeic dermatitis (there are more). Onycholysis is seen in psoriasis but not exclusively. Hair loss is often seen in scalp psoriasis but it is not scarring. Flakes of dandruff could be any of the above differentials and if the lesions were weeping then that would imply secondary infection. Beefy red lesions are characteristic; when scratched they often reveal blood vessels (Auspitz's sign).

34 a Although T/Gel is a coal tar preparation, the concentration is not enough to increase the risk of cancer (www.psoriasis-association.org.uk).

35 a See *MIMS Dermatology* 2011: 7(2): 33–5. Co-amoxiclav (augmentin) is usually reserved for a 10- to 14-day course if there is a recurrence of the impetigo. Topical agents are best avoided because of increasing bacterial resistance (although we are probably all prescribers in mild cases). Erythromycin resistance is increasing and also has more gastrointestinal side effects.

36 b A QT interval of greater than 0.44 seconds increased the risk of arrhythmias and sudden death. A normal corrected QT interval, the $QT_{C,}$ is 0.42 seconds. It is important to determine there is no other underlying cause for prolonged QT intervals (hypothermia, hypokalaemia, hypocalcaemia, hypomagnesaemia or medication). Maudsley guidance (tricky to get hold of but everyone refers to!) advocates regular checking of cardiovascular risk profiles, but raised levels are not a contraindication to treatment.

37 d This question is taken from the NICE guidance on depression (www.nice.org.uk/nicemedia/live/12329/45888/45888.pdf). Selective serotonin reuptake inhibitors (SSRIs) are not contraindicated with aspirin and non-steroidal anti-inflammatories, but it is advised that they are used with caution because of increased risk of gastrointestinal bleeds. The editorial 'SSRIs and gastrointestinal bleeding' (*BMJ* 2005; 331(7516): 529–30) explains the pathophysiological basis behind why SSRIs deplete platelet serotonin (so they are less likely to clot/more likely to bleed). Given SSRIs can cause gastrointestinal bleeding, some patients would benefit from gastroprotection. Where triptans are being used, it is suggested that you avoid SSRIs and offer mirtazipine, trazadone, mianserin or reboxetine (this is similar if patients are using mono-amine oxidase inhibitors such as selegiline). With flecainide or propafenon, sertraline is the preferred antidepressant. With warfarin the INR can be expected to increase. SSRIs are not usually used; mirtazipine could be considered.

38 e See *Hypertension in Pregnancy* (August 2010) (www.nice.org.uk/nicemedia/live/13098/50416/50416.pdf). First pregnancy, age >40 years, pregnancy interval of >10 years, BMI >35 kg/m^2 at booking, family history of pre-eclampsia and multiple pregnancies are all moderate risk factors for pre-eclampsia. High-risk factors include chronic kidney disease, hypertensive disease in a previous pregnancy, autoimmune disease such as systemic lupus erythematosus and antiphospholipid syndrome, type 1 and 2 diabetes and chronic hypertension.

39 a

40 c HER2 is a transmembrane protein that plays a part in cellular growth. It is overexpressed in 15%–20% of breast cancers and is usually associated with more aggressive disease. Herceptin is considered in women after surgery, adjuvant chemotherapy and radiotherapy where there is thought to be high risk of recurrence. It is recommended that patients with left ventricular ejection fraction <55% are excluded from treatment. The treatment is intravenous, 3-weekly for a year (or until disease recurs).

41 j Questions 41–45 are based on all the Royal College of General Practitioners' Faculty of Sexual Health and Reproductive Healthcare guidance and day-to-day experience in practice.

42 f (Don't forget that Implanon is now Nexplanon.)

43 e Dianette is not licensed as an oral contraceptive pill but it is effective.

44 i

45 f The emergency contraception choices are there as a red herring for this one. There is no need for emergency contraception when only one pill is missed in this instance.

46 a

47 e Although anterior uveitis may cause a retinal detachment, it is the detachment that causes the symptoms.

48 b Although it is probably a straightforward conjunctivitis, beware the sexually transmitted infections.

49 b A quinsy may be more common in unwell patients, with three out of four Centor criteria (fever >38°C, purulent tonsils, tender anterior cervical nodes and no cough). The incidence has been seen at 1 in 60 if these criteria are met, compared with 1 in 400 when not systemically unwell. It is worth offering antibiotics to patients who have been unwell for 48 hours and who fit the Centor criteria. If tonsils are touching in the midline there is a potential risk of obstruction, so, depending on the history, you may need an emergency referral.

50 e Recommendations are for an ACE inhibitor and either a diuretic or calcium channel blocker. Olmesartan is an ARB and would only be suggested if an ACE inhibitor was not tolerated. If there was a chance of pregnancy (i.e. female patient needing contraception) then the recommendation is to start with a calcium channel blocker.

51 d Although in option (a) the likelihood of diabetes is high, the World Health Organization definition as yet does not use HbA1c results. In options (b) and (c) the patients need referral for an oral glucose tolerance test.

52 c The level in men would be >2.5 mg/mmoL.

53 e See *Constipation in Children and Young People* (www.nice.org.uk/nicemedia/live/12993/48741/48741.pdf). NICE specifically states not to use any of these methods to help diagnose idiopathic constipation.

54 c This question is taken from a clinical review in the *BMJ*, 'Developmental dysplasia of the hip' (*BMJ* 2009: 339; b4454). It is worth remembering that there is some evidence that repeated Ortolani and Barlow testing may further increase the risk for the child, so unnecessary repetition of the test would be cautioned against.

55 c Both questions 55 and 56 are taken from the NICE guidance on neonatal jaundice (www.nice.org.uk/nicemedia/live/12986/48678/48678.pdf).

56 e

57 d Usually aged 6–7 years.

58 a Bow legs are often seen with out-toeing. Femoral anteversion is where the patellae point inwards and is common in children aged 3–8 years. Internal tibial torsion is where the patellae face forwards and the toes point inwards. Metatarsus adduction often resolves by the age of 6 years. Knock knees are common and are generally seen with in-toeing. For this question I used the review in Reports on the Rheumatic Diseases Series, *Hands On: practical advice on management of rheumatic disease* (Number 15, June 2008).

59 b Nosebleeds are rare under the age of 2 years and are more often associated with injury, although they can be an indication of severe disease. Haematoma after a routine vitamin K injection can be verified. A history of a bleed from the umbilical stump is a classical feature of factor XIII deficiency (1 in 2 million of the population) and is seen in some patients with haemophilia. The history of shin bruising in a 7-year-old is often unexplained specifically but secondary to playground and football-type play. This question is taken from 'Investigation of bruising in a child' (*BMJ* 2010: 341; 827–9).

60 b See *Attention Deficit Hyperactivity Disorder* (www.nice.org.uk/nicemedia/live/12061/42059/42059.pdf). Atomoxetine can be considered first line if the child also has tics, Tourette's syndrome, anxiety disorder or if there is stimulant misuse.

61 b At this stage consider either increasing the desmotabs to 400 μg or the desmomelts to 240 μg.

62 e The dose should already have been taken before bed. Routine lifting and delayed micturition are not encouraged as they are often not helpful in the long term. See *Nocturnal Enuresis* (www.nice.org.uk/nicemedia/live/13246/51367/51367.pdf).

63 b Pandemrix is recommended at any stage of the pregnancy, as it is a one-dose vaccine so it would confer immunity more rapidly. See section 23a of *The Green Book* (www.dh.gov.uk/prod_consum_dh/groups/dh_digitalassets/@dh/@en/documents/digitalasset/dh_129757.pdf).

64 a Some schools may force treatment prior to being allowed back because of the fear of spreading. Cold sores, athlete's foot and molluscum contagiosum are all cases where children can continue to attend school.

65 b The only exception to this would be if the gastroenteritis was caused by *Escherichia coli* O157, where two negative stools are required (if other forms of *E. coli*, then only one negative stool) prior to allowing back to school.

66 a Although the child may be off school because they are too ill to attend, there is no specific time placed on exclusion. If they have a *Haemophilus* meningitis they are not infectious within 24 hours of treatment but this is much less of a problem following the *H. influenzae* type B vaccination campaign.

67 g There are no reports of being infectious after day 5 of the onset of the rash, although most doctors advise 24 hours after the last lesion has dried. (b) – this would not be the correct answer.

68 b Option (a) is not necessarily abnormal; option (b), anxiety caused by the distress of obsessive thoughts; option (c) is not really an enlightening statement – a friend by definition usually understands; option (d) is avoidance, not compulsion; option (e) is not significant, although hording can be a trait.

69 e In obstetrics disseminated intravascular coagulation (DIC) can be caused by abruption of the placenta or pre-eclampsia (as well as all the non-obstetric causes for DIC). It may present with bleeding, bruising, prolonged oozing from venepuncture sites, or skin necrosis secondary to thrombosis, as DIC can present anywhere on the spectrum between bleeding and thrombosis. Other causes can include severe infection, trauma, burns, malignancy, severe pancreatitis and transfusion reactions. Diagnosis can be easily missed but you would see prolonged prothrombin time and activated partial thromboplastin time. Platelets and fibrinogen would be reduced, and D-dimers would increase if there was a clot.

70 True This question is from a Health Protection Agency circular (www.hpa.org.uk/Topics/InfectiousDiseases/InfectionsAZ/EscherichiaColiO157/). There is usually an increase in number in the spring, with symptoms lasting up to 2 weeks. It is a virulent disease but it only causes renal failure in 2%–7% of cases, so, because of their effect on the renal blood flow, non-steroidal anti-inflammatory drugs are best avoided. There is no evidence that antibiotics alter the clinical course of the infection and may increase the rate of haemolytic uraemic syndrome if given.

71 e It seems an easy answer! Cipro is unnecessary unless it is the only antibiotic the bug is sensitive to (quinolones are expensive). Ofloxacin is above and beyond what you would need. Trimethoprim would not used if septrin allergic. Nitrofurantoin is best avoided in renal impairment with an estimated glomerular filtration rate <60 mL/min/1.73 m^2.

72 d Crohn's, ulcerative colitis and coeliac disease are seen more frequently, it is suggested that screening for coeliac disease should take place every 2–5 years from the age of 8 years. Screening for liver disease should be yearly because of the risk of cirrhosis. Patients with Turner's are known to have congenital telangiectasia, which may present with iron deficiency anaemia if they bleed.

73 b With regard to evening primrose oil, placebo has been found to be better (*BMJ* 1994; 308(6927): 501–3). Tibolone increases breast cancer recurrence (*Lancet Oncol* 2009; 10(2): 135–46), and Kliovance and Premique are hormone replacement therapies that increase breast cancer risk.

74 c A quick breakdown: 30% male, 25% ovulatory, 25% unexplained, 20% tubal, 5% endometriosis, 5% coital problems, 3% cervical problems, <1% uterine causes. In 15% of cases there is more than one cause.

75 e Both the mother and the foetus would be at risk, especially for the foetus in the first 20 weeks where limb hypoplasia, microcephaly, skin scarring, mortality, premature delivery (foetal varicella syndrome) can all happen. Immunoglobulin can be offered if seronegative and exposed. Immunoglobulin can be administered within 10 days of exposure to reduce the risk of foetal and maternal infection. If a patient is found to be seronegative and is vaccinated, the advice is to avoid pregnancy for 3 months afterwards. See *MIMS Women's Health* article 'Management of chicken pox in pregnancy (2011; 16(2): 38–9).

76 e An ACE inhibitor and either a diuretic or a calcium channel blocker would be best current practice. If the patient is intolerant of an ACE inhibitor then an ARB could be substituted. If the case were different – i.e. a female with a chance of pregnancy – then you would start with a calcium channel blocker (as per NICE guidance).

77 a Note, for questions 77–83 regarding atrial fibrillation, it is important to differentiate between atrial fibrillation (sustained or paroxysmal) with or without valve problems, as well as those patients being warfarinised prior to cardioversion.

78 d Many trials have shown that warfarin is superior to aspirin (for both primary and secondary prevention) at reducing thromboembolism in non-rheumatic atrial fibrillation by up to 68% (compared with 28%). However, these studies are generally based on patients in secondary care with higher risks, the selected/excluded patient groups have been quite strict. Warfarin has also been compared with aspirin and clopidogrel used together, and has been found to be superior and to have less risk of bleeding.

79 i

80 h This is the newer antiarrhythmic, thought to be better than previous options but contraindicated in NYHA III-IV.

81 b

82 b

83 d

84 b A patient with epilepsy cannot drive passenger or large goods vehicles but they can drive a light goods vehicle if they have been fit-free for 12 months. If they have nocturnal seizures they can drive after a 3-year established period of asleep attacks with no daytime fits. Patients should not drive for 6 months after each change of medication, so long as they have remained fit-free. If there is only ever a single fit, patients can drive again after 6 months (5 years if large goods or passenger vehicle licence required) so long as they have been assessed as fit to drive.

85 e See *Colonoscopic Surveillance for Prevention of Colorectal Cancer in People with Ulcerative Colitis, Crohn's Disease or Adenomas* (www.nice.org.uk/nicemedia/live/13415/53592/53592.pdf).

86 c It can be treated with allergen avoidance, antihistamines, steroids or adrenaline, depending on severity.

87 g This is a type of eczema that usually requires strong steroid cream treatment.

88 e A dermatofibroma would not usually be itchy (i.e. excoriated). This is treated with strong steroids, moisturiser and habit awareness.

89 e Local honey, starting around 4 months before the pollen season, probably helps. Betterbar is the only complementary therapy that has been shown to be effective in trials, as compared with antihistamines. Immunotherapy can be done by injection or taken orally (Grazax) but it is very expensive and few primary care trusts will fund the cost. Montelukast is not licensed for hay fever, although it is licensed for rhinitis and asthma and there may be some crossover.

90 b Sotolol would be the most commonly used. Although amiodarone could be used it would not be the preference because of the risk of pulmonary fibrosis and hypothyroidism. Class I and III antiarrhythmics are both effective at reducing risk of recurrence, Class IA (disopyramide and quinidine) are associated with an increased mortality. This question was adapted from a clinical review article, 'Management of atrial fibrillation' (*BMJ* 2010; 340: 40–5).

91 c This is a 5-alpha reductase inhibitor that can stimulate hair growth. Hirsutism is terminal hair, so it is long, coarse and dark and in androgen-sensitive areas. It affects up to 15% of women.

92 f Recent NICE guidance has clarified that this is no longer thought necessary. These three questions were developed from a British Heart Foundation FactFile (May 2009) on prosthetic valves.

93 a

94 a The ball-and-cage valve is 2.5–3.5 but is less frequently used. Bioprosthetic valves, after 3 months, do not need warfarin, just 75 mg aspirin, unless there are associated risk factors such as atrial fibrillation or increased risk of venous thromboembolism, in which case anticoagulation to 2.0–3.0 is recommended.

95 a

96 g

97 c

98 e

99 d The most common bacteria are *Staphylococcus aureus* or beta haemolytic streptococci.

100 f

101 d Diuretics may not be possible to stop in cardiac failure or cirrhosis of the liver.

Is associated with adrenal insufficiency admission needs to be for intravenous corticosteroids; the low sodium could also be associated with tachycardia, hyperkalaemia or renal impairment in this cause. When coexistent with hyperglycaemia, correcting the glucose usually corrects the sodium. Urinary sodium levels = dietary intake – loss from the gastrointestinal tract. A low level strongly suggests a gastrointestinal cause (e.g. eating disorder, anorexia, alcoholism). This question was adapted from a *GP* clinical review on hyponatraemia (5 February 2010).

102 a You wouldn't expect a copper coil to be of any use. You would use a Mirena coil, and if there were no response to a Mirena coil, then that would be a risk factor. Specific cysts are not a risk but polycystic ovaries are. Hypothyroidism may cause heavy periods but is not a risk for endometrial carcinoma.

103 False The Mirena would be licensed for 5 years. In hormone replacement therapy progesterone cover it is licensed for 4 years.

104 False Tranexamic acid dose would be 2 × 500 mg = 1 gm three times a day. Mefenamic acid can also be used, but this is only really helpful for the pain.

105 True There is a great deal of evidence around the ability to reduce flow, also in Cochrane reviews. It can also be used on days 19–26, depending on severity. Some women choose to use it every day while awaiting surgery, because of the degree of haemorrhage.

106 e Hyperemesis occurs in around 1% of pregnancies as compared with morning sickness, which can occur in 50%–90%. Definition is vomiting in pregnancy, occurring usually weeks 6–8 (in the first trimester), with a 5% loss in weight. There is usually dehydration (note ketones in urine dipstick), electrolyte imbalance (hypokalaemia and hyponatraemia due to the vomiting). Wernicke's can occur – it can be precipitated by use of a high concentration of dextrose.

107 b Gilbert's is probable if >70% is unconjugated bilirubin. If there is no suspicion of haemolysis then no further testing would be needed. It can affect 5% of the population. Criglar–Najjar's syndrome is a rare autosomal recessive disorder of bilirubin. Pancreatic carcinoma would cause obstruction (post-hepatic) so increase in the conjugated bilirubin. Non-alcoholic fatty liver and autoimmune hepatitis rarely cause an increase in the bilirubin.

108 k

109 j

110 a

111 f

112 c This question is adapted from *Clinical GP* (21 May 2010) – 'Microcytic anaemia'. Anaemia of chronic disease occurs because of the effects of mediators of inflammation on bone marrow function, regulation or erythropoiesis and iron metabolism. Absorption seems to be reduced and can be trapped in macrophages. Option (a): in this instance you would need to recap over alcohol intake and consider checking B_{12}, folate and tumour necrosis factor levels. Option (b): this is an iron-deficient picture; there would usually be a reduced ferritin with increased red cell distribution width. Option (c): this is a normocytic anaemia seen in anaemia of chronic disease; it can become microcytic (e.g. in renal carcinoma, polymyalgia rheumatica, rheumatoid arthritis, hepatoma). Options (d) and (e): can happen in thalassaemis (option (e) specifically happened in an alpha thalassaemia patient with haemochromatosis).

113 b The application of cream needs to be every 2 hours (even on top of the P20 formulations available) and after swimming, with avoidance of midday sun (11 a.m.–3 p.m.). Silver sulphadiazine can be applied to sunburn to prevent infection but it is contraindicated in pregnancy. Other signs of sunburn include dehydration, syncope and hypotension. Sunscreen can be supplied on an FP10 (factor 30+), written as ABCS, for photodermatoses and abnormal cutaneous photosensitivities, e.g. vitiligo, lupus, porphyria and chronic herpes labialis.

114 d Dilated cardiomyopathies often present with sudden death; Marfan's syndrome can present with dilated cardiomyopathy. Brugada's syndrome has right bundle branch block on the ECG and ST elevation in V1–3 (occurs in 1 in 5000–10 000) (British Heart Foundation, FactFile, May 2009).

115 a With a small patch of alopecia, 80% of cases recover; if alopecia totalis, <10% will recover. Ophiasis also has a poor prognosis (a snake-like pattern of loss involving the hair around the edge of the hairline, behind the ears and the back of the head.

116 e Infection is intermittent, 25% of women have Group B *Streptococcus* in the vagina, one-third of people have Group B *Streptococcus* in the intestines, and 230 000 babies are born to Group B *Streptococcus*-positive women in the United Kingdom.

117 e Methicillin-resistant *S. aureus* colonisation has been slowly reducing since 2004. Screening is in place for inpatient admissions and chlorhexidine is part of the treatment to reduce colonisation (as is rifampicin and doxycycline). Antibiotics increase risk of carriage ×2 (*J Antimicrob Chemother* 2008; 61: 26–8) but quinolones triple the risk.

118 d CKD4 and 5 would be 3-monthly if not stable, 6-monthly if stable. CKD 3

6-monthly if you are not certain it is stable, and 12-monthly if stable. There are obviously reasons why you may need to check renal function much more frequently than this.

119 a Post coronary artery bypass surgery – patients may fly after 10 days unless there are complications. Post angiogram and stent – 2 days. Post ST-elevation myocardial infarction/non-ST-elevation myocardial infarction – 3 days if low risk, 10 days if medium risk, defer until stable if high risk. There are no restrictions on chronic heart failure.

120 b Human immunodeficiency virus (HIV) post-exposure prophylaxis was last updated in 2008 by the Department of Health (www.dh.gov.uk/prod_consum_dh/groups/dh_digitalassets/@dh/@en/documents/digitalasset/dh_089997.pdf). Although the quadruple approach is advocated in the UK (based on US studies showing that the triple approach seems to work more effectively), all medications used as post-exposure prophylaxis are being used out of licence and it is important to establish the degree of risk and to take samples where possible.

121 e That is 5 days after ovulation, which would be on day 14. The answers for questions 121–128 are taken from the Royal College of General Practitioners' Faculty of Sexual Health and Reproductive Healthcare guidance and the British National Formulary.

122 a

123 a

124 a She would still be covered by the 7-day pill-free week of her Microgynon.

125 b

126 f

127 g

128 a This is the middle week of her pill pack.

129 c As incidence is the measure of developing a condition in a period of time.

130 a Case fatality is the death rate in people who already have a condition defined in a period of time.

131 c This is fairly classic in appearance, given the surface.

132 c Diclofenac and fluorouracil are used for actinic keratoses. A wide local excision would probably not give the best cosmetic result.

133 b The rash described is a flexural psoriasis. Betnovate scalp application or Xamiol would be appropriate here.

134 e Alcoholism, chronic renal failure, acidosis and toxaemia of pregnancy all reduce excretion. Bendroflumethiazide can dehydrate, thereby it changes the circulating volume and cancer and chemotherapy causes an increase in production. Genetically Lesch–Nyhan's syndrome is associated with high uric acid. Cardiovascular disease and insulin resistance are also often associated with raised uric acid – the cause is talked about but not understood (?reactive or causative given the antioxidant properties of uric acid). Don't forget that a high level of uric acid can increase the risk of renal stones.

135 c The p-values give you a measure of significance. The confidence intervals are used alongside the tests used to analyse the data.

136 a This is very effective for skin that is oily and causing blackheads. It can be quite drying, so it tends to be used at night.

137 d Cyproterone is Dianette. Although Roaccutane is the best option, she would need very effective contraception while using the medication.

138 f Metrogel is a good option for rosacea. Lymecycline may be helpful if there is inadequate response.

139 e Diagnosis is based on four criteria: the urge to move your legs, with unpleasant sensation; symptoms made worse by rest; symptoms relieved by activity; and diurnal fluctuation, being worse at night. Iron deficiency may be a cause and it is probably sensible to do thyroid-function tests alongside routine bloods (and ?? a pregnancy test!). Reassurance may be all that is needed, with advice around alcohol and caffeine specifically. You can consider dopamine agonists as a treatment option.

140 a Atarax could be used for sedative effect at night but it would do nothing for the eczema. Synalar and Dermovate are really too potent for the face. Eurax, because of the urea component, is a good option, but given that we know that hydrocortisone has not been effective so far, it is probably a pointless choice at this stage.

141 e You would only use the antibiotic options if there were a superimposed infection. The important point to recognise is that a cholesteatoma will continue to erode and needs addressing surgically.

142 d If angina at rest, with emotion or at the wheel, you should stop driving until symptoms have stabilised, but you do not have to inform the Driver and Vehicle Licensing Agency (DVLA). Post surgery it needs to be established with the doctor when someone may be fit to drive, but you only need to inform the DVLA if it is likely to affect driving for more than 3 months. The patient would need to confirm things with their insurance, as there are certain procedures that have more specific rules. The issue around dementia is very difficult, as it is not a specific Mini Mental State Examination issue but more the functional ability. The DVLA needs to be informed and the licence may be subject to annual review. You can drive 6 months after an unprovoked seizure, assuming there is no recurrence.

143 b There is known to be a significant improvement in quality of life (PEACE Study, p=0.046). It reduces length of antibiotic therapy required and winter exacerbations by 21% (Cochrane review) by reducing activation of neutrophils, reducing goblet cell hyperplasia and reducing sputum viscosity.

144 c Currently there is no obligation to inform the patient, but the Department of Health states that you must inform the Information Commissioner's Office if a significant number of records have been breached. The new Data Protection Act will require that all breaches are reported to the Information Commissioner's Office and the patient. It is probably best practice to inform patients, in case the situation becomes public or if it may affect them in other ways. Similarly, the role of the police would need to be considered because there has been a break-in, and you should have a policy on breach of data records.

145 a A question on migraine management could easily come up in the Clinical

Skills Assessment. Dissolvable paracetamol and aspirin is a first-line treatment (trying to avoid codeine-based treatment, because of the risk of rebound headaches).

146 h If vomiting, this would be the only option to be absorbed.

147 c Propranolol will also help with the anxiety, alongside the prophylactic or PRN used for the migraine.

148 e Pizotifen is probably the best option; methysergide, topiramate and amitriptyline could be used, but probably not at this point. Clonidine may be of some help, but less so than all the other options – it is probably one to consider with menopausal flushing and hypertension.

149 d This type of problem would be under obstetrician care but I have included it because of the fallout that seems to occur because of general lack of ability to clarify things, causing significant amounts of stress in these women. It is relatively safe, and by stopping or changing you are running the risk of a significant flare-up, which would be a worse situation.

150 a Whereas previously people were not able to donate blood, from November 2011 they have been able to in the case of (a). Having had an HIV test is probably false reassurance, as there may not have been a seroconversion picked up by the test, depending on the timing of relationships.

151 a Chlamydia and bacterial vaginitis, although it may be uncomfortable, shouldn't preclude a speculum examination. Herpes simplex virus may prove too painful, depending on the position of the vesicles. Lichen sclerosis and lichen planus would usually be external and in an older age group, when extremely severe lichen sclerosis may cause narrowing of the introitus, making it impossible to pass a speculum.

152 b BuTrans is probably a bit above and beyond for initial management. Non-steroidal anti-inflammatory drugs are currently being shown to increase the risk of myocardial infarction, diclofenac being the worst culprit (although it is a very good analgesic).

153 d Further injection is probably not going to help, given the degree of calcification. If barbotage doesn't give improvement then orthopaedic involvement with a view to manipulation under anaesthetic may be worthwhile.

154 e The MMR vaccination is cultured in fibroblasts from chick embryos, the actual egg protein being minimal. In children aged 2–5 years there is a 1%–2% prevalence of egg allergy. The booster is important but under hospital supervision; similarly, if the child hasn't had an MMR at all, even the first vaccine would usually be done under hospital supervision in case of severe adverse reaction. The National Institute of Allergy and Infectious Diseases recommends that all children with egg allergy, no matter how severe, should still have their MMR vaccination as per the usual immunisation schedule (*BMJ* 2011; 343: 367–8).

155 c Because it gives a predisposition to folate deficiency.

156 e A haematocrit of >0.56 (56% in women) and >0.60 (60%) in men, hence 0.76 (76%) is the lowest of the available options. Remember to consider secondary causes (e.g. hypoxaemia, carbon monoxide, smoking) and remember to consider other bloods (e.g. whether someone is iron deficient).

157 d This is especially so if the haemoglobin is low. Folate deficiency and myelodysplasias can give a similar degree of macrocytosis. Alcohol abuse and hypothryroidism tend to give a mild macrocytosis in the region of 100–110. Don't forget drug causes such as methotrexate where someone is not taking their folic acid and hydroxycarbamide.

158 d This is from the meta-analysis (*BMJ* 2010; 341: 289) and it found that calcium supplements may increase the risk of myocardial infarction by up to 30% – you cannot tell this from the graphs.

159 a Aura is rare and the pain tends to be more periorbital in cluster headaches. Subcutaneous sumatriptan 6 mg is the drug treatment of choice, possible nasal triptans and oxygen therapy. Short-term prevention may include steroids (they give rapid relief) and methysergide (which has the risk of fibrosis). Long-term prevention would include use of verapamil, lithium, topiramate, valproate and gabapentin. This question is adapted from an article by Dr D Kernick in *GP*, 'Managing cluster headache' (28 May 2010).

160 b Ibandronic acid (Bonviva) is a once-monthly preparation but it is not the best choice (although you may need to come to that). Alendronic acid 70 mg is once weekly and it is the best choice, as the 10 mg would still be a daily dose. It is important to help patients to understand how to take their medication (30 minutes before breakfast, swallowed whole with plenty of water while upright, and remaining upright for at least 30 minutes after taking the medication) to minimise side effects. Although Calceos is a good option, it is usually twice a day (depending on dietary intake) and would not be adequate to help increase the bone strength in someone who is osteoporotic.

161 a This sounds like reflux. Adding Gaviscon to the formula would be a good first step, so long as there are no other concerns.

162 e This doesn't sound like you need to use anything for colic.

163 i This is sounding like a pyloric stenosis and a baby who is decompensating, although I haven't mentioned the word projectile(!). Admission is needed for urgent investigation with a view to surgery.

164 c In theory you could fluid restrict and go looking for a primary cancer but, realistically, at 124 (assuming it is not a chronic problem) you really need to be thinking of admission, especially if the mood is low, as there is a known risk/association with suicide.

165 c This is from the recent paper 'Xanthelasmata, arcus corneae, and ischaemic vascular disease and death in general population: prospective cohort study' (*BMJ* 2011; 343: d5497). Xanthelasmata are predictors of myocardial infarction, ischaemic heart disease and death; arcus corneae are not.

166 b Regular injections may be necessary but are certainly not ideal at this stage when a patient is still relatively able. A Scopoderm (hyoscine) patch is often used for motion sickness but it would be extremely helpful in this situation (they can be cut into quarters and titrated to give the desired effect).

167 b Antibodies against muscle-specific (tyrosine) kinase may also be positive but less frequently than acetylcholine receptor antibodies.

168 b Mycophenylate was used historically but is not used any longer, as it is not effective. Prednisolone and pyridostigmine are both first-line treatments; azathioprine and methotrexate second-line.

169 d This is due to the pressure on the optic chiasm.

170 e With this sort of issue the risk of osteoporosis is the last thing you are worrying about. Your prime concern is suppressing any stray thyroid carcinoma cells that, if you ran at a higher level of thyroid-stimulating hormone, may become active again.

171 b Chvostek's sign is the contraction of the corner of the mouth, nose and eye ipsilaterally to the tapping of the facial nerve. Tinel's sign is where tapping over the median nerve elicits irritability, and Phalen's is the forced flexion of the wrist, both of which are associated with carpal tunnel syndrome. Trendelenburg's sign is where when standing on one leg the pelvis drops to the opposite side of the stance leg, indicative of weak abductor muscles of the hip.

172 d This is a mid-luteal progesterone.

173 a The dates need to be pushed on by 8 days, as she will have ovulated on day 22 (not day 14).

174 d In the absence of hypoglycaemia a ROSIER score >0 is indicative of a stroke. Points are scored if any of the following issues are positive (−2 to +5).

Loss of consciousness	= −1
Seizure activity	= −1
New acute onset:	
asymmetric facial weakness	= +1
asymmetric arm weakness	= +1
asymmetric leg weakness	= +1
speech disturbance	= +1
visual field defect	= +1

175 g Questions 175–178 are adapted from the NICE guidance on *Management of Transient Loss of Consciousness in Adults and Young People* (http://guidance.nice.org.uk/CG109).

176 h

177 d

178 e

179 b This question is taken from the NICE guidance on management of fever in children. A cold bath and stripping a child off can vasoconstrict and cause core temperature to shoot up, thereby increasing the risk of fits; however, tepid sponging may help. Sweating out the fever in a child is not really wise. Paracetamol is recommended as first-line treatment and ibuprofen (because of renal effects) as second-line treatment; they can be used together or they can be alternated.

180 e Pinguecula is often similar in appearance but does not involve the cornea.

181 d

182 b Dendritic ulcers would not have such a painful globe.

183 d

184 c

185 c These questions apply to adults and are taken from the NICE guidance on obesity.

186 f More than 102 cm would be very high risk.

187 b Hypertension is classified as a co-morbidity, so starting treatment at a BMI of 28 is recommended. This would be 30 (Obesity I) if there were no co-morbidities.

188 h A waist circumference of more than 88 cm would be high risk.

189 e You could consider this first line if the patient had a BMI of 50 where considered appropriate.

190 a This question is taken from *The Green Book* and NICE guidance on tuberculosis. Option (b) is false – either under the age of 16 or 16–35 from sub-Saharan Africa or a country with a tuberculosis incidence of 50 per 100 000. Option (c) is false – only if no evidence of previous vaccination, younger than 35 years and Mantoux negative. Option (d) is false – this schedule was stopped in 2005.

191 d Febrile convulsions are seen in 3%–8% of children aged 6 months to 6 years, 30% of whom will have a recurrence. By definition, the temperature is at least 38°C.

The normal risk is 1.4%; risk after a febrile convulsion is 2.4%. Care needs to be taken, as peripheral vasoconstriction may increase core temperature. Using ibuprofen and paracetamol would form part of the ongoing management but if fitting, the child will be unable to take medication.

192 c Answers for this question are taken from a review article in the *BMJ* (2007; 334: 1211). It does not usually cross the midline. Meta-analyses have shown that if antivirals are started within 72 hours, they reduce pain severity and duration. Steroids do not seem to reduce post-herpetic neuralgia but it is worth considering the use of tricyclics to reduce pain from the acute attack in elderly patients. In fact there is some evidence that, used in the acute phase, it may reduce neuralgia.

193 d Haemochromatosis may lead to diabetes but papillary changes are unlikely. Horner's syndrome is not in itself a diagnosis, there is usually a cause; similarly, Holmes–Adie pupil (not syndrome) is an observation.

194 d This is a known side effect of calcium channel blockers.

195 d Prehn's sign is pain relieved on elevating the scrotum.

196 b

197 e

198 c These questions are developed from a clinical review article in *GP* (March 2008) written by Dr Rod Hughes. The risk of developing the disease over the age of 50 doubles every 10 years, with overall prevalence estimated at 5%. Bone biopsy is not essential but it can be useful to distinguish between Paget's and malignancy. Stress fractures occur because pagetoid bone is weaker than normal bone; skull bossing and jaw changes are often seen. Raised calcium is usually only seen if the patient is bed-bound/immobile. Osteosarcoma can occur, especially if untreated or long-standing.

199 d Tuberculosis is spread by respiratory droplets, and increase is because of immigration from Eastern Europe, sub-Saharan Africa and Asia. The Mantoux test is generally unhelpful; chest X-ray is a better investigation. There is no longer a routine vaccination. Drug resistance is still an increasing problem.

200 b Persistent lymphadenopathy, diarrhoea and sweats are a bit of a warning triad. Eczema isn't really increased but seborrhoeic dermatitis is. And if there was a pneumocystis you would be thinking AIDS, not HIV. You could also have a presentation with weight loss, oral hairy leukoplakia, shingles and arthralgia.

Clinical Skills Assessment: introduction

The Clinical Skills Assessment (CSA) is part of the MRCGP. It involves thirteen 10-minute consultations that test your ability as a general practitioner. You will be marked as a clear pass, marginal pass, marginal fail or clear fail.

The Royal College of General Practitioners' website goes through the issues that have been shown in past candidates who either passed or failed (www.rcgp-curriculum.org.uk/nmrcgp/csa.aspx). The table in this chapter summarises these points as presented by Drs Sue Rendel and Kamila Hawthorne, two senior examiners, and Professor Celia Roberts, a linguist expert.

Those candidates who did well showed good use of time, were fluent and created an interactive consultation, with the patient being very much a part of the consulting process. This interactivity included shared decision-making and was also demonstrated in areas of general uncertainty or where the candidate was unsure.

Those candidates who did less well were generally the opposite of this description. In part because of a lack of fluency, the history-taking process tended to come across as an interrogation, and comments were often seen as insincere and unknowledgeable.

	Passing	Failing
General Features	Fluent, interactive and relevant Is able to take patient into medical world as a shared partner Open about lack of knowledge or certainty and may use this constructively Active monitoring during consultation	Poor use of time Uneasy with or unable to acknowledge own ignorance or uncertainty More scripted summary than checking understanding Unaware of personal space
Data Gathering	Can take a focused history that includes all relevant information Embedding of questions in previous response	Formulaic questioning which can become interrogative Repetitive questioning Sequence of questions does not make sense
Clinical Management	Appears knowledgeable and refers to recognised algorithms or modes of practice Able to suggest solutions to problems or a range of reasonable management options likely to be agreeable to patient	Insufficient knowledge base, or ability to think of realistic and effective alternatives Fails to integrate and apply knowledge Puts off making clinical decisions or a clear diagnosis Doesn't appear to grasp the dilemma if there is one

(*continued*)

	Passing	Failing
Interpersonal Skills	Connects instantly with patient Non-judgemental Interested in the patient Reformulates explanations using helpful metaphors Can meet patient half way – picks up patient's agenda, accent, or cultural approach	Doctor-centred/patient's concerns not addressed Patronising Unable to explain effectively – may be wrong or not tuned to patient Inappropriate use of terms Overly patient-centred to the detriment of clinical outcome

The CSA cases presented in this chapter are written for at least two people working together, one playing the role of the GP and the other being the patient. If there are more of you then you have examiners to time keep and appraise, an important part of your CSA work for all roles. Your trainer will no doubt employ clinical observation tool surgeries and video analysis but these do have a different feeling to that of being judged and marked.

The person playing the role of the GP is to have the doctor information and is then expected to conduct a consultation. The patient can have the rest of the information so they are able to understand how to simulate the case.

Don't make the mistake of being afraid to formulate and commit to a management plan with prescriptions, referrals and safety netting in place before you run out of time. Similarly, take into account the comments outlined in the table and don't let yourself get too doctor centred (it may be a useful on-call technique when there aren't enough hours in the day but in some cases it can create unnecessary work further down the line). Be open and flexible and listen to the patient in front of you.

Don't forget the following:

- Introduce yourself.
- Your medical school history-taking skills form a good fallback framework.
- Not all patients want to shake hands!

If you would like more practice, please email me (gear@doctors.org.uk) and I will forward you the simulated cases from previous editions that you may also find helpful to work through.

Clinical Skills Assessment: cases and answers

Case 1

Doctor information

64-year-old, Mike McCredie
Past medical history: essential hypertension
Medication: felodipine 2.5 mg daily, ramipril 10 mg daily
Recent medication review with the practice nurse
CVD risk 10%
Cholesterol 3.9, eGFR >90
BP 132/76
Never smoked, alcohol 6 units/week

Patient information

You are going abroad for 6 months and, as you will be moving around Europe in your motorhome, you would like a 6-month prescription of your medication to take with you.

If asked, you are taking aspirin 75 mg, which you buy over the counter from the chemist, and there are no other problems or concerns.

Breakdown of important issues

This is a question that encompasses hypertension, patient safety and knowledge of NHS guidance around medicine management and writing of prescriptions.

Information to elicit

This would include:

- compliance/concordance with medication (presumable good given the patient information)
- side effects from medication – ask specifically about swelling of the ankles and dry cough
- the review – it may have been updated for 6 or 9 months (i.e. as per the Quality and Outcomes Framework), depending on local practice
- consider repeating the patient's blood pressure
- expectations – has this situation arisen before?

Specific management

- There is no medicolegal reason to refuse this request or to be uneasy about it. You would normally have updated this patient's prescription for at least 6 months anyway.
- There is no specific limit from the Department of Health on the number of scripts for travelling abroad. The decision is an individual one and is based on the medical history, types of medication and individual risks. Most primary care trusts agree that you can issue 3 months on an NHS script and then 3 months as a private script (not incurring a GP fee) to cover the period.
- It is important to safety net/educate on when to seek help: chest pain, shortness of breath, headaches, ankle swelling.
- Consider printing a medical summary for the patient to take with him as well.
- Consider discussing the purchase of a blood pressure machine, which can be checked when seen for his reviews at the practice against your sphygmomanometers.
- Consider discussing deep-vein thrombosis prophylaxis, checking vaccination history and enquiring after contact details/mobile telephone numbers that may be important to have available on the system.

Other ways this scenario may present

- Patients living abroad – these patients would be entitled to immediate and necessary treatment but, depending on the situation, they may not be eligible for other NHS services. On a private basis you may be able to help, but be aware of the medicolegal pitfalls if you don't have a reliable history.

Case 2

Doctor information

27-year-old woman, Pamela Jones
Past medical history: two normal vaginal deliveries (children now aged 2 and 6)
No medication or allergies recorded

Patient information

You have recently separated from your partner of 4 years (this has been on the cards for a couple of years now and is very much a positive decision for you and your children). You are concerned that your ex-partner is trying to get custody of both the children by proving that you are an unfit mother, specifically with regard to a broken arm your 6-year-old got while trying to learn to ride his bike – your ex-partner had been very keen for the stabilisers not to be removed. You are concerned that he is trying to get copies of the children's medical records but you also have an additional concern that he is not the father of your 2-year-old child and you would like paternity testing (note dates indicate that he is not the father of your 6-year-old either).

Breakdown of important issues

This is a question that involves an understanding of parental responsibility and, depending upon your experience so far, a degree of uncertainty covering the legalities of paternity testing.

It would be important to explore the following:

- The separation and psychological impact on both the patient and the children.
- That the patient has appropriate legal representation.
- Work out the dates, if possible, to try to work out the significance of the concern that the ex-partner may not be the father.
- Whether or not her ex-partner is named on the birth certificate(s). If he is, even if there is a question of paternity, he has parental responsibility unless deemed otherwise by the courts. If he did request the notes, he would need to show proof of identification and the children's birth certificates.
- Be clear with both birth certificates who is named as the father – it may be different for each child, do not assume.

Management issues

- You could flag up the children's notes to raise awareness, although if the father has parental rights he is legally allowed to request notes.
- If notes were requested you could inform the mother (defence unions often advise that this is done).
- It may be better for paternity issues to be dealt with by her solicitor and the courts. You can purchase paternity kits from the chemist, but the results of these would not be admissible in court.
- If you felt you had the experience to provide this service (Human Genetics Commission document, www.hgc.gov.uk and www.legislation.gov.uk) you would need to:

- council all parties appropriately as to the personal and wider, lifelong family implications
- obtain consent (statutory obligation, Human Tissue Act 2004) before taking samples (blood, saliva or hair). An adult with parental responsibility can authorise a test for their child, but it is advised that if they are old enough their view should be taken into account.

- If the sample is requested by the court then the clerk to the court would have a list of approved testers.

Be aware that you are taking the patient's word for this and that you are only getting one side of the story; you don't need to be defensive or obstructive, just cautious.

It isn't a right or wrong scenario; rather, it is an ethical discussion around certain difficult points. Be aware that the partner may also be your patient. If in doubt defer paternity testing decision and speak to your defence team (i.e. your legal advisors) and colleagues.

Case 3

Doctor information

52-year-old man, Trevor Wilton

Recent NHS health check: CVD risk 9%, BP 128/80, urine trace non-haemolysed blood

Patient information

You have been asked by the practice nurse to see the doctor because of your urine sample.

If asked, you have never had any blood in your water, you have no problems, you get up once in the night to pass urine and you don't do any exercise other than walking the dog. You have had no new sexual partners and your wife is going through the menopause so you are rarely sexually active.

There is no significant family history.

Breakdown of important issues

This question is based on a case of microscopic haematuria.

It would be important to enquire about the following issues:

- Genitourinary system:
  - any prostatic symptoms
  - any pain
  - any blood in the urine/frank haematuria
  - any new sexual partners.
- Dermatology – any suggestion balanitis/rash.
- Social issues – specifically exercise (can cause breakdown of myoglobin) – in relation to the sample being taken.
- What is his understanding of the situation so far?

Examination

- Examination would be appropriate in this situation.
- Abdominal examination is normal, PR apricot-sized prostate.

Management

- First, negotiate the need for further investigations to give you more information:
  - midstream urine/repeat dipstick
  - blood tests – prostate-specific antigen and urea and electrolytes, specifically
  - in other, similar cases you may need to request nucleic acid amplification testing for chlamydia.
- It is important to talk around the differentials – it may be a false-positive result, or it may be related to the prostate (role of prostate-specific antigen testing) or renal causes such as renal stones. The results will then help decide whether or not everything is clear enough for no further action to be needed, whether an ultrasound scan or further blood tests (e.g. immunology) may be needed or whether you need to use the 14-day cancer pathways to be able to have a look at the prostate and bladder wall.
- Follow-up with the results needs to be negotiated; a telephone call may be fine in

all of the scenarios listed to arrange further steps, but you need to have a safety net. For example, you might say something like 'I will have called you within a week of the tests being done. If you haven't heard from me by then, please contact us' (thinking you may have unforeseen circumstances where you need to be away from work).

Forty per cent of people with microscopic haematuria will have infection (which in itself may need further investigation). It is important in this type of case not to jump straight into cancer referral pathways but, rather, to adequately assess the situation and investigate appropriately.

Case 4

Doctor information

A 48-year-old woman, Anna Scott

Past medical history: anxiety and depression, alcohol abuse (abstinent for 20 years)

Currently: under psychiatry and the mental health nursing team

Medication: sertraline 100 mg, zopiclone 2 ≥ 7.5 mg nocte, clonazepam 0.5 mg three times daily, propranolol 40 mg as required

Patient information

This question looks at your understanding of insomnia and mental health in relation to alcohol dependence.

The main issue is lack of sleep – you can't get off to sleep until around 4 a.m. and then you wake up every hour or so. You really want to try melatonin because you have heard that it is very effective. You are so desperate that you are thinking of drink again; you used to go to Alcoholics Anonymous (AA) and you had worked through the 12 steps.

You feel guilty and flat that you aren't able to work to help support your family and that you spend all day in bed because you are so tired and exhausted.

Breakdown of important issues

Information to work through:

- Sleep is the main issue – explore sleep patterns, length of time that the patient has been suffering, how the patient is using current medication to help her sleep.
- Daytime routine – is the patient getting any exercise/fresh air? Is she getting out of bed at all?
- Consider mood, alcohol (possibly suggesting AA for support), anxiety issues, tobacco and drug use.
- Explore review of systems – is there any other reason that sleep could be affected (e.g. hyperthyroidism, diabetes, urinary problems meaning being woken to go to the toilet, and so forth).

Management

The management options are very individual and patient/doctor dependent, but consider the following:

- A re-look at a sleep diary.
- Relaxation techniques, self-hypnosis and other self-help tools, the UK Sleep Council.
- Look at daytime routine.
- Reconsider the use of AA to help prevent a relapse.
- Review medication use, timing of zopiclone 30 minutes before going to bed, consider if there is a possibility to reduce clonazepam, do you need to reconsider antidepressants and change to trazadone (as an example)?
- Other psychological options may be needed: cognitive behavioural therapy, psychotherapy, a local well-being service (usually CPN-based).
- Finally, you need to address the melatonin question. It is probably not appropriate

to talk about it being incredibly expensive, but it would be appropriate to readdress all of the options discussed before moving on to melatonin.

Case 5

Doctor information

82-year-old woman, Phyllis Lockett
Past medical history: NAD
Medication: nil

Patient information

You attend with your daughter, who kindly does most of the talking in a gentle and concerned way. She is someone you trust and defer to. You keep fiddling with your hands and rings, sometimes looking up at the doctor and smiling, but not really engaging.

Your daughter explains about her concerns over memory and your ability to find words. There is poor short-term memory, worsening over the last 5 years. Food and housing circumstances are all sorted – social services would not be acceptable to you. Things are coming to a head because of safety and external doors being left open, worry about falls, although this hasn't happened yet.

Friends still visit but they are all becoming increasingly frail.

Breakdown of important issues

This is a memory deficit and cognitive impairment assessment question.

Take a thorough history, trying to engage the patient.

- Duration
- Type of memory problems
- The specific concerns and reason for presenting now
- Nutrition, weight and social circumstances
- Continence
- Social issues, including smoking and alcohol intake (occasional with dinner)
- Review of systems, enquiring about reversible causes of memory problems

Examination

- BP 136/88 with a regular pulse.
- Mini-Mental State Examination:
  - Orientation: day of the week, date (day/month/year), season *(3/5 (forgets day and month)).*
  - Orientation: what town/city, what county, country, what building and what floor *(4/5 (forgets county)).*
  - Registration: recall three objects (apple, coin, shoe), repeat up to six times for recall *(3/3).*
  - Attention and calculation: subtract 7 from 100, then subtract 7 from your answer, then subtract 7 from your new answer, and so on and so forth (stop after five answers); alternatively, spell WORLD backwards *(2/5 (manages 93 and 86)).*
  - Recall: the three objects asked to remember *(1/3 (only remembers apple)).*

- Language naming and repeating:
  - show a watch – name and describe function *(1/1)*
  - repeat 'no ifs, ands or buts' *(1/1)*.
- Reading: write CLOSE YOUR EYES and ask the patient to do what it says *(1/1)*.
- Ask the patient to write a short sentence that makes sense *(1/1)*.
- Three-stage command: take this piece of paper in your right hand, fold it in half and put it on the floor *(3/3)*.
- Copy the following diagram *(0/1 (keeps making them squares on the side))*.

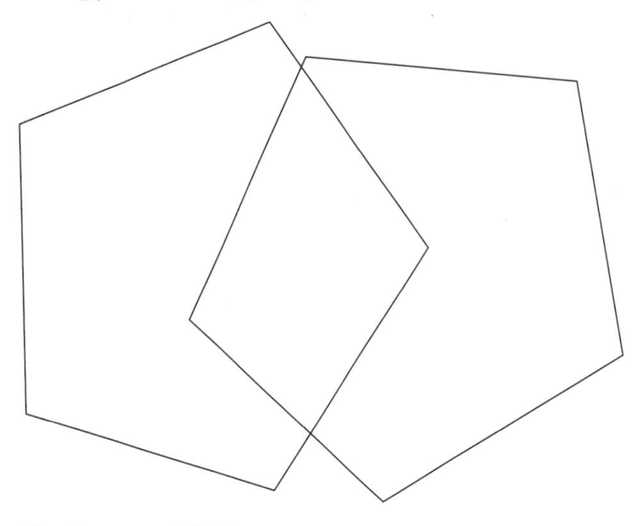

Total score = 20/30.

Discussion of management options

- The need for investigation/dementia blood tests, to ensure there is no reversible cause – probably unlikely.
- Consider input social services as help for the family as well as the patient.
- Follow-up – telephone or in person with the blood results to talk through referral to memory clinic (can deal with at this consultation, if appropriate).
- Consider updating next of kin details on the records, ensuring you have the daughter's contact details.
- Talk about care call in case of falls, and key safe options, although these may not be acceptable or may not even work practically for some people.
- Talk though housing situation – is it a manageable situation with what the family are able to offer?
- Have they considered lasting power of attorney may be appropriate to consider as going through the process of looking into dementia.

The elderly health cognitive assessment may come in many forms. Be sensitive – rarely are family members anything other than helpful and caring.

Case 6

Doctor information

22-year-old female, Nula Key
There are no past records – this patient is new to the practice

Patient information

You have recently, 6 weeks ago, moved to the area for work, having completed university. You had an upper respiratory tract infection 3 months ago and have had a persistent cough since, which gets worse with exercise.

You do not produce sputum, and you smoke socially on occasion (3–5 cigarettes a week at most but sometimes none). You have no skin problems and occasionally get hay fever. There is no significant family history.

Breakdown of important issues

This question is about a new presentation of asthma, exploring your understanding of investigation needed to prove the point.

In the history be certain to touch upon the following:

- current symptoms including reversibility, sputum, noctural and exercise-related symptoms
- smoking history
- past history, atopy, family history of problems, pets and review of symptoms.

Examination would be normal but don't forget to do the peak flow and look at the skin. If you are very keen, also check the shins for erythema nodosum (signs of sarcoid).

In the negotiation of diagnostic tests and management:

- Investigations that could be considered: pulmonary function tests (usually in-house), serial peak flow readings to determine whether there is diurnal variation and the need for a chest X-ray.
- Trial of treatment with a salbutamol inhaler – don't forget the volumatic option and seeing the nurse to teach technique. Preferably with a peak flow reading before and 20–30 minutes afterwards to look for reversibility.
- Smoking advice should be covered but probably not in too much depth – encourage, don't lecture!
- Plan for review, ideally 2 weeks down the line.
- Safety net this case around what to do if symptoms get worse.

This is based on a diagnosis of asthma having been sensitised by a viral infection. There is a history of hay fever. The chest X-ray case could be argued either way, but I'm not sure it is really worth the radiation at this point, despite fitting the guidelines. It could be something you agree to come back to if symptoms don't improve.

Case 7

Doctor information

48-year-old, Frank Lane
Past medical history: NAD
Medication: nil

Patient information

Your friend at work has recently died of prostate cancer and you would like a prostate cancer blood test. You otherwise have no problems; you eat a good, varied diet but have red meat every day and drink around 20 units of alcohol a week.

Breakdown of important issues

This question is about a request for prostate cancer screening when there is no formal screening programme in the NHS.

Information to consider

Assessing risk factors:

- **Family history**: it is thought that there may be a 5%–10% risk of inheriting a genetic cause. It is important to ask about family history, including ages, as a slight increase in risk is seen with close relatives (father, brother) who have had prostate cancer under the age of 60 years. There is also thought to be a link with female members of the family who have had a breast cancer under the age of 40 years.
- **Diet**: a diet high in animal fats, including dairy products and high in calcium (possibly linked to dairy) contributes to a higher risk. A diet low in fruit and vegetables is similarly linked. If people eat a lot of tomatoes (including ketchup) there is a protective effect from the lycopene. Selenium may be protective if taken as a supplement.
- **Ethnicity**: Afro-Caribbean men are seen to be at higher risk, whereas Asians seem to have a reduced risk.
- International Prostate Scoring System score for further clarity.

Management discussion

Be aware of the argument that surely it is better to know so that we can make an informed decision about what we are dealing with, and also the question 'what would you do?'

The rest of the consultation will be a discussion about risk.

- There is no evidence that screening healthy men for prostate cancer improves mortality; it may do more harm than good (of 100 men with a raised prostate-specific antigen (PSA) level, 30 will have prostate cancer).
- In the United States, screening is suggested for men over the age of 50 who have a 10-year life expectancy.
- Results from trials (PROTECT, ERSPC and PLCO) are awaited to clarify whether there is a benefit to screening and the role of early treatment (again, the best course of action is not known).

- PSA level will be normal in one in five men with prostate cancer (i.e. false negatives would be falsely reassuring).
- Biopsies as part of assessing a raised PSA level may lead to bleeding or infection of the prostate gland.
- Prostate cancers grow very slowly, and investigations and treatments may be worse than the cancer.
- A recent study suggests that a single PSA measurement at 60 years of age may predict the lifetime risk (i.e. younger patients with a higher PSA level are the patients who need more focus).

If the patient has no family history and is under 50 years of age you should probably be encouraging them to go away and think about things (until he is at least 60 or develops symptoms).

Possibly suggest downloading the leaflet from the NHS cancer screening website (in short, discouraging them without saying no). The NHS also provides answers online to frequently asked questions regarding the Prostate Cancer Risk Management Programme (www.cancerscreening.nhs.uk/prostate/faqs.html). Another useful website you could direct them to is the National Cancer Institute (www.cancer.gov/), where they can select prostate cancer for further information.

Case 8

Doctor information

18-year-old male, Richard Centor
Past medical history: tonsillitis
Medication: nil
You have a request for a telephone consultation

Patient information

You are having tonsillitis every 1–2 months and would like to be referred for a tonsillectomy.

Sometimes you go to the doctors for antibiotics because the anti-inflammatories aren't helping enough. You know it is your tonsils because you can see them in the mirror when they are inflamed. Although you don't always go to the doctor, the symptoms are severe enough to have to take time out of college and you are on a warning because of the number of days you have been absent.

You are otherwise fit and well and you have never smoked.

Breakdown of important points

This is a telephone consultation about a referral request for recurrent tonsillitis.

The information to consider is as follows:

- First, believe the patient; don't come across as doubting him.
- Enquire as to how he knows it is the tonsils and not a sore throat, and ask about the duration of symptoms.
- Explore why he is calling now (i.e. what is the importance/urgency?).

National Institute for Health and Clinical Excellence: referral practice, May 2000

In recurrent episodes of acute sore throat in children aged up to 15 years the following should be considered:

- Outcomes are likely to be improved if the parent, child and health professional decide on a treatment in partnership; communication is key.
- Agree on analgesia that can be used (ibuprofen and/or paracetamol).
- Avoid prescribing antibiotics if acceptable (children issued antibiotics may be at increased risk of further infection and attend more frequently).
- Issue antibiotics if there are:
  - features of systemic upset
  - peritonsillar cellulites
  - a history of rheumatic fever
  - increased risk from infection (e.g. a child with immunodeficiencies or diabetes mellitus).
- A specialist referral should be considered:
  - acutely if there is suspicion of a quinsy, airway obstruction or swelling causing dehydration
  - routinely if there is a history of sleep apnoea, failure to thrive, five or more

episodes of infection in the last 12 months for the previous 2 years (Paradise criteria) or they have guttate psoriasis caused by recurrent tonsillitis.

A quinsy may be more common in unwell patients with three out of four Centor criteria (fever >38°C, purulent tonsils, tender anterior cervical nodes and no cough). The incidence has been seen at 1 in 60 if these criteria are met, compared with 1 in 400 when not systemically unwell. It is worth offering antibiotics to patients who have been unwell for 48 hours and fit the Centor criteria.

Negotiation of management plan

- You are going to want to help this chap out with a referral, but professionally it might be prudent to see if the next time it flares up for absolute confirmation.
- You could offer emergency slots, and if there is appointment difficulty he could call as a back-up (you would be able to know where you are able to extend your surgeries).
- You could discuss over-the-counter preparations. Confirm that he is taking adequate doses that will tide him over until he can get to see you.
- You should discuss the procedure of a tonsillectomy in brief, so he understands the implications.

Your safety net here is the review with a view to referral at the next infection.

Case 9

Doctor information

76-year-old female, Joan Lyles
Past medical history: fractured right wrist 6 weeks ago
Medication: Calceos, one tablet twice a day on repeat, not yet ordered

Patient information

You fell on wet leaves as you went to peg out the washing. You have not had any previous fractures and you are otherwise well, coping with the pain and using paracetamol.

Your dietary calcium intake is around 800 mg per day (1 pint skimmed milk, yoghurt and lots of fruit and vegetables) without the supplement, so you can't understand why you need it.

You have never smoked, and you walk regularly with the ramblers and for about 30 minutes each day to get your newspaper. You drink around 2 units of alcohol a week and you have no significant family history.

If not discussed, question the need for a bone density scan.

Breakdown of important issues

This question looks at fragility fractures and secondary prevention in relation to probable osteoporosis.

Information to be clear about:

- Mechanism of injury – a fragility fracture is a fall from standing height or below at walking speed or less.
- Risk factors.
- What the calcium intake is – don't jump to accusing someone of not taking their medication without understanding the issues behind why, in this case the calcium intake and exposure to sunlight (30 minutes per day from April to October, if pigmented skin or elderly may need more).

Royal College of Physicians Guidelines 2000 Osteoporosis (also steroids and osteoporosis)

Smoking history – if she is a smoker you can assess the need and acceptability of intervention at this point.

Alcohol use – should be less than 14 units in women.

Family history of maternal hip fractures.

Exercise undertaken: it is recommended that patients should undertake 20 minutes of bone loading exercise three times a week. The improvement in muscle tone helps with balance but there is no evidence that walking alone reduces falls.

Diet – 1200 mg calcium/day is recommended in those over 51 years of age. It is difficult to assess this just from a review conversation but it may be worth considering a food diary to look at in more detail (i.e. the patient could drop it in for you to look at and you could call her back if inadequate amounts are shown and she needs calcium supplement dose adjusting).

Falls prevention – this would be a real bonus if you could find the time to incorporate.

If the patient had fallen in the past you need to try to assess further:

- Does she know why she fell/was there loss of consciousness?
- Are there environmental elements? If so, consider occupational therapy.
- Was the patient able to get up? If not, consider physiotherapy.
- Are the falls recurrent or unexplained? Consider specialist falls referral.
- Don't forget to review treatment and blood pressure.

Management issues to negotiate

- Given calcium intake, consider one Calceos tablet a day (patient may still decline).
- Given she is over 75 years old, she would be eligible for a bisphosphonate without a DEXA scan. Again depending on the patient it is sometimes sensible to do the bone density scan. Be prepared to talk around this subject.
- Specifically with the bisphosphonate the most used is alendronic acid 70 mg once a week. You should explain how to take this: at least half an hour before food with a pint of water and try to stay upright to reduce the risk of dyspepsia.
- Consider the role of blood tests (FBC, UE, LFT, bone, TFT, immunoglobulins) to look for secondary causes of a fragility fracture.
- Consider pain control and function if right hand dominant.
- You should arrange review to determine acceptance of the bisphosphonate.
- If you truly are OK for time then you could consider other health promotion issues such as blood pressure check and so forth (although falls outside the age range for the NHS Health Check).

The Leicester Medicines Management Strategy Group has a good summary available online (www.lmsg.nhs.uk/LMSGDocs%5CGuidelines%5CG_OsteoporosisGuidelinesFinal200812.pdf). Other sources of useful information are Age UK (www.ageuk.org.uk/), which provides services funded by local councils aimed at reducing isolation, and Later Life Training (www.laterlifetraining.co.uk), which provides gait and balance training and lists of qualified instructors and balance exercises available to download.

Case 10

Doctor information

A 32-year-old woman, Helen Daniels
Past medical history: nothing of note
Medication: Femulen

Patient information

You had a cold 3 weeks ago that has left you hoarse.

You work as a lecturer at the university, and you haven't had time off work (if you are offered a sick note, decline, as you have a 3-month sabbatical coming up in 2 weeks' time).

You have had no sputum, fever or other problems. You are an ex-smoker of 10 years, having smoked occasionally at university. If asked about pets, you only have a corn snake.

Breakdown of important issues

This is a question around presentation of a hoarse voice in a patient who would not be considered to be in an at-risk group.

It would be important to enquire about the following:

- The chronology of events, in particular whether the hoarse voice is intermittent, progressive or associated with any other symptoms.
- You can look at family and social history, and pack-years if possible. Regarding her pet (thinking allergy, *Chlamydia psittaci*), there is unlikely to be anything related to her problem, but you could double-check what she feeds her snake on.
- Examination would be important but normal in this case (in real terms there may be some resolving cervical lymphadenopathy) and if it was in an at-risk patient then consider doing a weight to see if there has been any unrecognised loss. Similarly, a peak flow rate would be normal.

Discussion of the management plan

- You can explore her ideas as to what the problem might be. This takes some skill and sometimes, if not understood by the patient, you get back 'you tell me, you're the doctor'.
- The issue around a chest X-ray and further investigations can be discussed. Depending on the consultation you could go either way, but the case is written as a low-risk case in a person who needs to rest their voice.
- You could discuss a sick note either for time off or for amended duties, to allow the patient to rest her voice.
- General advice would involve avoidance of smoke, alcohol, caffeine, throat lozenges (which can dry the throat), straining of the voice and repetitive throat clearing. Try to rest the voice (and yourself), try humming (relaxes the voice box) and keep well hydrated. The Voice Care Network UK (www.voicecare.org.uk) is a good source of information.
- Safety net for the possibility that things may not improve and that the patient may need further investigation.

This case has been adapted using the information from clinical practice on a day-to-day basis and the 10-minute consultation article 'Hoarse voice' by Judd and Colvin (*BMJ* 2010; 340: c522). It is important to identify risks as a tool to use when considering whether an X-ray is needed (over 50 years of age, smoker, alcohol to excess and hoarseness for more than 3 weeks) as well as other differentials such as reflux, asthma, rhinitis/postnasal drip and use of inhaler. All of these would require a different focus in the management of symptoms.

Case 11

Doctor information

46-year-old male, Ivor Payne

Past history: was seen 2 weeks ago with a painful right first metatarsophalangeal joint

Alcohol 28 units/week, BMI 32, BP 130/74

Medication: colchicine as required

Results from last week: full blood count, normal; urea and electrolytes, normal; estimated glomerular filtrated rate, 82 mL/min/1.73 m^2; liver function tests, normal, Gamma GT 52; urate, 498 µmol/L

Patient information

You have come for your blood test results.

With regard to the pain, it is now not bad. You have had to stop using the colchicine, as it was giving you diarrhoea, and you are just taking an occasional paracetamol.

You have a sedentary job in pharmaceutical sales; it would be difficult to reduce your alcohol intake because of the relationship this has to your job. Your diet is very good, with lots of fish such as mackerel, shrimp, crab and good-quality meats.

Breakdown of important issues

This is a question relating to hyperuricaemia and first presentation of gout.

Further information to qualify:

- That this was the first attack and there have been no other episodes.
- The type of job and some colour explaining this man's lifestyle and diet.
- The degree of pain and how things have gone with the colchicine. Don't forget to clarify whether he is using any other medications. Is the use of the joint/foot now back to normal?

Discussion of management

- Here there are no reference ranges with the blood tests. It would be a little unlucky in the exam if they weren't provided, but try not to get used to relying on them being there for you. The urate is up a little (214–494 µmol/L) and the estimated glomerular filtration rate is under 90 but probably not significant as a one-off.
- You may be discussing these results prior to clarifying the issues around lifestyle, depending on how the patient wants the consultation to go. They are in keeping with gout, but recognise that a urate may be normal and the diagnosis can still be gout. You can explain that gout is either too much uric acid being produced or not enough being excreted, causing the crystals to be deposited in the joint space.
- As this is a first attack, allopurinol is probably not indicated and your management will be directed towards reducing the risk of recurrence.
- Look at weight and diet; although the fish is good from a cardiovascular point of view, the ones outlined are purine rich (as are liver, heart, sweetbreads and kidney). He should try to look at incorporating more vegetables and white fish into his diet.

- Look at alcohol – recognise and sympathise with the difficulties around the job. Explain the current guidance is 21 units a week for men but that if he really can't change, to try to avoid red wine, port and stout – all of which contain purines/oxypurines.
- Look at fluid intake and try to aim for an intake of 2 L a day (3 L in an acute attack) to reduce recurrence.
- If there is a recurrence you can talk through fluids and over-the-counter anti-inflammatories; alternatively, you can re-discuss the use of colchicine (2 × 500 μg tablets initially and then one every 2–3 hours, a maximum of 6 mg per course – that is, 12 tablets – with 3 days between courses).
- Safety net when to review things: if three attacks in a year, if attacks are getting more frequent, if getting residual pain in the joint (as it may be affecting the cartilage and may warrant allopurinol to reduce recurrence). If there was doubt around the diagnosis you could arrange joint aspiration with the next flare-up. Finally, the repeat of the blood tests, given the estimated glomerular filtration rate, would be sensible a few months down the line after the gout attack has resolved.

Case 12

Doctor information

72-year-old man, Jack Bower

Past medical history: ischaemic heart disease; myocardial infarction 10 years ago; last review with the nurse was 5 months ago and last blood tests 11 months ago

Medication: simvastatin 40 mg nocte; aspirin dispersible 75 mg daily; bisoprolol 5 mg twice a day; ramipril 10 mg daily; glyceryl trinitrate spray as required

Patient information

You have been starting to get light-headed when doing the gardening and occasionally when standing up. It can be any time but usually it is in the morning.

You have had no vertigo or neurological features

You have had no chest pain or shortness of breath but you are left feeling tired/exhausted for several hours afterwards.

Examination

- BP sitting 136/88, standing 112/60, pulse 62/minute.
- Chest is clear, heart sounds normal and there is no ankle swelling.
- There is no nystagmus (other cranial nerves don't really warrant being examined but are normal if they are).

Breakdown of important issues

This is a question around postural/orthostatic hypotension.

The following points are important.

- Ensure with your history taking that you elicit this is postural and that there are no other cardiovascular, neurological or ENT problems.
- Confirm that angina control remains good, with no suggestion of heart failure.
- Look at review of systems to clarify there is no reason why this patient would be anaemic.
- Enquire about medication – has there been a break or has he started taking it in a different way? Do the episodes correlate with the timing of the medication (in this case it is mainly in the morning, so probably related to the dose of tablets in the morning)?
- I would usually discuss whether the patient had any specific concerns above what he has already described.
- Don't forget to examine this patient – sitting and standing blood pressures as well as pulse, cardiovascular system, ankles and chest (for heart failure).

Management options

- With the results this is a fairly clear case of postural hypotension and something you can solve by adjusting medication.
- Consider further investigations such as repeating the bloods (including a full blood count). As they are about due anyway you may as well do the complete cardiovascular set. Consider an electrocardiogram, to compare with older electrocardiograms to see if there are any underlying changes developing.

- You don't have to wait for the results before making changes and there are several ways the problem can be managed. The pulse is OK, so he is not over beta-blocked. Similarly, the exhaustion seems to only be related to episodes of hypotension. Leave the bisoprolol alone – this will give him a lot of protection in the future.
- Consider the ramipril: either stop, reduce the dose into 5 mg twice a day or take the dose at night (note there isn't a history of hypertension here). My preference would be to split the dose, given the half-life and that the symptoms are relatively mild with the drop in blood pressure still being above 100 mmHg.
- Arrange review with regard to the result having changed the medication at 1–2 weeks. Decide whether it will be with yourself or the nurse; I would normally suggest the nurse if symptoms have all resolved for further postural blood pressure checks. If in doubt, always review yourself.
- Further issues to double-check if you have time would be his glyceryl trinitrate spray and whether it is still in date, and also the use of a proton pump inhibitor to cover the aspirin use and reduce the risk of long-term peptic ulceration.
- Consider your safety net and what to do if symptoms get worse if he starts to get more angina, particularly if associated with features of heart failure.

There was a very good overview article, 'Postural hypotension', published recently in the *BMJ* (2011; 342: d3128). It is not a difficult consultation and it is a good feeling to be able to do something that should make an immediate difference to the patient's symptoms. Just be thorough, don't jump to conclusions, and get to the bottom line/ management within the 10 minutes.

Case 13

Doctor information

A 22-year-old female, Louise Franklin
Past history: acne
Medication: Marvelon

Patient information

You have unpleasant acne over your chest and back, which makes you very self-conscious (e.g. with your partner and when swimming).

You are not happy with the PanOxyl and antibiotics you have tried over the last few years (erythromycin and tetracyclines) and you would like to see a dermatologist about Roaccutane, which you have heard of. You had a slight improvement in the severity of your acne when you started the Marvelon (having been on Microgynon).

You can ask about skin hygiene and different ranges as well as dietary effects on skin.

Breakdown of important issues

This question is about acne, contraception and negotiation of effective management plans without the need for referral (you need to work within your level of competence; be aware of your limitations but remember you are a doctor, not a triage system).

Further issues to explore

- How long has she had the acne and what has previously been tried?
- Do any issues flare it up, such as the pill-free week, alcohol and so forth?
- What skin-care regime does she use?
- Was there any improvement in her skin when she started the Marvelon, and has she tried any other methods of contraception?
- Has there been any scarring?
- How does it affect her life? Are there any things she avoids doing because of her skin?

Examine the skin if you are able specifically to grade the acne, pustules, comedones and scarring.

Negotiation of the management plan

- Recognise the impact that this is having on the patient's life.
- Explain that there is one significant alternative treatment that would be worth trying before a referral.
- Discuss Roaccutane as an effective treatment but with significant side effects such as lip cracking, which may be more unpleasant than what she has now, as it would be more visible. It is certainly something you can consider, but there are other options that may be effective and more acceptable.
- Talk through Dianette and ensure that you mention that, although it works as a contraceptive, it is not a licensed indication. Ensure you do the risk-factor check,

blood pressure and weight. Ensure you talk through the change from one pill pack to another, taking, missed pills, issues that reduce effectiveness and so forth.

- Explain that it takes 3–6 months to begin to get maximal effect but that you would be hopeful that she would start to see changes before this.
- Consider using Dalacin T or Duac as an additional topical agent.
- Negotiate a review date for around 3 months, and with yourself rather than the nurse. It is important to get across that you are not being obstructive; a referral is always an option, but there is a lot more you could achieve for this patient.
- Give permission/safety net that if things are getting worse she should come straight back to see you.

Beyond the MRCGP

Exams and courses to consider while doing your training

While going through your hospital you will have a study allowance and grants that can be used for different courses (relevant to general practice, not necessarily the subspecialty you may be doing as part of the rotation at that time).

Use the study-leave time and money wisely, bearing in mind that if you want to go on revision courses this will use a lot of your registrar allocation and that certain courses will be free in certain posts (e.g. advanced life support).

Diplomas to consider

DRCOG (Diploma of the Royal College of Obstetricians and Gynaecologists)

This is not necessary for general practice, but if you look at job advertisements some practices stipulate that they would like applicants to have the diploma.

If you want to give it a go, request the information from the college early. If you can, time it with your obstetrics and gynaecology attachment; by doing this you will probably find it easier to be motivated, and you will get significantly more out of the teaching on rounds from your seniors.

Royal College of Obstetricians and Gynaecologists
27 Sussex Place, Regent's Park, London NW1 4RG
Tel. +44 (0)20 7772 6200
www.rcog.org.uk

DFSRH (Diploma of the Faculty of Sexual and Reproductive Healthcare) and Letters of Competence

This, again, is not essential for being a GP unless you want to do family-planning sessions or fit coils and implants. You can do ad hoc family-planning sessions once you have the diploma, while you are still doing either hospital posts or a GP registrar year, which may help keep your skills up to date.

Once you have completed the DFSRH you can then do the coil training for the intrauterine device letters of competence and the implant training. The syllabus and logbook can be viewed on the faculty website (www.fsrh.org.uk/) (under General Training Committee).

Faculty of Sexual and Reproductive Healthcare
27 Sussex Place, Regent's Park, London NW1 4RG

DCH (Diploma of Child Health)

This is a detailed diploma involving practical-based sessions as well as the exam. These sessions may be possible to do while in your paediatric job.

Only a few practices seem to request this diploma, but as with all things, it may be something that tips the balance in your favour when applying for the post of your choice.

Royal College of Paediatrics and Child Health
5–11 Theobalds Road, London WC1X 8SH
Tel. +44 (0)20 7092 6000
www.rcpch.ac.uk/

Courses to consider

Advanced life support

Ensure this is up to date before your registrar year and that you have a signed form confirming that you are qualified in advanced life support. If you are thinking of taking the MRCGP you have to have proof of basic life support competency, which the advanced life support training incorporates. Most trusts give this training free of charge for trust employees.

Acupuncture

Many hospital trusts will fund acupuncture courses. Acupuncture is as relevant to general practice as you want to make it. The courses tend to be held at weekends, which means getting study leave is not part of the ordeal. A good basic course to ensure you are competent to practise would take around 4 days.

Information can be found in *BMJ* advertisements. See also:

British Medical Acupuncture Society
BMAS House, 3 Winnington Court Northwich, Cheshire CW8 1AQ
Tel. +44 (0)1606 786 782
www.medical-acupuncture.co.uk

Other courses

Some half-day release courses (or within your post-graduate region) will offer the following courses to GP registrars:

- alternative medicine
- ENT
- ophthalmology
- dermatology
- GP management issues
- communication skills.

All of these courses and more would be time well spent. It is all about developing your own interest and deciding what kind of a service you would like to be able to offer your patients.

Minor surgery

You can pay to go on a minor surgery course while doing your hospital training. GP registrars can usually go on the course without having to use any of their allowance. If you want to be signed up by your primary care trust for minor surgery, so that you can be eligible to perform minor surgery under your contract (which attracts a payment for each individual case), then you need to do this course. The theoretical course is not how you will become competent in minor surgery. You will learn this through either your trainer or other colleagues (e.g. dermatologists, surgeons, rheumatologists and so forth) in hospital posts.

Child health surveillance

It is important to check your regional policy as to what is required and whether you have to be on a named list to carry out any child health surveillance work. Child health protection (especially the recognition of problems) is an important part of work in primary care, so if you have the opportunity to attend one of these courses it would be worthwhile.

Palliative care

Most regions are now running palliative care courses. Again, usually no payment is required for GP registrars. Although palliative care is unlikely to be a huge part of day-to-day life, it will be something that, if you do it well, you will be remembered and respected for. The courses teach the knowledge base as well as the practical issues (e.g. setting up a syringe driver).

After you qualify

Preparing your curriculum vitae

There are many acceptable themes and variations when preparing your curriculum vitae; whatever your approach, make it easy for an employer to navigate, don't write that your hobby is shopping and do write a sound covering letter to go with it.

Matt Green's 'Preparing the perfect medical CV' was published in the *BMJ* (Careers, 3 September 2011, p. 61). It is worth reading or cross-checking with your CV before getting your trainer to proofread it with you and offer their advice.

Self-employment as a GP/locum

We have a self-employed, independent contractor status.

Good records are essential. Outgoings that are tax deductible are also essential to keep receipts for.

Once you have qualified as a GP you need to register with HM Revenue and Customs as being self-employed. If you do not register within 3 months of starting work, you will probably be fined. You will find some information as well as a selection of relevant publications online (www.inlandrevenue.gov.uk). There is a helpline available for the newly self-employed (tel. +44 (0)8459 15 45 15). You can call this helpline to register or, alternatively, you can complete a CWF1 form.

By registering as self-employed you will pay Class 2 National Insurance. At the end of the tax year, when you send in your self-assessment, the amount of National Insurance contributions you owe will be calculated. This is then payable as Class 4 National Insurance at the same time as you pay your income tax bill.

You also have to ensure you are registered with a primary care trust on the supplementary list.

Expenses that will probably be tax deductible

- Professional subscriptions: General Medical Council, *BMJ*, Diploma, Medical Defence Union and so forth.
- Mileage: for visits, not to and from work (unless there is a visit on the way). As a locum, all mileage is tax deductible because you are working from home.
- Office at home: running costs, rates, electricity, gas and so forth are worked out as a proportion depending upon the number of rooms in your house or square footage.
- Computer: if you use it for work.
- Stationery: used for work (e.g. paper, envelopes, stamps and postage, equipment).
- MRCGP exam fees: this is necessary if you want to be involved in training.
- Courses: if you pay for them (if reimbursed you must declare this).

- Telephone expenses: if using your home phone for work, then ensure that you get an itemised bill to be able to calculate the amount. Alternatively, your accountant may use estimates.
- Internet: links from home and anti-virus packages.
- Miscellaneous: digital camera if used for work purposes/teaching/publications (if also used for home, then a proportion of the cost); books and equipment if necessary for your job.

Keep up-to-date records of all incomings and outgoings.

Speak to your accountant or the business advisors at Inland Revenue. You are self-employed as a GP, and they are an excellent source of information and will help you with your tax return if needed. If speaking to a revenue advisor it is prudent to remember whom they work for!

Remember that you will have to declare all incoming monies (e.g. cremations fees, DS1500s, disabled badge reports) from private work. Even if you have not filled in a tax return while doing your hospital jobs you could still be investigated. This is especially likely if your first tax return is as a GP. Get used to doing them early, when the figures are easier! And always keep all your receipts.

Applying for locum jobs

- Negotiate pay before doing a job; ask around and find out what other people are charging.
- Negotiate what work is to be done (length of surgery, number of appointments, visits and so forth).
- Invoice the practice once the job is complete, or on a weekly or monthly basis.
  - If you don't do this, you are unlikely to get paid.
  - If you take the invoice with you on the final day, apart from it saving on postage, your records will be up to date, and there is less chance of forgetting what you have claimed for.
- Locums can contribute to the superannuation scheme. Your primary care trust will have the relevant information. If you ask them, they will send you the forms (you will need the practice you are temporarily working in to complete these) to prove what your earnings have been.
- Information is also available from the NHS Pensions (tel. 0845421 4000).
- Try to save around 40% of your income in a high-interest account for:
  - income tax
  - Class 4 National Insurance
  - superannuation
  - Medical Defence Union subscriptions for next year.

Considerations when looking for a GP post

When making any major decision it is important to work out the things that are fundamentally important to you and the things you would be prepared to compromise on.

Don't feel you have to rush into anything. There are always jobs and, in the interim, locum work is not only lucrative but also it may help you develop your idea of how you want to work.

The following are some of the things to consider when choosing a post:

- Full-time or part-time?
- Personal Medical Services or General Medical Services practice?
- Salaried, partnership or retainer?
- Portfolio career options.
- Outside work:
  - clinical assistant post
  - family planning
  - private health screening
  - obesity clinics
  - local medical committee (LMC) involvement
  - post-marketing surveillance work
  - forensic work.
- If considering a partnership:
  - Rural or inner city?
  - Where in the country?
  - How many partners would you be comfortable with?
  - How many sessions do you want to work?
  - Do you want to be involved in training or with medical students?
  - Do you want a dispensing practice?
  - How involved do you want to be in antenatal care, child health, minor surgery, practice development?
  - Do other members of the primary healthcare team have a base at the practice?
  - What computer system is used?
  - Who does the auditing?
  - What role do the practice nurses have (is there a nurse practitioner, triage and so forth)?
  - What are the premises like (owned, rented, new or ageing)?
  - What is car parking like (small problems can become very irritating)?
  - How do the appraisals work and who does them?
  - What are the local hospitals, educational meetings and out-patient waiting times like?
  - What security measures are there?
  - What meetings are there (weekly business, nurse, practice, in-house educational and so forth)?
  - Does the practice have social events?
- Other issues:
  - What are the local schools like (comprehensive and public)?
  - What are house prices like in the area?
  - What are the road/motorway links like (remember your family and social commitments!)?

Partnership agreement

If you are a member of the British Medical Association, request a copy of *Medical Partnerships under the NHS*. This should get you oriented as to what issues a practice agreement should cover. You should be thinking towards signing a written mutual agreement at the end of your period of mutual assessment. It is foolhardy to enter into a partnership with no written agreement in place. In such an instance this is a partnership at will, which can be brought to an end as quickly as it is formed.

It is advisable to take specialist independent legal (and accountancy) advice before signing. You need to protect yourself, no matter how well you think you know your partners.

What should a partnership agreement cover?

- All parties' names and addresses.
- Commencement date.
- Declaration relating to termination of partnership, retirement, a party wishing to move, gross misconduct and so forth.
- Capital assets.
- Sale and purchasing of shares.
- Valuation methods, especially in relation to cost rent scheme.
- Occupation of premises by non-owning partners.
- Expenses – individual and partnership.
- Income – individual and partnership, especially notional/cost rent income, outside work (is it to be pooled?).
- Schedule of profit shares from commencement date to parity.
- Partners' obligations to one another.
- Partnership accounts (drawings, tax reserve, year end, accountants).
- Superannuation.
- Holiday and study leave.
- Sickness, maternity and paternity entitlement.
- Effect of retirement or death – restrictive covenant.
- Arbitration of provisions.
- Declaration about patients.

Things to consider in detail, prior to accepting the partnership

There will be things to negotiate and this will involve compromise.

- Commitment to the practice:
  - number of sessions to be worked
  - earning from outside interests/work (will this be pooled?).
- Finances.
- Determine the cost of buying in and the time to parity.
- Profit-sharing distribution.
- Voting rights.
- Some matters should only be acted on with a unanimous agreement (e.g. appointment of a new partner).

- One vote per partner is ideal.
- Part-time partners should have equal voting power, as they buy into a share of the profits but are 'jointly' liable and have the same professional interest in the business.
- Maternity leave and paternity leave clauses – time allowed must be fair.
- Determine what will happen to drawings and who will cover the locum costs and what happens to funds reimbursed by the primary care trust.
- Expulsion clauses. This may be important if you have any existing conditions. Don't presume it will never happen to you (e.g. lengthy incapacity, gross misconduct).
- Expenses. This includes all things (e.g. phones, subscriptions, courses and travel, equipment, books and so forth). It needs to be explicit about what will be covered in the practice and what will be paid for personally.

Accounts

When considering buying in to a practice, it is necessary to look over and to understand (to a certain degree) the practice accounts.

I am not an accountant, and I certainly make no claim to be expert on the subject. Having been through the process and having to put your name to the yearly accounts will make you learn quickly. I hope you find this Noddy-like guide a useful starting point.

The things you are looking at are:

- Is the practice solvent?
- How much will you be drawing?
- Have there been any major changes from one year to the next, and why?
- Where could the practice potentially improve?

When you receive the accounts they will probably be in a summarised format (i.e. they will not include every single transaction but, rather, sections will be lumped together).

Look at the year of the accounts that you are given. Some run from 6 April to 5 April (i.e. the tax year), others run from 1 January to 31 December. It doesn't really matter. Be aware that you may be looking at accounts well over 12 months old.

In the accounts you should see two columns of figures: the current year and the previous year, for easy comparison.

Look at each of the following.

- The layout – is it a logical format?
- Is it clear where the numbers are from? If not, ask.
- How were the figures calculated?
- How did performance compare with previous years?
- How does it compare with the national average (often represented graphically at the end of the accounts using information from the Medeconomics database)?
- What areas can be improved?

- Are the following shown clearly?
  - value and ownership of property
  - fixed assets (fixtures, fittings, computers, furniture, drug stock)
  - investments and running costs.
- Is seniority pay and so forth kept personally or pooled?
- Does the practice pay for General Medical Council, Medical Defence Union and professional subscriptions and so forth?
- How much profit was made and was this shared fairly in line with the partnership agreement?
- Is there a partnership tax account?
- How much tax and National Insurance are you likely to pay?
- Is there an accountant's report (a summary of the important features of the accounts)?

Also consider the following:

- Are the partners' current accounts drawn up by the accountant (i.e. not a separate account, as if each partner had their own account within the business)? It is likely to include things such as seniority pay areas where one partner may assume all responsibility and so forth. It is recommended that these accounts are zeroed each year. If a substantial amount builds up, the practice could go into the red if a partner was to leave and want that money reimbursed.
- Getting professional help to go through the accounts with you (a specialist in GP finance and accountancy).
- Sources of private income (insurance certificates, medicals, sick notes and so forth).
- If a practice is doing well above average, or below, why is this? Remember that if fraud is committed (i.e. incorrect claims) money will have to be reimbursed to the primary care trust and Inland Revenue. There may be criminal proceedings. In this situation, all partners are liable.

Useful websites and references

Many journal articles, guidelines and online sites have been referenced through the text. The following is a list of additional sources used to check and verify information to enable this book to be brought together reliably.

Bandolier
 www.medicine.ox.ac.uk/bandolier/

Centre for Evidence-Based Medicine
 www.cebm.net

Clinical Evidence
 www.clinicalevidence.com

Cochrane Library
 www.thecochranelibrary.com

The Condensed Curriculum Guide: for GP training and the new MRCGP, by Ben Riley, Jayne Haynes and Steve Field

Doctors.net.uk
 www.doctors.net.uk

eGuidelines.co.uk
 www.eguidelines.co.uk

General Practice Notebook
 www.gpnotebook.co.uk

GP-training.net
 www.gp-training.net/

NHS Clinical Knowledge Summaries
 http://cks.library.nhs.uk

NHS Evidence Journals and Databases
 www.evidence.nhs.uk/nhs-evidence-content/journals-and-databases#

Patient.co.uk (many printable leaflets available)
 www.patient.co.uk

Trainer (common consultation models)
 www.trainer.org.uk

Index